Critical Topics in an Aging Society

Editorial Adviser, Toni C. Antonucci, PhD

- *Using Technology to Improve Care of Older Adults*
  Diane Chau, MD, FACP, and Thomas F. Osborne, MD, Editors
- *Homeless Older Populations: A Practical Guide for the Interdisciplinary Care Team*
  Diane Chau, MD, and Arnold P. Gass, MD, FACP, Editors
- *The New Politics of a Majority-Minority Nation: Aging, Diversity, and Immigration*
  Fernando M. Torres-Gil, PhD, and Jacqueline L. Angel, PhD
- *Social Isolation in Later Life: Strategies to Bolster Health and Well-Being*
  Lenard W. Kaye, DSW, PhD, and Cliff Singer, MD, Editors
- *Elder Justice, Ageism, and Elder Abuse*
  Lisa Nerenberg, MSW, MPH

Using Technology to Improve Care of Older Adults

Diane Chau, MD, FACP, is an associate professor of health sciences medicine at the University of California, San Diego (UCSD), and former geriatrics division chief at the University of Nevada School of Medicine. She has practiced medicine in the field of aging (geriatrics, palliative, and hospice care) since 1997 and held numerous academic program directorships of aging-related training programs for the University of Nevada and UCSD. She currently serves as project director of the San Diego Geriatrics Education Center/Geriatrics Workforce Enhancement Project. Dr. Chau is medical director of several elderly skilled nursing care settings including a Program of All Inclusive Care for the Elderly. Throughout her career, she has successfully created innovative curricula and has implemented transformative aging-related training programs for both graduate education and continuing education for interprofessional health learners. She has been grant-funded as principal investigator in over $5 million of geriatrics education grants. Dr. Chau holds an MD from Drexel University College of Medicine, and sits on the board of directors for the American Geriatrics Society as well as the California Geriatrics Society. Dr. Chau continues as a trailblazer as the principal in cross-discipline projects involving grants-funded telehealth, augmented reality, and simulation technology in geriatrics training.

Thomas F. Osborne, MD, is the director of medical informatics at Virtual Radiologic, a national radiology practice providing telemedicine services to over 2,100 hospitals and clinics in all 50 states as well as multiple different countries. He is also the director of research at MEDNAX, a national multispecialty medical group which comprises the nation's leading providers and is reshaping the delivery of care with evidence-based solutions. Dr. Osborne is a forward-thinking leader who excels at the collaborative intersection of medicine, technology and business. He is known for his ability to anticipate industry trends and has been nationally recognized as the top physician to watch in his field. His teams are currently focused on a variety of healthcare quality and process improvement initiatives which are positively impacting the care of millions of patients around the world. Additional active projects and research include the design and development of enterprise infrastructures for clinical collaboration, engagement, education, and workflow efficiencies. Dr. Osborne graduated from Dartmouth Medical School and went on to complete his residency in diagnostic radiology at Harvard Medical School's Mount Auburn Hospital. Dr. Osborne also completed advanced fellowship training in neuroradiology at Harvard Medical School's Massachusetts's General Hospital.

Using Technology to Improve Care of Older Adults

Diane Chau, MD, FACP
Thomas F. Osborne, MD
Editors

SPRINGER PUBLISHING COMPANY
NEW YORK

Springer Publishing Company, LLC
11 West 42nd Street
New York, NY 10036
www.springerpub.com

Acquisitions Editor: Sheri W. Sussman
Compositor: Exeter Premedia Services Private Ltd.

ISBN: 978-0-8261-4242-9
Ebook ISBN: 978-0-8261-4243-6

17 18 19 20 21 / 5 4 3 2 1

Library of Congress Cataloging-in-Publication Data

Names: Chau, Diane, editor. | Osborne, Thomas F., editor.
Title: Using technology to improve care of older adults/Diane Chau and Thomas F. Osborne, editors.
Description: New York, NY: Springer Publishing Company, LLC, [2018] | Includes bibliographical references and index.
Identifiers: LCCN 2017023014 | ISBN 9780826142429 | ISBN 9780826142436 (e-book)
Subjects: | MESH: Health Services for the Aged | Biomedical Technology | Monitoring, Physiologic—instrumentation | Attitude to Health | Aged
Classification: LCC RC952.5 | NLM WT 31 | DDC 618.9700285—dc23
LC record available at https://lccn.loc.gov/2017023014

Printed in the United States of America.

Contents

Contributors

Roxana Aminbakhsh, MD, Clinical Assistant Professor of Medicine, Division of Geriatrics, University of California, San Diego, San Diego, California

Bryan T. Arkwright, MHA, Managing Consultant, Schumacher Clinical Partners, Charlotte, North Carolina

Jeremy Bellay, PhD, Cyber Innovations, Battelle Memorial Institute, Columbus, Ohio

Jessica C. Cate, PharmD, BCPS, Clinical Geriatric Pharmacist for Home Based Primary Care, Veterans Affairs Sierra Nevada Healthcare System, Reno, Nevada

Diane Chau, MD, FACP, Associate Professor of Health Sciences Medicine, University of California, San Diego, San Diego, California

Kelly Conright, MD, CMD, Clinical Assistant Professor of Medicine, Division of Geriatric Medicine, University of Nevada, School of Medicine, Veterans Affairs Sierra Nevada Healthcare System, Reno, Nevada

Lauren Cook, MEd, CCC-SLP, Del Mar, California

Dawn R. Currie, PharmD, CGP, Clinical Geriatric Pharmacist for the Community Living Center, Veterans Affairs Sierra Nevada Healthcare System, Reno, Nevada

David A. Friedenberg, PhD, Principal Research Statistician, Battelle Memorial Institute, Columbus, Ohio

Leonid A. Gavrilov, PhD, Senior Research Associate, National Opinion Research Center, University of Chicago, Chicago, Illinois

Gavin W. Hougham, PhD, Director, Battelle Seattle Regional Center, Advanced Analytics and Health Research, Seattle, Washington

Jessica L. Kalender-Rich, MD, CMD, Associate Professor, Internal Medicine, University of Kansas Medical Center, Kansas City, Kansas

Kevin M. Krcmarik, MD, Attending Hospitalist and Assistant Professor of Clinical Medicine, San Diego Veterans Affairs and University of California, San Diego, San Diego, California

Andrew J. Landgraf, PhD, Research Statistician, Battelle Memorial Institute, Columbus, Ohio

T. J. McCallum, PhD, Associate Professor of Psychology, Case Western University, Shaker Heights, Ohio

Bruce A. McClelland, PhD, Senior Research Scientist, Battelle Memorial Institute, Charlottesville, Virginia

Nancy J. McMillan, PhD, PMP, Research Leader/Manager, Battelle Memorial Institute, Columbus, Ohio

Renee Melton, MS, RD, LD, Austin, Texas

Andrew Michael, MD, Chief Medical Officer, Pacific Clinical Research, San Diego, California

Ramin Motarjemi, MD, FACP, Assistant Professor of Medicine, University of California, San Diego, San Diego, California

Ian C. Neel, MD, Medical Director for Senior Behavioral Health Consultation Service, Assistant Clinical Professor, Department of Geriatric Medicine, University of California, San Diego, San Diego, California

Thomas F. Osborne, MD, Director of Medical Informatics, Virtual Radiologic; Director of Research, MEDNAX

Aroop K. Pal, MD, Associate Professor and Hospitalist, Internal Medicine, University of Kansas Medical Center, Kansas City, Kansas

Amir M. Rahimi, PhD, Principal Research Scientist, Battelle Memorial Institute, Columbus, Ohio

Joel J. Reich, MD, FACEP, MMM, Chief Medical Officer, Eastern Connecticut Health Network, Glastonbury, Connecticut

Ashley Reynolds, PhD, RN, ACSM-HFS, Chief Operating Officer, Kaviva, Jacksonville, Florida

Ender Ricart, PhD, Research Scientist, Battelle Seattle Regional Center, Advanced Analytics and Health Research, Seattle, Washington

John Russo, Jr., PharmD, Managing Editor, *Telehealth and Medicine Today*, Candler, North Carolina

Adriana J. Salas, MSN, RN, CNS, ANP-BC, Veterans Affairs San Diego Healthcare System, Lemon Grove, California

Jürgen P. Schulze, PhD, Associate Research Scientist, University of California, San Diego, San Diego, California

Michael A. Schwemmer, PhD, Research Statistician, Advanced Analytics and Health Research, Battelle Memorial Institute, Columbus, Ohio

Colin M. Thomas, MD, MPH, Clinical Professor of Medicine, Division of Geriatric Medicine, University of California San Diego School of Medicine, San Diego, California

John Waggoner, MAS, MA, University of California, San Diego, San Diego, California

Victor H. S. Wang, MS, CEO, care.coach, Millbrae, California

Muhammad A. Waqar, MD, Assistant Professor, Department of Internal Medicine & Oncology, Aga Khan University, Karachi, Pakistan

Preface

Using Technology to Improve Care of Older Adults is part of the Critical Topics in an Aging Society series that began as a spark among geriatrics colleagues from different disciplines. These providers were inspired to address critical gaps in knowledge dissemination among those passionate in the care of older adults. Currently, adoption of technology among the aging services community is limited even though it holds the potential to solve some of the greatest challenges we face. This book serves as a catalyst in the technological transformation of aging services through the organized presentation and evaluation of these tools for a broad health care audience.

Geriatrics interprofessional care is a fundamental part of older adult clinical practice, which is modeled on a team approach inclusive of various fields, among them social work, pharmacy, nursing, rehabilitation, administration, and medicine. All clinicians who treat older adults, from the independent to the frail, are engaged in geriatrics team care, which is continually adapting and evolving for individuals based on functional status changes, new treatment paradigms, and different settings of care. The authors and topics of this book have been assembled to reflect this holistic care model.

The need for advanced technology is clearly evident as one enters a hospital, nursing home, or geriatric care setting, including the patient's home. Older adults have limited abilities to adapt to the changes across these care locations, and thoughtfully implemented technology may eliminate these obstacles while also providing safer, more enjoyable, and cost-effective care. This book presents some of the latest medical technological innovations and discusses options to help improve not only transitions of care, but also independence and quality of life for older adults. Readers will benefit from reading current literature reviews, insights from key opinion leaders, and clinical practice experts about how the latest and most practical advanced technological tools can be used in the care of older adults.

The chapters in this book are organized into four main sections. Section I presents two foundational chapters that provide both an overview of how emerging technology may be utilized to solve major challenges in aging, and how to best design and implement solutions for successful adoption. Section II includes three chapters that detail some of the most compelling location-based perspectives, tools, and strategies for the incorporation of medical technology to the care of older adults. In Section III, we focus on specific conditions and challenges that may benefit the most from the use of medical technology, with special attention to frailty, cognitive impairment, general medication management, and pain management. The last section details some of the most exciting emerging medical technologies for the care of older adults, including wearable devices, social robots, artificial intelligence, and advanced medical educational tools for both patients and providers.

Diane Chau
Thomas F. Osborne

I: Foundation

1

Current Major Challenges in Aging and Targets for Technology

Ender Ricart, Thomas F. Osborne,
Leonid A. Gavrilov, and Gavin W. Hougham

Increasing numbers of people are living longer with multiple chronic conditions and diminished ability to remain independent. Our current tools and strategies are not well aligned to providing high-quality health care to this aging population. Therefore, there is a critical need for improvement in the areas of health care, services, and support, such as resource allocation, service delivery, continuity of care, and chronic disease management, for the elderly adult population. Fortunately, these components of care and others may all be enhanced with thoughtfully designed and implemented technology. This chapter provides insight into the demographics of aging, and an overview of potential benefits and challenges of using technology to help older adults.

THE AGING POPULATION—A NATIONAL AND GLOBAL CHALLENGE

It is estimated that the U.S. population aged 65 years and older will more than double to nearly 90 million by 2050 (Figures 1.1 and 1.2; U.S. Census Bureau, 2014), with 21% of the population over the age of 65 years by 2050, nearly a quarter of which will be over the age of 85 years (Figure 1.3). To complicate the challenge, from 2010 to 2030, the proportion of the U.S. population in the prime caregiving years is expected to increase by only 1%, while the number of people 80 years and older who are in need of long-term services and support (LTSS) is projected to increase by a staggering 79% (Redfoot, Feinberg, & Houser, 2013).

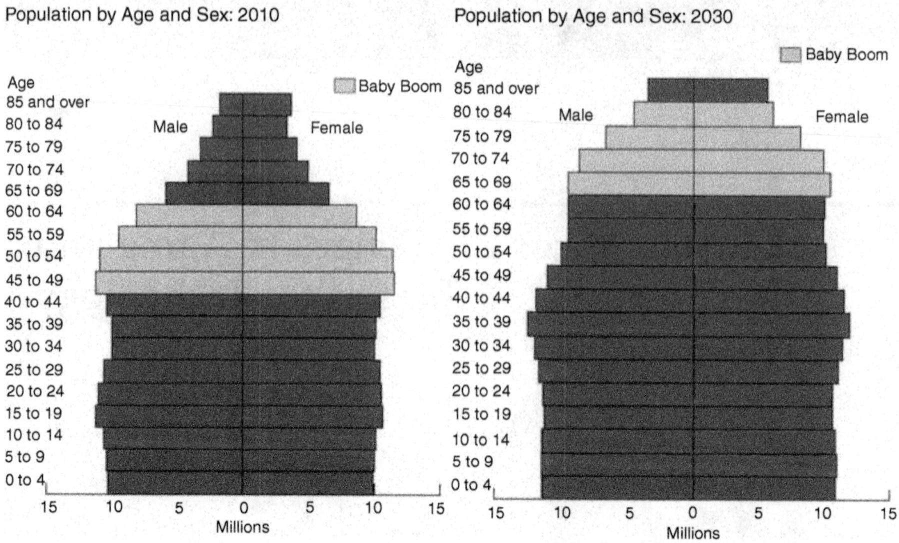

FIGURE 1.1 U.S. population by age and sex in 2010 and 2030.

Source: U.S. Census Bureau (2014).

This phenomenon is not unique to the United States, as both developed and developing nations worldwide face, or will face, the challenges of aging populations. On a global scale, the number of elderly will increase

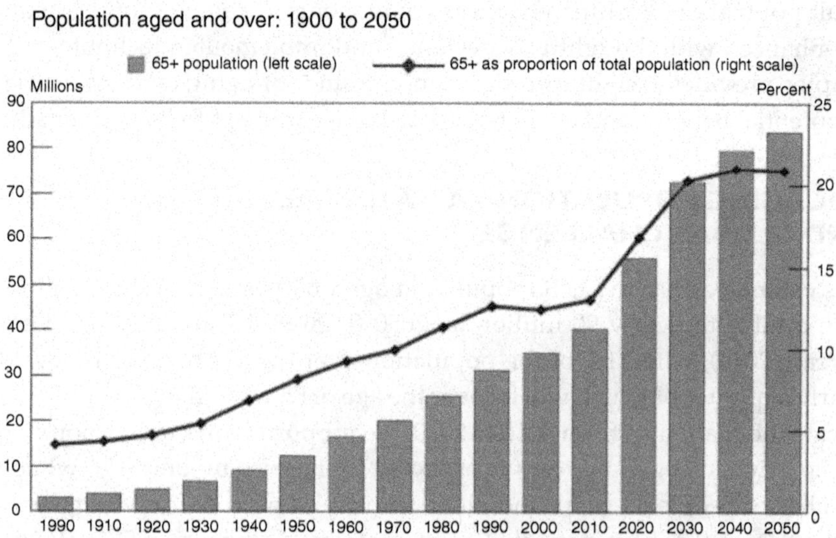

FIGURE 1.2 Population aged 65 and over: 1900 to 2050.

Source: U.S. Census Bureau (2014).

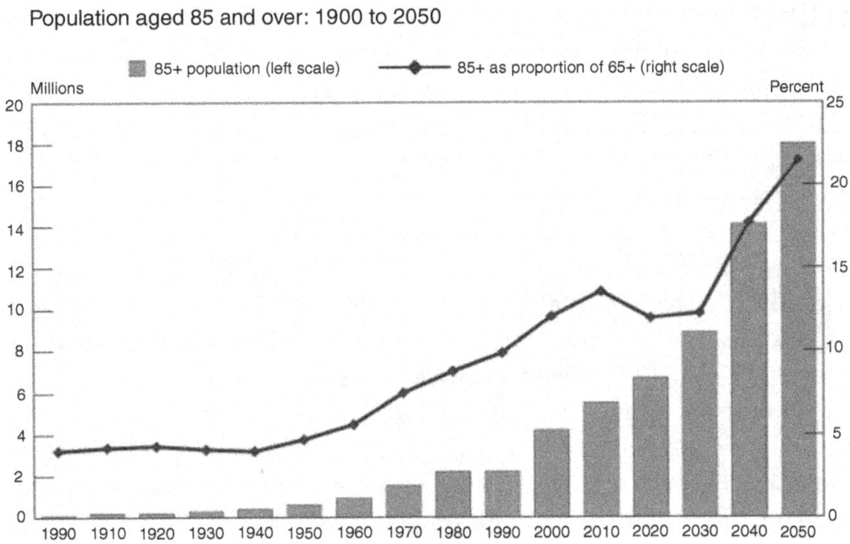

FIGURE 1.3 Population aged 85 and over: 1900 to 2050.

Source: U.S. Census Bureau (2014).

from 8.5% of the population in 2015 to a projected 16.7% in 2050 (U.S. Census Bureau, 2016).

Population aging results from a combination of decreased fertility rates and increased life expectancy. As the number of children born decreases, the relative number of people of working age and older in the population proportionally increases. As they age, so does the population. By 2047, the number of persons aged 60 years and over in the world is expected to exceed the number of children (United Nations, Department of Economic and Social Affairs Population Division, 2013, p. xii). In the past, such demographic shifts tended to occur over the course of a century or more (as was the case with France), but more recently, the pace has accelerated, leaving some countries with just a few decades to adjust to these tectonic demographic pressures (Brazil, China, and India being some examples of the latter; World Health Organization [WHO], 2015, p. 43; WHO et al., 2011, p. 4). Consequently, major shortages are projected in the number of health professionals available to care for older adults, both in the United States and worldwide, which, if not augmented by technological solutions, may result in poorer patient outcomes.

World population aging will bring about great changes. Whether these changes are for the better or worse depends on what can be done to ensure active and healthy aging. Some society-level benefits that could result from population aging include economic productivity related to seniors serving as a strong and experienced component of the labor force, not to mention the sheer numbers of older prime consumers in the marketplace (Fried, 2016, p. S167). However, at the moment, the pendulum is swinging in a less favorable direction. In the United States, for example, 70% of Americans over the age of 65 years are expected to require some form of long-term care for at least 3 years (Bowser, 2013), along with an estimated 91% of older adults with at least one chronic condition, and many more with functional limitations and disability (Dessem et al., 2013, p. 2). Worldwide, close to a quarter of the global death and illness burden is concentrated in people aged 60 years and over (WHO, 2014b). With strong associations between aging and morbidity, public spending on health and social care for aging populations is expected to proportionally accelerate, possibly threatening worldwide economic stability (Prince et al., 2015, p. 549). With limited time, infrastructure, and resources available (Institute of Medicine, Committee on the Future Health Care Workforce for Older Americans, 2008), far-reaching and scalable changes are needed to be designed and implemented on a population level to meet this challenge.

Disability can impact individuals of any age, but is much more prevalent in older populations. In efforts to better understand disability, it can be organized into intrinsic attributes and changes at the individual level (e.g., genetics, behavioral, or lifestyle choices) and extrinsic or environmental factors (e.g., access to public transportation, health care, and basic amenities; WHO, 2015, p. 50). To address the latter, part of a proposed response to an aging population lies in expanding responsibility for health and treatment to a societal infrastructure approach (Beard, Officer, & Cassels, 2016, p. S164). This social model of disability has, for example, been adopted by WHO in the holistic approach recommended for building age-friendly cities that support active aging (Bauman, Merom, Bull, Buchner, & Fiatarone Singh, 2016; WHO, 2007).

Another framework for organizing the goals and needs of population health is the Triple Aim. This ambitious strategy was developed by the Institute for Healthcare Improvement (IHI) a decade ago in its effort to redesign the U.S. health care system, and has since been adopted by more than 150 organizations around the world (Lewis, 2014). The three intertwined goals of the Triple Aim are to improve the individual experience of care; improve the health of populations; and reduce the per capita costs of care for populations (Berwick, Nolan, & Whittington, 2008). This outline for delivering higher value care can be utilized as a guiding force in the design and development of solutions to match the many needs of our growing older population. With these shifts in conceptualization and need, we can expect the development and application of technologies of care to broaden beyond the individual to include the surrounding environment, caregivers, and health care systems.

FOUR CHALLENGES OF AN AGING POPULATION AND THE ROLE OF TECHNOLOGY

The following sections outline four interconnected challenges of an aging population. With the expected increase in care needs that coincides with an aging population, the first challenge presented here is the question of how to provide relevant high-quality care to older persons. Second, with fewer caregivers available in relation to the growing population in need, we can expect that the relative burden of care experienced by caregivers—including both physical and emotional—will increase. We explore how caregiver burden can be reduced through the use of technology. The third challenge is to increase the relative number of healthy and independent seniors by taking a more proactive approach with prevention and health maintenance strategies. The final challenge addressed here concerns the development of health care systems and policy changes that are more inclusive of needed assistive technologies and medical devices.

First Challenge: How to Provide Care to an Aging Population

As the number of older people in need of care has risen, there has been a simultaneous shortage of skilled labor and resources available to provide health care services (Redfoot et al., 2013; Stone & Harahan, 2010). More specifically, the *old-age support ratio*—the number of people of working age (ages 20–64 years) per persons aged 65 years or above—has been declining. By 2050 this ratio is expected to drop below the threshold of two working-age persons per every one 65+ person for 7 Asian countries, 24 European countries, and 4 countries in Latin America and the Caribbean (United Nations, Department of Economic and Social Affairs Population Division, 2015, p. 7). While this has broader implications for the global economy, unfavorable support ratios, such as this, will put pressure on countries' health care systems, the ability to deliver high-quality care, and other core aspects for these societies.

In the past, family members, usually a daughter or daughter-in-law, provided care to older parents (Beard & Bloom, 2015, p. 659; Stone & Haraham,

2010, p. 111; WHO, 2015, p. 130). However, worldwide, women are entering the workforce in greater numbers, generations are more likely to live in separate households, and seniors increasingly live alone. In 2010, 28% of all noninstitutionalized older persons lived alone in the United States. Among persons aged 85 years and over, almost half (48%) lived alone in 2010 (U.S. Census Bureau, 2014). This trend is not just an artifact of necessity, living alone in the home has been demonstrated to be a preference by many seniors, with more than 40% of women aged 65 years and over in European countries electing to do so (WHO, 2011, p. 22). This trend extends even to countries with strong traditions of joint family households and family caretakers, such as Japan (WHO, 2011, p. 23).

This rise in the number of seniors who remain in their own homes for the latter years of their lives is a phenomenon popularly referred to as *aging in place*. The sustained need to provide them with in-home support presents a challenge of how we can support independent living even in the face of physical and/or cognitive decline. The potential solutions that technology can offer are manifold—some of the more promising options include mobile health monitoring, telehealth, and various assistive technologies.

Remote patient-monitoring technologies have the potential to provide regular or even continuous real-time information about those who use them. While some older adults have resisted monitoring devices out of a concern for invasion of privacy and loss of autonomy (Garcon et al., 2016), these options are increasingly welcomed by seniors because they promote independence with the added sense of safety that if something went wrong they could receive timely assistance (Center for Technology and Aging, 2009; Fischer David, Crotty, Dierks, & Safran, 2015, p. 4; Pol et al., 2016). This remotely obtained health information can be shared electronically with medical providers or family. Remote patient monitoring and communication technologies include a variety of specific solutions such as glucose monitoring devices, activity-tracking wearables, medication management tools, fall detection technology, and global positioning system (GPS) tracking devices. These tools may be mobile or represent solutions that are directly built into the living environment. A number of chapters in this book provide in-depth review of these types of technological solutions.

While many remote patient–monitoring technologies are stand-alone devices, they are also being integrated with other technologies, or a network of devices and "smart appliances," to monitor and regulate the home environment. The potential goals of these integrated systems include environmental control such as temperature and lighting, as well as appliance activity monitoring, thereby promoting efficiency and safety

(Coughlin, 2014). Sensor data may be integrated into on-site software or processed off-site with specific computer algorithms to assess and mitigate potential adverse events, such as falls. These same tools can alert medical providers, emergency services, caregivers, or family members when appropriate to expedite care (Center for Technology and Aging, 2009). As such, "smart homes" are an important step for effective health monitoring at one's residence, enabling older adults to remain independent and in the home. Companies such as Samsung, Amazon, Intel, and Motorola have seen a market in these types of services and have invested significantly in research and development of smart homes (Center for Technology and Aging, 2009, p. 22). Major barriers to greater incorporation of smart devices and smart home innovations are cost, safety, and reliability (Lee, 2014). Growing public conversation, as well as investment in integrative smart devices, is reflective of shifts in health care approaches, from curing chronic diseases and disability to supporting persons with such conditions (Beard et al., 2016, p. S164).

Other interrelated technologies that can be applied to help seniors remain independent in the home and reduce the need for outside care include e-Health or *telehealth* technologies (see Chapters 4, 10, and 11) that digitally connect older adults with care providers, health education, and emergency services (Garcon et al., 2016, p. S295). Telehealth technologies allow older adults to interact with health professionals using a variety of interfaces, most popularly through video teleconferencing. As a result, health care providers can assess a patient's health condition at a distance to allow remote diagnosis, recommend a course of treatment, coordinate care, and collaborate with other remote providers (Thomas & Applebaum, 2015). Additionally, for seniors with limitations that keep them home bound, for those who live in rural hard-to-reach settings (see Chapter 5), and for those who have limited access to transportation, e-Health and telehealth provide convenient and more equitable access to quality medical care. The use of such information and communication technologies offers an opportunity for more timely intervention and care for many conditions and illnesses that, if left unmanaged, may lead to more permanent and costly complications. Telehealth technologies also reduce exposure to nosocomial infections, increase convenience, and lower transportation costs (Boots, Widdicombe, & Lipman, 2016; Dunn, Hongyung, Almagro, Recla, & Davis, 2000). Research has shown that with these solutions, the number of in-person visits made to medical care providers and overall expenditure decrease while contact hours between provider and patient increase (Thomas & Applebaum, 2015, p. 59).

Although the focus of this book is advanced health technology, relatively simple but effective traditional assistive devices should not be overlooked when implementing a holistic care strategy. For example, research has demonstrated that basic assistive technologies such as those that aid in vision and hearing (glasses and hearing aids), mobility (canes, walkers, and walking frames), toileting, hygiene, and comfort (cushions for adjusting beds and furnishings), are invaluable contributors to quality of life and health (Garcon et al., 2016, p. S295; Marasinghe, Lapitan, & Ross, 2015; WHO, 2014a; WHO, 2015, p. 111). Additional analogue interventions include ramps, rails, stair lifts, retexturing of floors, and bathroom modifications. Research has shown a drop in reliance of in-person home service by seniors when multiple traditional assistive devices and home modifications are incorporated into the home (Anderson & Wiener, 2015, p. 430; Hoenig, Taylor, & Sloan, 2003; Hong, 2010, p. 96; Wolff, Agree, & Kasper, 2005, p. 1140, 1148).

Perhaps not surprisingly, the adoption rate of newer "smart" technologies is low in comparison to traditional assistive devices (Lee, 2014, p. 14). There are several potential explanations for this observation, including the relative affordability of basic assistive devices (Garcon et al., 2016; Schulz, Wahl, et al., 2015; Wolff et al., 2005), awareness among caregivers and receivers of such devices, ease of use (Kramer, 2014), perceived use value, and their coverage by health insurance. Chapter 2, "Promoting Technology Adoption and Engagement in Aging," explores these topics with the ultimate goal of improved care at a lower cost.

Second Challenge: Increased Caregiver Burden

As noted earlier, the proportional numbers of individuals available to provide care, both formally and informally, is projected to decrease (Anderson & Wiener, 2015, p. 429; Institute of Medicine, Committee on the Future Health Care Workforce for Older Americans, 2008; Redfoot et al., 2013; Stone & Haraham, 2010). The continued decline of the dependency ratio increases the burden of care carried by fewer individuals. Earlier, we outlined the application of technology for keeping seniors independent in the home and reducing the need for care; another important application of technology is to help reduce the burden of care that the provider experiences. Caregivers are a relatively neglected market for the development of technologies that will assist in care (Schulz, Beach, et al., 2015), while caregivers may even be a more receptive market for purchasing assistive technologies than older adult end users (Schulz, Beach, et al., 2015). To that point, job-related injuries among caregivers are high, especially back injuries, as direct care workers help disabled seniors in and out of beds and chairs, for example (Brannon, Barry, Kemper, Schreiner, & Vasey, 2007; Kemper et al., 2008). Institutional-based caregivers have emotionally taxing and physically demanding jobs. These issues are particularly problematic for home nurses who are noted to work more hours than nurses in nearly any other setting (U.S. Department of Health and Human Services, Health Resources and Services Administration, 2010). Importantly, it has been shown that improved managerial support of nursing practice and better relations with physicians, can translate to improved morale and patient outcomes (Flynn, Dickson, & Moles, 2007; Lake & Friese, 2006). Therefore, technological communication and collaboration tools that bridge these gaps may also provide alternate or additional paths to improved patient care.

Informal caregivers are typically untrained and unpaid family or friends of the patient. Unfortunately, this group is more likely than the general population to experience mental health and financial issues because of the demands of caregiving (Hughes, Giobbie-Hurder, Weaver, Kubal, & Henderson, 1999, p. 534). More specifically, for those caring for someone with dementia, caregiver burden is linked to higher rates of depression (Hughes et al., 2004; Sugihara, Sugisawa, Nakatani, & Hougham, 2004). These issues may, in part, be compounded by a lack of training among informal caregivers, the often personal and intensive nature of care, and a lack of supporting care infrastructure for the challenging tasks they are burdened with (Yates, Tennstedt, & Chang, 1999). It is important to acknowledge and account for the specific needs of informal caregivers who may benefit from technological solutions that are configured to their level of understanding and ability.

Appropriately designed and implemented technology can extend the reach of caregivers, ultimately offsetting the cost of care and need for skilled labor. Examples of such technologies include remote patient–monitoring technologies such as wearable devices and teleconferencing, which have been discussed earlier. Another related, and sometimes overlapping, technology is the *relational agent*. Relational or companion devices have been popularly referred to by several names, such as *carebots*, *robot caregivers*, and *social robots*, but their intent is the same—they are designed to build a care relationship with a patient or to perform care duties in order to promote quality health care at a lower cost. Some of the more popularly known products in this category include PARO the robot seal, Robobear, and Polly the talking parrot, all of which are companion devices intended to interact with the recipient. Preliminary research among seniors with dementia who interact with these robots has demonstrated an objective reduction in stress hormones, as seen by decreased cortisol levels. Other fundamental benefits of relational agents include companionship for lonely and/or socially isolated seniors (Bursack, 2016), as well as an alternative interface for remote care interaction, health education, encouragement, and monitoring. Chapter 11 provides an in-depth review of the different types of relational agents as well as their application and value.

Typical relational agents available today are only able to mechanically support themselves with their internal architecture and machinery. However, more robust robotics are under development to assist in the movement of patients or objects in the environment. For example, Robina is a recent robotic caregiver developed by Toyota that is intended to provide direct medical and nursing care and perform other physical activities such as housework (Toyota, n.d.). There are also mechanical exoskeletons in development that can be worn by physically impaired individuals to promote mobility, or be worn by caregivers to assist in physically demanding tasks. Examples include Toyota's Walk Assist Robot (Toyota, 2011, Care Assist Robot Technical Presentation) and Cyberdyne's HAL (Cyberdyne, n.d.). However, these futuristic solutions are projected to be cost intensive (Schulz, Beach, et al., 2015). It may be difficult to justify replacing more standard but less glamorous assistive devices such as electronic lifts and chairs, which are typically used to move bedridden or disabled patients.

In the future, technologically enabled senior care is likely to progress in the direction of a "global, immersive, ambient computing environment with advanced connectivity between devices, systems and services that will alter everyday life for individuals of all ages" (Schulz, Wahl, et al., 2015, pp. 728–729). This medical sensor and Internet of Things (IoT)-enabled vision for health care brings with it challenges and opportunities that are further discussed in Chapter 10. Artificial intelligence and electronic medication management strategies will also play an important role in the future development and design of these solutions to improve the delivery of care for both provider and patients. Chapter 12 provides an extended discussion of the many developing applications of artificial intelligence in health care, and Chapter 8 provides information about the latest advances in medication management and compliance innovations. Finally, with increased time pressures on caregivers, there is a critical need to provide educational resources in a more efficient way. Chapter 13 provides an overview of some of the exciting technological advances in education that are available or currently under development.

Third Challenge: Health Promotion and Prevention

The third challenge is to efficiently and effectively provide health promotion and prevention measures to our older population. The following section provides an overview of how these concepts are relevant to older adults, followed by specific examples.

As outlined earlier, our older population is growing, and research has shown most age-related illnesses are known to develop after the age of 75 years (Shinkai, 2013). The most rapid growth of our older population is occurring in the oldest age groups. In other words, population aging is becoming "deeper" with preferential accumulation of particularly old and frail people who are prone to additional disability. Of particular concern in the United States is the accelerated growth of the population aged 85 years and over, which will occur after 2030 owing to the large size of the Baby Boomer generation (U.S. Census Bureau, 2014; Figures 1.2 and 1.3). Because the prevalence of disability and chronic diseases increases and accelerates with age, there is an imperative to use cost-effective measures to promote health in this group now in order to prevent illness and disability later. This type of intervention may take several forms, but typically involves tailored, population-specific, prevention and health promotion programs. Research has demonstrated that health promotion and lifestyle intervention is effective in compressing morbidity—that is, reducing the time spent in one's life suffering from age-related diseases or disability—and the prevention of some diseases (Fried, 2016; WHO, 2015). Various forms of technology hold great potential for application in prevention and health promotion, helping to personalize treatment to individual older adult's lifestyle and needs. Two common examples of age-related conditions that respond positively to health promotion and prevention with technological applications in this area are discussed in the following paragraphs.

Frailty is a multidimensional medical condition typically marked by a loss of muscle mass and bone density. One's susceptibility increases with age, and research has demonstrated a correlation between a decline in physical activity and an increased risk of developing frailty (Shinkai, 2013). Seniors are among the least physically active of all age groups, and relatively simple steps can be taken to prevent and even reverse the development of frailty. Common examples include musculoskeletal strength and dexterity training and dietary changes. Some examples of technologies currently being applied to encourage physical activity and better nutrition among older adults include consumer health technologies such as the FitBit, Apple watch, and other devices and smartphone applications that track and monitor health. These tools are particularly empowering and powerful because they have the potential to provide immediate feedback and a sense of control over one's own health (Chapter 10 continues the discussion about personal health and wearables, providing an in-depth review of the available options).

The use of mechanical exoskeletons to reduce some of the physical burden of care was discussed earlier. However, these same technologies can also be applied to empower seniors with physical limitations. Even simple mobility assistance devices such as a walkers and canes are examples of technologies that encourage seniors to be active, thereby strengthening their musculoskeletal system so that they may more easily navigate standard living environments and return to a former level of relative physical activity (Chapter 6 offers specific discussion of frailty).

However, there is an important balance to be made in the use of these technologies; assistive devices that oversupport mobility may become too convenient or helpful, leading to the erosion of skills and abilities through their continued use, undermining the very goal of health promotion and prevention (Schulz, Wahl, et al., 2015, p. 732). This underlines the need for appropriate assessment, application, and monitoring of these types of technology.

Increased physical activity has also been linked to the improvement of a variety of other health conditions in old age, including lowered risk for developing chronic diseases, improved psychological status, improved reported well-being, and improved social engagement (U.S. Department of Health and Human Services, 2008). Depression is common among older adults, and research has shown that active seniors who regularly socialize are less likely to develop depression (Shinkai, 2013). Simply encouraging older adults to leave their homes and participate in some form of social engagement, including running errands, can help reduce their risk of developing depression (Shinkai, 2013). In addition to mobility assistance devices that help seniors safely leave their houses, within-the-home information and communication technology can also help facilitate socialization by providing opportunities for talking with friends and family, access to continued education, and stimulate new hobbies and interests, thereby elevating mood and overall psychological well-being (Schulz, Wahl, et al., 2015, p. 725). The discussion in Chapter 11 about relational agents offers further insight into potential technological solutions to mitigate loneliness and isolation.

Finally, home telehealth services offer a virtual extension of a caregiver into a senior's home. This not only provides a way to receive care with a decreased risk of nosocomial infections, but also provides a convenient forum to consume preventive health education as well as health maintenance monitoring. Dedicated discussion about the many facets of home telehealth can be found in Chapter 4.

Fourth Challenge: Develop Service Delivery System Inclusive of Assistive Technologies

The fourth major challenge of an aging society is to effectively deliver advanced assistive technologies to those who need them. Meeting this challenge will involve a fundamental change in how health care is viewed, as well as how patients, caregivers, and health care insurers interact. The following section highlights some of the major challenges and opportunities for successful integration of advanced health care technologies.

Although most older adults and their caregivers feel that assistive technologies should be comprehensively covered by health insurance or paid for by the government, such a responsive health insurance system has yet to be enacted in the United States (Schulz, Beach, et al., 2015, p. 11). Medicare-approved assistive technology is limited to durable medical equipment (DME), which includes medical supplies, medical devices, and assistive devices, but limits it to those that are "reusable, medically necessary, and ordered by a physician for use in the client's home. This definition excludes assistive technology that are obtained without medical authorization, designed for use outside of the home (e.g., portable wheelchairs), and environmental modifications used mainly to enhance functioning or safety" (Kitchener, Ng, Yuol Lee, & Harrington, 2008, p. 182). Recently, the Food and Drug Administration Safety and Innovation Act (FDASIA) endeavored to broaden the scope, especially as it relates to devices that may have health IT functionality (U.S. Food and Drug Administration, 2014). Currently, Medicaid (which provides medical coverage for low-income individuals of all age groups) provides payment for some assistive technologies through its waiver program. However, to complicate matters, what is offered under Medicaid varies from state to state. More evidence of the cost saving and improved care potential of advanced assistive technologies, such as telehealth and robotic caregivers, will be needed before the Centers for Medicare & Medicaid Services will consider paying for them (Schulz, Beach, et al., 2015, p. 12; Schulz, Wahl, et al., 2015, p. 732). There is some hope, however, as already industrialized countries, with more comprehensive service delivery programs, already have policies that offer incentives and subsidies to increase adoption of assistive technologies by insurance providers (Lee, 2014, p. 16).

Despite the challenges of reimbursement and coverage policy, evidence supports the need for a comprehensive health care system that provides coverage for the purchase of assistive medical technology in aging populations. For example, standard assistive device use climbs from 20% at age 70 years to a staggering 90% by age 90 years (Ivanoff & Sonn, 2005 in Garcon et al., 2016, p. S293). Furthermore, advanced medical technologies offer opportunities to lower cost, improve the standard of care, and, in some cases, prevent or even reverse debilitating conditions (Illes, de Grey, & Rae, 2007). Therefore, there is an imperative to build a supportive environment for the innovation and application of assistive technologies and medical devices. An important element of developing a service delivery system inclusive and supportive of assistive technology is to increase the accessibility, affordability, and availability of safe and effective assistive technology and medical devices (WHO, 2014a, p. vi). One proposed strategy to meet these aims can be broken down into four primary initiatives: (a) providing funding mechanisms for the research and development of assistive and medical devices; (b) raising public awareness and building market capacity for assistive technologies and medical devices; (c) putting policy supportive of assistive technology into practice; and (d) fostering service networks and suppliers to bring these technologies into the hands and homes of the older adults and caregivers who need them (Garcon et al., 2016, p. S300) and ensure that they are properly maintained (Coughlin, 2014). Assistive health technologies and medical devices hold the potential of cost-effective care for both individuals and health care systems (Kitchener et al., 2008; Lee, 2014, p. 14). Creating the kinds of technologies that demonstrate value requires both investment as well as the collaborative insight of multiple different types of expertise. For example, technology developers and entrepreneurs need the insight of both caregivers and patients to deliver relevant products to improve health quality, efficiency, and safety. Without dedicated attention to these key elements, health technology and/or the implementation of technology will not be embraced. Chapter 2 provides an in-depth review of these concepts, as well as specific considerations for successful technology design and adoption.

CONCLUSION

While population aging represents a success story of human progress, it also presents profound challenges for health care as well as for society as a whole. Fortunately, the acceleration in technological advances holds the promise of providing improved care more equitably and efficiently. It is important to keep in mind that technology by itself is not the solution, but rather another tool to enhance the quality and delivery of care and the abilities and reach of caregivers. Bringing about successful technology development and deployment requires the collaboration of a variety of different participants including, but not limited to, clinicians, engineers, statisticians, computer scientists, social scientists, political scientists, policy makers, and patients themselves. Insightful leadership and management will need to understand the requirements and perspectives of these stakeholders to meet the growing demands of our rapidly aging population. The chapters in this book present some of the most exciting solutions available to not only adapt, but also lead new paradigms in the effective delivery of high value health care.

REFERENCES

Anderson, W., & Wiener, J. (2015). The impact of assistive technologies on formal and informal home care. *The Gerontologist, 55*(3), 422–433. doi:10.1093/geront/gnt165

Bauman, A., Merom, D., Bull, F., Buchner, D., & Fiatarone Singh, M. (2016). Updating the evidence for physical activity: Summative reviews of the epidemiological evidence, prevalence, and interventions to promote "active aging." *The Gerontologist, 56*(S2), S268–S290. doi:10.1093/geront/gnw031

Beard, J., & Bloom, D. (2015). Towards a comprehensive public health response to population ageing. *The Lancet*, 385, 658–661.

Beard, J., Officer, A., & Cassels, A. (2016). The world report on ageing and health. *The Gerontologist, 56*(S2), S163–S166.

Berwick, D. M., Nolan, T. W., & Whittington, J. (2008). The triple aim: Care, health, and cost. *Health Affairs, 27*(3), 759–769.

Boots, R., Widdicombe, N., & Lipman, J. (2016). Applications of telemedicine in the intensive care unit. *Quality Management in Intensive Care: A Practical Guide*, 235–246. doi:10.1017/CBO9781316218563

Bowser, B. A. (2013). Why long-term care for U.S. seniors is headed for 'crisis.' *PBS Newshour*. Retrieved from http://www.pbs.org/newshour/rundown/americas-looming-long-term-care-crisis-and-what-can-be-done

Brannon, D., Barry, T., Kemper, P., Schreiner, A., & Vasey, J. (2007). Job perceptions and intent to leave among direct care workers: Evidence from the better jobs better care demonstration. *The Gerontologist, 47*(6), 820–829. doi:10.1093/geront/47.6.820

Bursack, C. (2016). I, caregiver: Do robots have a place in elder care. Retrieved from https://www.agingcare.com/Articles/robots-in-elder-care-170581.htm

Center for Technology and Aging. (2009). *Technologies for remote patient monitoring in older adults*. Paper presented at the SCAN Foundation and Public Health Institute, Oakland, CA.

Coughlin, J. (2014). Technology, innovation, and developing a NexGen aging services workforce. *Public Policy & Aging, 24*, 6–9. doi:10.1093/ppar/prt009

Cyberdyne. (n.d.). Other HAL series. Retrieved from http://www.cyberdyne.jp/english/products/supporting.html

Dessem, E., Walsh, M., Beattie, B., Kulinski, K., Lachenmayr, S., & Boutaugh, M. (2013). *Monograph: Evidence-based programs and resources for changing behavior in older adults.* Retrieved from http://www.healthandtheaging.org/wp-content/uploads/2011/12/Evidence-Based-Programs-and-Resources-for-Changing-Behavior-in-Older-Adults-final-11-23.pdf

Dunn, B. E., Hongyung, C., Almagro, A., Recla, D. L., & Davis, C. W. (2000). Telepathology networking in VISN-12 of the Veterans Health Administration. *Telemedicine Journal and e-Health*, 6, 349–354.

Fischer, S., David, D., Crotty, B., Dierks, M., & Safran, C. (2014). Acceptance and use of health information technology by community-dwelling elders. *International Journal of Medical Informatics, 83*(9), 624–635. doi:10.1016/j.ijmedinf.2014.06.005

Flynn, L., Dickson, G., & Moles, D. J. (2007). Focus on caregiving. Enhancing the nursing workplace: In a recent study of long term care nurses, key organizational factors emerge as most important in supporting a productive work environment. *Provider, 33*(1), 35–39.

Fried, L. (2016). Investing in health to create a third demographic dividend. *The Gerontologist, 56*(S2), S167–S177. doi:10.1093/geront/gnw035

Garcon, L., Khasnabis, C., Walker, L., Nakatani, Y., Lapitan, J., Borg, J., . . . Velazquez Verumen, A. (2016). Medical and assistive health technology: Meeting the needs of aging populations. *The Gerontologist, 56*(S2), S293–S302. doi:10.1093/geront/gnw005

Hoenig, H., Taylor, D., & Sloan, F. (2003). Does assistive technology substitute for personal assistance among the disabled? *American Journal of Public Health, 93*, 330–337.

Hong, S. (2009). Understanding patterns of service utilization among informal caregivers of community older adults. *The Gerontologist, 50*(1), 87–99. doi:10.1093/geront/gnp105

Hughes, S., Giobbie-Hurder, A., Weaver, F., Kubal, J., & Henderson W. (1999). Relationship between caregiver burden and health-related quality of life. *The Gerontologist, 39*(3), 534–545.

Illes, J., de Grey, A., & Rae, M. (2007). Ending aging: The rejuvenation breakthroughs that could reverse human aging in our lifetime. *Nature*, 450(7168), 351–352.

Institute of Medicine, Committee on the Future Health Care Workforce for Older Americans. (2008). *Retooling for an aging America: Building the health care workforce.* Washington, DC: National Academies Press.

Ivanoff, S. D., & Sonn, U. (2005). Changes in the use of assistive devices among 90-year-old persons. *Aging Clinical and Experimental Research, 17*, 246–251. doi:10.1007/BF03324604

Kemper, P., Heier, B., Barry, T., Brannon, D., Angelelli, J., Vasey, J., & Anderson-Knott, M. (2008). What do direct care workers say would improve their jobs? Differences across settings. *The Gerontologist, 48*(1), 17–28.

Kitchener, M., Ng, T., Yuol Lee, H., & Harrington, C. (2008). Assistive technology in Medicaid home- and community-based waiver programs. *The Gerontologist, 48*(2), 181–189.

Kramer, B. (2014). Dementia caregivers in Germany and their acceptance of new technologies for care: The information gap. *Public Policy & Aging Report*, 24, 32–34.

Lake, E. T., & Friese, C. R. (2006). Variations in nursing practice environments: Relation to staffing and hospital characteristics. *Nursing Research, 55*(1), 1–9.

Lee, C. (2014). Adoption of smart technology among older adults: Challenges and issues. *Public Policy & Aging Report, 24*, 14–17. doi:10.1093/ppar/prt005

Lewis, N. (2014). A primer on defining the Triple Aim. Retrieved from http://www.ihi.org/communities/blogs/_layouts/ihi/community/blog/itemview.aspx?List=81ca4a47-4ccd-4e9e-89d9-14d88ec59e8d&ID=63

Marasinghe, K. M., Lapitan, M. J., & Ross, A. (2015). Assistive technologies for aging populations in six low-income and middle-income countries: A systematic review. *BMJ Innovations, 1*(4), 182–195. doi:10.1136/bmjinnov-2015-000065

Pol, M., Van Nes, F., Van Hartingsveldt, M., Buurman, B., De Rooij, S., & Krose, B., (2016). Older people's perspectives regarding the use of sensor monitoring in their home. *The Gerontologist, 56*(3), 485–493. doi:10.1093/geront/gnu104

Prince, M., Wu, F., Guo, Y., Gutierrez Robledo, L., O'Donnell, M., Sullivan, R., & Yusuf, S. (2015). The burden of disease in older people and implications for health policy and practice. *The Lancet, 385*, 549–562.

Redfoot, D., Feinberg, L., & Houser, A. (2013). The aging of the baby boom and the growing care gap: A look at future declines in the availability of family caregivers. *AARP Public Policy Institute* (Insight on the Issues 85), 1–12.

Schulz, R., Beach, S., Matthews, J., Courtney, K., De Vito Dabbs, A., & Mecca, L. (2015). Caregivers' willingness to pay for technologies to support caregiving. *The Gerontologist, 56*, 817–829. doi:10.1093/geront/gnv033

Schulz, R., Wahl, H. W., Matthews, J., De Vito Dabbs, A., Beach, S., & Czaja, S. (2015). Advancing the aging and technology agenda in gerontology. *The Gerontologist, 55*(5), 724–734. doi:10.1093/geront/gnu071

Shinkai, S. (2013). *Kōreisha no Jyaka wo Yobō Shi Kenkō Yomei wo Ennshinn Suru Shakai Shisutemu no Kaihatsu* [Development of a social system or preventing frailty in old age and extending remaining years of healthy life]. Research Institute of Science and Technology for Society (RISTEX), Ministry of Education, Culture, Sports, Science and Technology. Retrieved from http://www.ristex.jp/korei/02project/prj_h23_07.html

Stone, R., & Harahan, M. (2010). Improving the long-term care workforce serving older adults. *Health Affairs, 29*(1), 109–115. doi:10.1377/hlthaff.2009.0554

Sugihara, Y., Sugisawa, H., Nakatani, Y., & Hougham, G. W. (2004). Longitudinal changes in the well-being of Japanese caregivers: Variations across kin relationships. *Journals of Gerontology, Series B: Psychological Sciences and Social Sciences, 59*(4), P177–P184.

Thomas, K. S., & Applebaum, R. (2015). Long-term services and supports (LTSS): A growing challenge for an aging America. *Public Policy & Aging Report, 25*, 65–62. doi:10.1093/ppar/prv003

Toyota. (2011). Care assist robot technical presentation. Retrieved from http://www.toyota-global.com/innovation/partner_robot/technical_presentation

Toyota. (n.d.). Partner robot family. Retrieved from http://www.toyota-global.com/innovation/partner_robot/family_2.html

United Nations, Department of Economic and Social Affairs Population Division. (2013). *World population ageing 2013*. New York, NY: United Nations Publication.

United Nations, Department of Economic and Social Affairs Population Division. (2015). *World population prospects: The 2015 revision*. New York, NY: United Nations Publication.

U.S. Census Bureau. (2014). *65+ in the United States: 2010*. Washington, DC: Government Printing Office.

U.S. Census Bureau. (2016). *An aging world: 2015*. Washington, DC: Government Printing Office.

U.S. Department of Health and Human Services. (2008). Physical activity guidelines for Americans. ODPHP publication. Retrieved from http://health.gov/paguidelines/guidelines

U.S. Department of Health and Human Services, Health Resources and Services Administration. (2010). *The registered nurse population: Findings from the 2008 national sample survey of registered nurses.* Chicago, IL: Author.

U.S. Food and Drug Administration. (2014). *FDASIA health IT report: Proposed strategy and recommendations for a risk-based framework*. Washington, DC: The Office of the National Coordinator for Health Information Technology.

Wolff, J. L., Agree, E. M., & Kasper, J. D. (2005). Wheelchairs, walkers, and canes: What does Medicare pay for, and who benefits? *Health Affairs, 24*(4), 1140–1149. doi:10.1377/hlthaff.24.4.1140

World Health Organization. (2007). *Global age-friendly cities: A guide*. Geneva, Switzerland: Author.

World Health Organization. (2014a). *Survey of needs for assistive and medical devices for older people in six countries of the WHO Western Pacific Region: China, Japan, Malaysia, the Philippines, the Republic of Korea and Viet Nam.* Chuo-ku, Kobe: Author.

World Health Organization. (2014b). "Ageing well" must be a global priority. Retrieved from http://www.who.int/mediacentre/news/releases/2014/lancet-ageing-series/en

World Health Organization. (2015). *World report on ageing and health*. Geneva, Switzerland: Author.

World Health Organization; National Institute on Aging, National Institutes of Health; U.S. Department of Health and Human Services. (2011). *Global health and aging*. Bethesda, MD: National Institutes of Health.

Yates, M. E., Tennstedt, S., & Chang, B. H. (1999). Contributors to and mediators of psychological well-being for informal caregivers. *Journals of Gerontology, Series B: Psychological Sciences and Social Sciences, 54*(1), P12–P22.

2

Promoting Technology Adoption and Engagement in Aging

Ashley Reynolds and Thomas F. Osborne

Digital tools are becoming an integral part of the health care system. According to a Healthcare Information and Management Systems Society (HIMSS) survey, 90% of health care organizations use some form of digital health tool to engage patients, with 73% using application-enabled patient portals, 62% using telehealth services, 57% using text communications, and 49% using remote patient–monitoring technologies (HIMSS, 2015). Rapid advances in technology are providing many new tools that are designed to allow older adults to manage their health, stay connected with their providers and social groups, and maintain their independence longer (Goldwater & Harris, 2011). Older adults are using digital health tools with increasing frequency (Entertainment Software Association, 2011; Fox, 2012; Gerling, Schild, & Masuch, 2010; Pew Research Center, 2010) and over half of adults aged 65 years or older would be willing to use wireless health monitoring devices in their homes (Barrett, 2011). Although older adults may benefit the most from using health technology, many, particularly frail, low-income, or poorly educated adults, may not use these devices owing to lack of training, technophobia, shortage of resources, and physical or cognitive impediments (Kim et al., 2009). As a generational cohort, older adults possess similarities that may impact their perceptions about technology, thereby influencing their preferences and use of digital tools (Reynolds, 2013). Fortunately, there are ways practitioners can encourage health technology adoption and sustained engagement by their patients.

Many technologies hold great promise for improving the quality of life in an aging population; however, these benefits will only be realized if they are embraced. It is necessary for patients to establish and maintain engagement with these tools in order to benefit themselves, their caregivers, and care team. From the viewpoint that use of technology for health can be considered a type of health behavior, practitioners may rely on established health behavior theories and other models of technology adoption to implement interventions supporting patient engagement with digital tools.

In this chapter, we explore the functionality necessary to promote older adults' engagement with digital health tools, health behavior concepts that may be used to promote adoption, and suggest interventions to promote usage. The primary focus is on addressing factors that are within the practitioner's ability to influence, such as digital health tool user education and proper selection of technology, while recognizing that some barriers to adoption, such as lack of high-speed Internet connections in rural areas, will require federal, state, and local community involvement. In addition, we explore practical considerations when deploying technologies to diverse groups of older users and their caregivers. Finally, we examine methods in which providers may seek reimbursement for digital health services within their practices.

ADOPTION OF HEALTH TECHNOLOGY

On a population level, the adoption and diffusion of a new technology over time can be illustrated and described with a bell-shaped curve. This type of representation may use various terms for the different population subgroups, but the general concepts of stratifying the demographics is similar. Everett M. Rogers is perhaps the most cited expert on the topic and has described five population categories based on their innovativeness and rate of adoption. In his model, from most adoptive to least, are the innovators, early adopters, early majority, late majority, and laggards (Rogers, 2010).

The diffusion of a new technology is highly dependent on the types of adopters in the cohort, as well as the perceived relative cost benefit of the innovation. As such, many of the factors influencing the adoption of a technology are intimately related to the concepts of engagement discussed earlier. More specifically, innovations that are disruptive to routine workflows, complex to learn, or otherwise difficult to use may not be adopted even when they provide significant advantage. Likewise, health technologies that cost-effectively solve problems, make tasks easier, incorporate support from other users, facilitate engagement, and are generally enjoyable to use are more likely to be rapidly adopted (Aubert & Hamel, 2001; Dobbins, Cockerill, & Barnsley, 2001; Rogers, 2010).

The opinions of individuals may also have a significant impact on the rate of adoption and diffusion of a new technology. However, not all individuals exert the same amount of influence as others. In this sense respected key opinion leaders may exert their influence in spreading either positive or negative information about an innovation (Katz & Lazarsfeld, 1970; Rogers, 2010). In health care, this influence can be imparted to different groups through various routes. For example, patients may be positively influenced by the experiences of friends, family, directed advertising, and by the opinions of health care providers. Health care providers may likewise be positively influenced by similar factors, personal practice experience, as well as the objective results published in respected peer-reviewed journal articles.

At an institutional level, medical practices and hospitals face more complex adoption possibilities because organizations are both the aggregate of its individuals, as well as its own goals, process, and procedures. There are two major types of decisions that impact the adoption of a new technology: collective decisions and authority decisions. However, both of these may be influenced by a "champion" who may enthusiastically break through opposition (Greenhalgh et al., 2004; Howell & Higgins 1990; Rogers, 2010).

In health care, the factors influencing adoption of a new technology are further complicated by the additional needs and perspectives of larger groups such as health insurance providers, as well as federal influences in the form of mandates and regulations. With this level of intertwined influences, barriers to adoption may arise when the vested interest or needs of each of these distinct groups are not in alignment. However, when the needs of each stakeholder are addressed, widespread adoption may occur rapidly.

AGE-RELATED DIFFERENCES IN TECHNOLOGY USE

Age-related differences have been observed in the use of various types of technology such as Internet use (Chu & Mastel-Smith, 2010; Cohall et al., 2011; McInnes, Gifford, Kazis, & Wagner, 2010; McMillan & Macias, 2008), online health programs (Bickmore, Caruso, Clough-Gorr, & Heeren, 2005), social networks (Fukuoka, Kamitani, Bonnet, & Lindgren, 2011), video games (Gerling et al., 2010; Nitz, Kuys, Isles, & Fu, 2010; Pearce, 2008), and self-monitoring devices (Beaudin, Intille, & Morris, 2006; Svensson & Lagerros, 2010), although the reasons for these differences are varied. Generally speaking, technology use declines with advancing age, especially after age 75 years. However, older adults tend to utilize technology for health more frequently than their younger counterparts (Olson, O'Brien, Rogers,

& Charness, 2011; Pew Research Center, 2014; Reynolds, 2013). Ostensibly, these differences are due, in part, to increased illness burden or cognitive and physical changes; however, it should be noted that these changes do not occur for every individual, and providers must take care to assess the suitability of a particular digital health tool on a case-by-case basis. According to the Center for Technology and Aging (2011), 11% of adults over the age of 50 years use mobile devices to track health metrics such as blood glucose, physical activity levels, or blood pressure. Finally, use of online e-Health tools by older adults peaks at ages 65 to 69 years, before decreasing as age reaches the oldest old (McInnes et al., 2010; McMillan & Macias, 2008; Pew Research Center, 2014).

For seniors who do not use digital tools, 48% agree that not using them puts them at a disadvantage. A significant majority of older adults (77%) agree that they need assistance when learning to use digital tools, compared to just 18% who are comfortable learning on their own (Pew Research Center, 2014). Although older adults tend to lag behind the general population in their use of technology, once comfortable using the tools, they tend to use them frequently and perceive them as being important to their everyday lives (Pew Research Center, 2014).

Older adults tend to prefer certain technologies over others and this information can be useful when considering which digital health tools to use. For example, tablet and e-reader ownership is much higher (27%) than smartphone ownership in older adults (Pew Research Center, 2014). Additionally, while 77% of older adults own some form of mobile phone, just 18% of these devices are smartphones. In one study, Mercer et al. (2016) found that a majority of older adults aged 50 to 84 years old, who were diagnosed with a chronic illness, perceived wearable activity devices as useful. Participant technology acceptance scores for this study were high, ranging from 55.7 to 67.6 on a 95-point scale for each device studied, thereby indicating increased perceived usefulness (Mercer et al., 2016).

DIGITAL TOOL FUNCTIONALITY

The first step in promoting user engagement with clinical digital tools by older adults is ensuring that the proposed instrument functions in a way that supports health. With the advent of health technology software, wearable devices, mobile platforms such as the smartphone, and the ease with which developers are able to create new functionality, there is a glut of digital health resources available that are not evidence based. However, even though there were estimated to be over 165,000 mobile health applications in the app stores in 2016, only about 24% possess features necessary for disease and treatment management (IMS Institute, 2015; Mottl, 2015). In many instances, developers failed to integrate evidence-based clinical or behavioral concepts when constructing digital health tools (Masterson Creber et al., 2016). Unfortunately, this can happen because well-intended developers may work in a vacuum without clinical guidance or oversight, leading to reduced value of their tool and limited patient engagement.

If a digital tool is used for wellness, disease management, remote monitoring, or to improve health literacy, but is not evidence based or does not meet a clinical need, it may impede user engagement with the digital health tool, negatively affect self-efficacy, produce untoward outcomes, or not support health in the way the practitioner or the patient intends. Therefore, it is important to assess proposed digital health tools to ensure that they are meeting evidence-based standards of care prior to adding them to a treatment plan. Broadly speaking, digital health tools should be designed to meet one or more of the following defined needs (Reynolds, Rubens, King, & Machado, 2016): facilitate communication, improve health literacy, increase social interaction, create awareness of risk(s), support condition management, enable user self-monitoring of behavior, and generate actionable data that can be used to further refine both population-wide and individual interventions.

In other words, the selected tool should provide a discernable benefit to the user while contributing to the treatment plan. User interfaces should be designed so that older users may interact easily with them. If the digital health tools are complicated, confusing, or expensive, with little or no perceived benefits for use, they become a barrier rather than an enhancement to care. Digital health tools should be designed to promote patient and caregiver engagement, provide information to improve health literacy, help guide treatment decisions, and foster communication.

PATIENT ENGAGEMENT

Engaging patients in their own care has been recognized for decades as a key component of care delivery (Choi & Dinitto, 2013; Hibbard & Greene, 2013; James, 2013). According to the World Health Organization (WHO; 2007), the goals for general engagement in older adults include social participation, employment and volunteerism, and access to information and resources. While there is not a single, consistent definition of patient engagement in health, most include variants on the concepts of shared decision making, promotion of health literacy, and individual empowerment (Reynolds et al., 2016). Poor engagement has been linked to negative outcomes for older adults. For example, decreased health literacy is associated with increased mortality in older adults (Bostock & Steptoe, 2012).

Digital tools offer many opportunities to improve patient engagement. For example, using glucose self-monitoring tools, such as wireless glucometers, in conjunction with automated feedback, provider-alerting integration, and targeted decision-support education can be useful in promoting diabetes self-management. Embedded video content and interactive tools such as online tutorials, risk assessments, and learning libraries can improve health literacy. Furthermore, social network use by older adults, especially those who are unable to easily travel or leave their homes, can facilitate social interactivity, which has been associated with improved physical and mental health (WHO, 2007).

CAREGIVER ENGAGEMENT

The incorporation of digital tools into the health care of older adults often requires collaboration from multiple different stakeholders. Therefore, acceptance and endorsement of the technology from a variety of key participants is a critical but sometimes neglected feature of success (NORC at the University of Chicago, 2012). These health care collaborators are varied and include professional caregivers, nonclinical support staff, administrators, and, in some cases, family and friends (Cimperman, Brenčič, Trkman, & Stanonik, 2013). The incorporation of family and friends is particularly important for older adults because they may be intimately involved in a patient's health care. Therefore, when appropriate, these additional caregivers can provide added value in the implementation, use, and troubleshooting of these technological tools (Reich & Osborne, 2016).

Failure to properly address the needs and perspectives of important contributors may result in dissatisfaction or even the perception that technology has become a substitute rather than an enhancer of quality patient-centered care (Reich & Osborne, 2016). Thoughtfully designed user interfaces that are tailored to the various contributing caregiver needs promotes a more effective, intuitive, and enjoyable experience, which also decreases the need for extensive training and elaborate change management strategies. As an example, a recent research study demonstrated marked health care efficiency and return on investment from a communication and collaboration health care platform based on user-centered design methodology (Osborne et al., 2017). These positive results, coupled with improved communication tools, create a natural path to engagement for caregivers, and the positive attitude that this fosters can translate to increased patient engagement as well. Alternatively, when technological tools are developed without the direct consultation or understanding of a caregiver's perspectives, the results are typically suboptimal. As a minimum requirement, digital solutions should not hamper the abilities of those involved. However, for successful acceptance and engagement, these additional features should improve upon an existing framework (Liker, 2004; Reich & Osborne, 2016). More specifically, health technology tools may be more efficient and embraced to a greater degree when integrated into an established care workflow and when data are transmitted automatically to information systems such as an electronic health record (EHR; Singh, Mathiassen, Stachura, & Astapova, 2011). Unfortunately, this level of interoperability is uncommon.

These issues are particularly pertinent to home caregivers who may already be overworked; home health nurses work more hours than nurses in nearly any other setting (U.S. Department of Health and Human Services, Health Resources and Services Administration, 2010). Importantly, it has been shown that improved managerial support of nursing practice and better relations with physicians can translate to improved morale and patient outcomes (Flynn, Dickson, & Moles, 2007; Lake & Friese, 2006). Therefore, technological communication and engagement tools that bridge these gaps may also provide nonlinear paths to improved patient care (Osborne, Reich, Arkwright, & Russo, 2016).

BEHAVIORAL MODELS

Adoption and use of digital tools by older adults can be viewed as an action that may be influenced by various concepts within health behavior frameworks. Using these concepts, practitioners can develop strategies influencing these variables, thereby influencing the intended action. There are many different health behavior theories, and this section does not cover them all. Rather, this section is meant to provide an overview of commonly used evidence-based health-behavior concepts, along with suggestions for utilization, in order to improve older adults' engagement with digital health tools. Leveraging digital tools with older adults may require a commitment of practitioner time and resources; however, this effort is needed in order to fully realize the benefits these technologies provide.

Social Cognitive Theory (Behavioral Model)

Social cognitive theory (SCT) is deeply rooted in the study of human learning and behavior. SCT is a theoretical framework used throughout psychology and health education that states that learning and behavior can be attributed to various influences such as social influences or a sense of personal self-confidence. According to Bandura (1997), individual behaviors can be influenced through direct observation and modeling, expected outcomes, presence of barriers, self-efficacy, and through intrinsic or extrinsic rewards. SCT has been widely used to explain a variety of health behaviors such as exercise and tobacco use.

A principal component of SCT is the concept of self-efficacy. Bandura (1997) defines self-efficacy as one's personal belief in one's capability to perform an action. Bandura adds, "Perceived self-efficacy is concerned not with the number of skills that you have, but with what you believe you can do with what you have under a variety of circumstances" (Bandura, 1997, p. 37)—simply put, how confident a person is in his or her ability to complete a task, given a variety of stressors.

Some authors also suggest how e-Health support may influence social cognitive variables, such as self-efficacy (Anderson-Bill, Winett, Wojcik, & Winett, 2011; Bandura, 2004; Song, Peng, & Lee, 2011), outcome expectations (Anderson-Bill et al., 2011; Bandura, 2004), and barriers to exercise (Boschman, 2010; Center for Technology and Aging, 2011). According to Reynolds (2013), increased self-efficacy for health technology use is related to increased use of digital tools in older adults. Based on social cognitive theory, there are four ways self-efficacy can be influenced to promote adoption and engagement with digital health tools in older adults. According to Bandura (2004), self-efficacy can be affected by mechanisms such as mastery experiences, vicarious learning, verbal persuasion, and overcoming physiological/affective states.

Mastery Experiences

Of the four mechanisms to increase self-efficacy, *mastery experiences* provides the greatest influence on personal efficacy beliefs (Bandura, 1997). As an individual experiences continued successes with a task, the confidence in his or her ability to perform increases. Practitioners can influence digital health tool use by providing mastery experiences for older adults so that they can become more confident in their use of digital tools. Offering staged training and building from basic tasks toward more complex ones can improve older users' confidence, thereby influencing their efficacy beliefs and promoting use. In one study, Howard, Jacobson, and Kriplani (2013) found that utilizing the teach-back method was effective at promoting health literacy, although only 22% of practitioners actually used it.

Vicarious Learning

Another key component of SCT is the concept of vicarious learning. According to Bandura (1997), human beings learn by observing another's behaviors.

This is an effective way to influence self-efficacy. Humans tend to emulate those who appear most like themselves. The more a person observes another similar person completing a task or behaving a certain way, the more likely that person will attempt to repeat that behavior (Bandura, 1986, 1997). In order to influence the concept of vicarious learning to foster digital tool adoption, practitioners can use teaching groups of similarly situated older adults who can share their experiences and successes with each other and their caregivers. Providers can support vicarious learning through a variety of ways including provision of peer technology champions, social learning experiences, and peer demonstrations of health technology usage.

Verbal Persuasion

Feedback in the form of verbal communications also has an impact on self-efficacy beliefs (Bandura, 1997). Affirmative statements given to individuals regarding their capabilities support their beliefs that they possess the characteristics needed to be successful in their endeavors. Practitioners should provide ongoing verbal encouragement and feedback when promoting digital tool engagement. This can be accomplished during clinical interactions, training classes, or through outreach and communications. Unfortunately, these can be expensive and time consuming. New advances in digital interactions, including in the development of digital relational agents, virtual teaching environments, and cognitive computing, offer opportunities to enable automated, conversational digital teachers who would be able to assist and encourage older adults in learning how to use digital health tools. More data are needed to determine whether these approaches will be effective and inexpensive enough to justify their use.

Other Behavioral Models

In addition to health behavior theories that can be leveraged to support the intended behavior of technology use by patients and caregivers, other models provide insight into ways providers can promote digital tool use within their practices. The Accelerating Diffusion of Proven Technologies (ADOPT) model is a framework that identifies factors that affect older adults' use of technology and recommends ways to promote diffusion (Wang, Redington, Steinmetz, & Lendeman, 2011). *Diffusion* is defined as the speed with which new technologies are adopted (Rogers, 1995). Diffusion models attempt to explain the factors that influence technology adoption within certain groups. In their model, Wang et al. (2011) identify several key factors that influence technology adoption in older adults. These factors include coaching users and collaborators on the use of the technology, and establishing technology champions who can promote technology within practices or in the home, establish the value technology provides for the user, and design user-friendly interfaces that make interaction easier.

ADDITIONAL FACTORS INFLUENCING ENGAGEMENT

Computer technology has existed since the late 1930s, although most individuals did not see or interact with these machines until much later. Prior to 1976, computers were often large, bulky devices that could not be used in the home (Computer History Museum, 2006). It was not until the advent of the personal computer in 1977 with the Apple II, the first widely adopted personal computer, that exposure to computers became widespread. Experiential timing can influence how older users perceive technology. For example, as older adults' first exposure to digital technology was not until much later in life compared to younger users, they may tend to view them as work tools rather than health supports (Reynolds, 2013). The cost of digital tools at the time of older adults' first exposure may influence their perceptions of technology being expensive and therefore costly to purchase or replace if they break it. In addition, many older adults may have not experienced newer tools such as smartphones and wearable devices until recently, if at all. Thus, it is important to note that some older adults may never have seen these digital health tools in use, and therefore may be fearful or unable to intuit any real benefit from their use (Czaja et al., 2006).

Older adults view electronic resources differently from their younger counterparts in that they tend to be more fearful in their use, and are slower to adopt new technologies (Reynolds, 2013). While both Millennials (24%) and Generation X (12%) view their use of technology as the defining characteristic of their respective generations, Baby Boomers cite work ethic (17%) and the Silent Generation cite the Depression and World War II (14%) as theirs (Pew Research Center, 2010). These viewpoints are not surprising when one considers the emergence of various technologies and the differences when they were first experienced and adopted.

BARRIERS TO ADOPTION

Adding technology to an older adult's treatment care plan requires thoughtful consideration to ensure that the right tools are being leveraged, and that they enhance the user experience rather than complicate it. Adoption and use of technology for health varies within diverse populations.

Privacy Concerns

Protecting health information is a fundamental component of health programs. Federal laws, combined with state regulations and various accreditation bodies, have prioritized the concept of protected health information (PHI). However, the rapid emergence of new mobile technologies and their adoption within the health management model pose significant challenges and, in some instances, well-known regulations such as the Health Insurance Portability and Accountability Act (HIPAA) have failed to keep up. For instance, wearable devices or mobile applications may collect data from users that would be traditionally considered PHI, yet they are often not explicitly addressed in privacy rules. Furthermore, in many instances, personal health data collected via mobile applications and wearable devices are poorly protected (Healthcare Business Tech, 2014). As evidenced by recent wearable device data breaches, more work is needed to improve privacy and security protections within these types of emerging mobile health technologies (Mangan, 2016).

Lack of Interoperability

Another key consideration is the potential lack of interoperability among technology systems (President's Council of Advisors on Science and Technology, 2016). User-generated health data may be contained within several disparate systems that often lack integration, resulting in siloed data, which can result in medical errors and decreased efficiency. For example, electronic medical records may not be integrated with remote patient–monitoring data, telehealth platforms, or mobile application databases, thereby making a holistic view of the patient difficult. In addition, requiring providers to access information in multiple systems presents a barrier to workflow and creates inefficiencies in an already busy work environment. Therefore, decision makers should seek partnerships with technology providers who are willing and have the resources to integrate their tools and the data they generate into the primary workflow and information systems such as an EHR (Wang et al., 2011).

Digital Divide

Regardless of the quality and ubiquity of digital tools, gaps remain in their use owing to a variety of factors. This gap is often termed the *digital divide* and is commonly related to lower education, lower socioeconomic status, or advanced age (Kreps & Neuhauser, 2010). Environmental access to technology is a function of infrastructure (availability) and resources (affordability).

The digital divide refers to the limitations of some populations to receive digital services because of reduced access or affordability (Kreps & Neuhauser, 2010; Noar & Harrington, 2012). According to Zickuhr and Smith (2012), one in five adults do not have access to the Internet. Older adults, those of lower socioeconomic status, non-English speaking, and less-educated adults lead this disconnected group in the United States.

Practitioners should assess potential users of health technology to determine whether or not they possess the necessary infrastructure, financial means, or cognitive capacity to use digital tools successfully. For instance, digital tools requiring broadband Internet connectivity are clearly not appropriate for those who do not have Internet access. In these situations, alternative tools that allow delayed information transfer can be achieved asynchronously in a "store-and-forward" process. A sometimes less-obvious consideration is device data usage because data consumption can be a hidden cost for programs or patients who use mobile applications or wearable device integrations.

Technology Design

How a digital tool is constructed can greatly impact its usability for older adults, thereby impacting technology engagement. According to McCloskey (2006), older adults' perceptions about technology, as well as its ease of use, are important factors influencing adoption. Various changes typically associated with aging require development of user interfaces that recognize the specific needs of the older user and do not require them, or their caregivers, to perform actions outside of the scope of their physical or cognitive capabilities (Czaja, et al., 2006; Fisk, Rogers, Chamess, Czaja, & Sharit, 2009; Reynolds, 2013).

According to Or and Tao (2012), health technology should be designed to meet a defined patient or caregiver need in order to be perceived as useful. As older adults often struggle with keyboard entry, especially on smartphones, practitioners should consider tools that reduce data entry burden, such as wearable monitoring devices, which passively acquire and automatically transfer the data to the appropriate destination (Correia de Barros, Leitao, & Ribeiro, 2014). For example, wearable activity monitors that are connected to a technology platform allow activity data from older users to be automatically captured without requiring unneeded interactions with technology interfaces.

PROMOTING USE

There are several interventions, from selecting the appropriate digital health tool to providing user education, that practitioners can utilize to promote digital tool use in older adults. These techniques include clearly defining the benefits of technology use, how the information will be used to support the treatment plan, and how users can provide feedback regarding their experiences with these tools. As described earlier, a significant majority of older adults are not comfortable learning to use technology without some assistance (Pew Research Center, 2014). This concept is further supported by recommendations from the President's Council of Advisors on Science and Technology (PCAST), which states that technology training is a critical component in fostering digital tool adoption in older adults (President's Council of Advisors on Science and Technology, 2016).

Practitioners can use the *sentinel effect* to promote digital tool use. According to Kvedar (2014), the sentinel effect is the effect in which performance of a particular behavior improves when a person is aware that the behavior is being evaluated. In practical terms, the practitioner should inquire about the digital tools during patient interactions, review logs, and discuss the data collected from the digital health tools while integrating the knowledge gained from the tools into the treatment plan. This feedback loop helps patients see that digital tool use is valuable and important to the practitioner, thereby increasing its perceived value and importance for themselves.

Providers should identify digital technology champions within their organizations, as well as enlisting caregivers as in-home supports (Rogers, 1995; Wang et al., 2011). These individuals may include staff members within the practice, or the providers themselves. Technology champions are often a key component to successful adoption of digital tools by acting as a resource, reinforcing the value these tools provide, while serving as a teacher and guide when needed. Champions should believe in the value of using the digital tool and consistently act by supporting the user and caregivers.

TEACHING TO PROMOTE TECHNOLOGY USE AND SELF-EFFICACY

Experiential learning, coupled with individualized support, mastery experiences, and opportunities for social interactions can aid in skill development and acquiring the understanding necessary to promote self-efficacy, thereby leading to adoption (Bandura, 1997). Training may take different forms and can be as simple as demonstrating how to place and remove wearable sensors, to complex, such as ongoing educational sessions in which the patient and caregiver learn how to navigate a web-based online portal. It is important to note that training should be individualized to meet the unique needs of each patient and caregiver. Providers should break up learning tasks into simple exercises, building in complexity and length in order to promote user confidence.

When presenting new information such as how to use a digital tool, providers should recognize age-related, cultural, and linguistic differences in processing new information and adjust their training accordingly. For example, older adults may find it difficult to process new information quickly, infer information from instructions, manipulate different types of data simultaneously, or focus on important information when presented with extraneous details (National Institute on Aging, 2008). The National Institute on Aging recommends providing information in a clear and concise way in order to promote understanding, which includes being specific, limiting the number of key points, offering manageable action steps, using positive statements, using active voice, supporting instructions with real-world examples and relatable stories, using images and demonstrations to communicate ideas, and repeating main points several times. It is also important to provide materials such as training guides and handouts, as well as online learning opportunities for both patients and their family to review at a later date. Again, these are guidelines and not all aging patients will require these techniques, therefore it is incumbent upon the practitioner to tailor these training opportunities to specifically meet the needs of each patient.

COST

As mentioned previously, many older adults live on fixed incomes and therefore may not be able to afford computers, Internet access, smartphones, or wearable computers or mobile devices. Based on their prior exposures to technology, older adults may view digital health tools as an unnecessary expense and, therefore, out of reach given their limited incomes. While the cost of some digital health tools such as wireless scales, wearable devices, and smartphones may be high in some instances relative to older adults' incomes, many are becoming more affordable. Practitioners should be aware of the potential financial implications when including digital health tools in their treatment plan, and they should seek reimbursement models that unburden the end user from bearing the majority of the cost. This may be accomplished through the development of technology-enabled interventions that may be supported through health insurance reimbursement or by seeking funding such as research grants or small-business innovation research grants.

Digital tools are gaining acceptance as mechanisms to promote and maintain health. Mounting evidence supports the use of digital tools as effective methods for reducing costs while improving outcomes, for example, early detection of warning signs that suggest exacerbating conditions and the need for treatment, thereby reducing the incidence of readmission in heart failure treatment (Hale, Jethwani, Kandola, Saldana, & Kvedar, 2016), diabetes management (Quinn et al., 2008), and preventing diabetes in prediabetic patients (Sepah, Jiang & Peters, 2015). In some instances, tools such as diabetes management mobile applications are being prescribed and reimbursed under commercial insurance (Pai, 2015).

CLAIMS-BASED REIMBURSEMENT FOR DIGITAL HEALTH

The Centers for Medicare & Medicaid Services (CMS) has created or adapted several current procedural terminology (CPT) codes that may be enabled or enhanced by digital health technology. As of October 2015, CMS has required providers to transition from the former code set ICD-9 to the updated ICD-10 set. During this period, several codes were added or updated. Examples of these codes include Chronic Condition Management (CCM) (99490), Telehealth Codes, Transitional Care Management (99495 and 99496), and Diabetes Prevention Programs (98969 and 99412). This section of the chapter is intended to illustrate examples and is therefore for informational purposes only. It is the practitioner's responsibility to ensure that any programs developed for reimbursement comport with the requirements set forth by various payers.

CONCLUSION

Digital health tools are expanding the reach and capability of health care for older adults. From providing remote monitoring capabilities to supporting independence, these technologies offer ways to improve the quality of life and clinical outcomes for older adults and their caregivers. Practitioners play a key role in the success of these technologies by selecting the right tools for their patients, educating them on their use, and incorporating the data they provide into their treatment plans. Emerging evidence supports the efficacy of digital tools for promoting health, maintaining independence, improving health outcomes, and preventing avoidable events; however, these benefits will not be achieved if the patient and caregiver do not use these digital tools. While practitioner efforts to promote adoption represent additional work, the benefits of patient engagement, coupled with opportunities for reimbursement, may make the effort worthwhile for all stakeholders. Although digital health technology is not a panacea, it is becoming an integral part of the health care delivery system, and practitioners must be ready to capitalize on the benefits in order to improve the lives and outcomes of their older patients. In order for these tools to be successful, providers must consider the intended users and adjust the types of tools to reflect their needs and preferences.

REFERENCES

Anderson-Bill, E., Winett, R., Wojcik, J., & Winett, S. (2011). Web-based guide to health: relationship of theoretical variables to change in physical activity, nutrition and weight at 16-months. *Journal Medical Internet Research, 13*(1), e27. doi:10.2196/jmir.1614

Aubert, B. A., & Hamel, G. (2001). Adoption of smart cards in the medical sector: The Canadian experience. *Social Science & Medicine, 53*(7), 879–894.

Barrett, L. (2011). Healthy @ Home 2.0: Full report. Retrieved from http://assets.aarp.org/rgcenter/health/healthy-home-11.pdf

Bandura, A. (1986). *Social foundations of thought and action: A social cognitive theory*. Englewood Cliffs, NJ: Prentice Hall.

Bandura, A. (1997). *Self-efficacy, the exercise of control*. New York, NY: W. H. Freeman.

Bandura, A. (2004). Health promotion by social cognitive means. *Health Education and Behavior, 31*(2), 143–164. doi:10.1177/1090198104263660

Beaudin, S. J., Intille, S. S., & Morris, E. M. (2006). To track or not to track: User reactions to concepts in longitudinal health monitoring. *Journal Medical Internet Research, 8*(4), e29. doi:10.2196/jmir.8.4.e29

Bickmore, T. W., Caruso, L., Clough-Gorr, K., & Heeren, T. (2005). It's just like you talk to a friend, relational agents for older adults. *Interacting with Computers, 17*(6), 711–735. doi:10.1016/j.intcom.2005.09.002

Boschman, L. R. (2010). *Exergames for adult users: A preliminary pilot study*. Paper presented at the Proceedings of the International Academic Conference on the Future of Game Design and Technology, Vancouver, BC, Canada.

Bostock, S., & Steptoe, A. (2012). Association between low functional health literacy and mortality in older adults: Longitudinal cohort study. *British Medical Journal, 344*, e1602. doi:10.1136/bmj.e1602

Centers for Medicare & Medicaid Services. (2015). Telehealth. Retrieved from https://www.cms.gov/Medicare/Medicare-General-Information/Telehealth

Center for Technology and Aging. (2011). mHealth technologies: Applications to benefit older adults. Retrieved from http://www.phi.org/resources/?resource=position-paper-mhealth-technologies-applications-to-benefit-older-adults-discussion-draft

Choi, N., & Dinitto, D. (2013). Internet use among older adults: association with health needs, psychological capital, and social capital. *Journal of Medical Internet Research, 15*(5), 97.

Chu, A., & Mastel-Smith, B. (2010). The outcomes of anxiety, confidence, and self- efficacy with Internet health information retrieval in older adults: A pilot study. *Computers, Informatics, Nursing, 28*(4), 222–228.

Cimperman, M., Brenčič, M. M., Trkman, P., & Stanonik, M. D. L. (2013). Older adults' perceptions of home telehealth services. *Telemedicine and e-Health, 19*(10), 786–790.

Cohall, A. T., Nye, A., Moon-Howard, J., Kukafka, R., Dye, B., Vaughan, R. D., & Northridge, M. E. (2011). Computer use, Internet access, and online health searching among Harlem adults. *American Journal of Health Promotion, 25*(5), 325–333.

Computer History Museum. (2006). Timeline of computer history. Retrieved from http://www.computerhistorysokol.org/timeline/?category=cmptr

Correia de Barros, A., Leitao, R., & Ribeiro, J. (2014). Design and evaluation of a mobile user interface for older adults: Navigation, interaction and visual design recommendations. *Procedia Computer Science, 27*, 369–378. doi:10.1016/j.procs.2014.02.041

Czaja, S., Charness, N., Fisk, A., Hertzog, C., Nair, S., Rogers, W., & Sharit, J. (2006). Factors predicting the use of technology: Findings from the center for research and education on aging and technology enhancement. *Psychology and Aging, 21*(2), 333–352.

Dobbins, R., Cockerill, R., & Barnsley, J. (2001). Factors affecting the utilization of systematic reviews. *International Journal of Technology Assessment in Health Care, 17*, 203–214.

Entertainment Software Association. (2011). Essential facts about the computer and video game industry. Retrieved from http://www.theesa.com/wp-content/uploads/2015/04/ESA-Essential-Facts-2015.pdf

Fisk, A. D., Rogers, W. A., Charness, N., Czaja, S. J., & Sharit, J. (2009). *Designing for older adults: Principles and creative human factors approaches*. Hoboken, NJ: CRC Press.

Flynn, L., Dickson, G., & Moles, D. J. (2007). Focus on caregiving. Enhancing the nursing workplace: In a recent study of long term care nurses, key organizational factors emerge as most important in supporting a productive work environment. *Provider, 33*(1), 35–39.

Fox, S. (2012). What's the future for self-tracking? Retrieved from http://www.pewinternet.org/presentations/2012/sep/medicine-x.aspx

Fukuoka, Y., Kamitani, E., Bonnet, K., & Lindgren, T. (2011). Real-time social support through a mobile virtual community to improve healthy behavior in overweight and sedentary adults: A focus group analysis. *Journal Medical Internet Research, 13*(3), e49. doi:10.2196/jmir.1770

Gerling, K. M., Schild, J., & Masuch, M. (2010). *Exergame design for elderly users: The case study of SilverBalance*. Paper presented at the Proceedings of the 7th International Conference on Advances in Computer Entertainment Technology, Taipei, Taiwan.

Goldwater, J., & Harris, Y. (2011). Using technology to enhance the aging experience: A market analysis of existing technologies. *Ageing International, 36*, 5–28. doi:10.1007/s12126-010-9071-2

Greenhalgh, T., Robert, G., Macfarlane, F., Bate, P., & Kyriakidou, O. (2004). Diffusion of innovations in service organizations: Systematic review and recommendations. *The Milbank Quarterly, 82*, 607–610.

Hale, T. M., Jethwani, K., Kandola, M. S., Saldana, F., & Kvedar, J. C. (2016). A remote medication monitoring system for chronic heart failure patients to reduce readmissions: A two-arm randomized pilot study. *Journal of Medical Internet Research, 18*(5), e91. doi:10.2196/jmir.5256

Healthcare Business Tech. (2014). Mobile health apps create privacy risk, study says. Retrieved from http://www.healthcarebusinesstech.com/mobile-health-apps-privacy

Healthcare Information and Management Systems Society. (2015). 2015 HIMSS mobile technology survey. Retrieved from http://www.himss.org/2015-mobile-survey

Hibbard, J., & Greene, J. (2013). What the evidence shows about patient activation: Better health outcomes and care experiences; fewer data on costs. *Health Affairs, 32*(2), 207–214. doi:10.1377/hlthaff.2012.1061

Howard, T., Jacobson, K. L., & Kripalani, S. (2013). Doctor talk: Physicians' use of clear verbal communication. *Journal of Health Communication: International Perspectives, 18*(8), 991–1001. doi:10.1080/10810730.2012.757398

Howell, J. M., & Higgins, C. A. (1990). Champions of technological innovation. *Administrative Science Quarterly, 35,* 317–341.

IMS Institute. (2015). Patient adoption of mHealth: Use, evidence and remaining barriers to mainstream acceptance. Retrieved from http://www.imshealth.com/files/web/IMSH%20Institute/Reports/Patient%20Adoption%20of%20mHealth/IIHI_Patient_Adoption_of_mHealth.pdf

James, J. (2013). Health policy brief: Patient engagement. Retrieved from http://www.healthaffairs.org/healthpolicybriefs/brief.php?brief_id=86

Katz, E., & Lazarsfeld, P. (1970). *Personal influence: The part played by people in the flow of mass communications.* New Brunswick, NJ: Transaction Publishers.

Kim, E., Stolyar, A., Lober, W., Herbaugh, A., Shinstrom, S., Zierler, B., . . . Kim, Y. (2009). Challenges to using an electronic personal health record by a low-income elderly population. *Journal of Medical Internet Research, 11*(4), e44.

Kreps, G. L., & Neuhauser, L. (2010). New directions in eHealth communication: Opportunities and challenges. *Patient Education and Counseling, 78*(3), 329–336. doi:10.1016/j.pec.2010.01.013

Kvedar, J. (2014). Making health addictive: Use the sentinel effect. Retrieved from https://chealthblog.connectedhealth.org/2014/05/29/making-health-addictive-use-the-sentinel-effect

Lake, E. T., & Friese, C. R. (2006). Variations in nursing practice environments: Relation to staffing and hospital characteristics. *Nursing Research, 55*(1), 1–9.

Liker, J. K. (2004). *The Toyota way.* New York, NY: McGraw-Hill.

Mangan, D. (2016). There's a hack for that: Fitbit user accounts attacked. Retrieved from http://www.cnbc.com/2016/01/08/theres-a-hack-for-that-fitbit-user-accounts-attacked.html

Masterson Creber, R. M., Maurer, M. S., Reading, M., Hiraldo, G., Hickey, K. T., & Iribarren, S. (2016). Review and analysis of existing mobile phone apps to support heart failure symptom monitoring and self-care management using the Mobile Application Rating Scale (MARS). *Journal of Medical Internet Research Mhealth and Uhealth, 4*(2), e74. doi:10.2196/mhealth.5882

McCloskey, D. (2006). The importance of ease of use, usefulness, and trust to online consumers: An examination of the technology acceptance model with older consumers. *Journal of Organizational and End User Computing, 18*(3), 47–65.

McInnes, D. K., Gifford, A. L., Kazis, L. E., & Wagner, T. H. (2010). Disparities in health-related internet use by US veterans: Results from a national survey. *Informatics in Primary Care, 18*(1), 59–68.

McMillan, S. J., & Macias, W. (2008). Strengthening the safety net for online seniors: Factors influencing differences in health information seeking among older Internet users. *Journal of Health Communication, 13*(8), 778–792. doi:10.1080/10810730802487448

Mercer, K., Giangregorio, L., Schneider, E., Childana, P., Li, M., & Grindrod, K. (2016). Acceptance of commercially available wearable activity trackers among adults aged over 50 with chronic illness: A mixed methods evaluation. *Journal of Medical Internet Research, 4*(1), e7. doi:10.2196/mhealth.4225

Mottl, J. (2015). Despite increase in mHealth apps, functionality is problematic. Retrieved from http://www.fiercemobilehealthcare.com/story/despite-increase-mhealth-apps-functionality-problematic/2015-09-16?utm_medium=nl&utm_source=internal

National Institute on Aging. (2008). Making your printed materials senior friendly. Retrieved from https://www.nia.nih.gov/sites/default/files/making_your_printed_health_materials_senior_friendly.pdf

Nitz, J. C., Kuys, S., Isles, R., & Fu, S. (2010). Is the Wii Fit a new-generation tool for improving balance, health and well-being? A pilot study. *Climacteric, 13*(5), 487–491. doi:10.3109/13697130903395193

Noar, S., & Harrington, N. (2012). *eHealth applications: Promising strategies for behavior change*. New York, NY: Routledge.

NORC at the University of Chicago. (2012). *Health IT and health disparities: Patient provider telehealth network-using telehealth to improve chronic disease management*. Bethesda, MD: Author.

Olson, K. E., O'Brien, M. A., Rogers, W. A., & Charness, N. (2011). Diffusion of technology: Frequency of use for younger and older adults. *Ageing International, 36*(1), 123–145.

Or, C., & Tao, D. (2012). Usability study of a computer-based self-management system for older adults with chronic diseases. *Journal of Medical Internet Research, Research Protocols, 1*(2), e13. doi:10.2196/resprot.2184

Osborne, T. F., Clark, R. H., Williamson, P. J., Blackowiak, J., Werb, S. M., & Strong, B. W. (2017). Efficiency analysis of an interoperable healthcare operations platform. *Journal of Medical Systems, 41*(4), 52.

Osborne, T. F., Reich, J. J., Arkwright, B. T., & Russo, J. (2016). On the digital road to improved home healthcare. *Telehealth and Medicine Today*, 2016, *1*(3). Retrieved from http://www.telhealthandmedtoday.com/on-the-digital-road-to-improved-home-healthcare

Pai, A. (2015). WellDoc raises $22M for its BlueStar mobile-enabled diabetes management offering. *MobiHealthNews*. Retrieved from http://mobihealthnews.com/content/welldoc-raises-22m-its-bluestar-mobile-enabled-diabetes-management-offering

Pearce, C. (2008). The truth about baby boomer gamers: A study of over-forty computer game players. *Games and Culture, 3*(142), 142–174. doi:10.1177/1555412008314132

Pew Research Center. (2010). MILLENNIALS: Confident. Connected. Open to change. Retrieved from http://pewsocialtrends.org/files/2010/10/millennials-confident-connected-open-to-change.pdf

Pew Research Center. (2014). Older adults and technology use. Retrieved from http://www.pewinternet.org/2014/04/03/older-adults-and-technology-use

President's Council of Advisors on Science and Technology. (2016). Report to the President: Independence, technology, and connection in older age. Retrieved from https://www.broadinstitute.org/files/sections/about/PCAST/2016%20pcast-independence-tech-ging.pdf

Quinn, C., Sysko Clough, S., Minor, J., Lender, D., Okafor, M., & Gruber-Baldini, A. (2008). WellDoc™ mobile diabetes management randomized controlled trial: Change in clinical and behavioral outcomes and patient and physician satisfaction. *Diabetes Technology & Therapeutics, 10*(3), 160–168. doi:10.1089/dia.2008.0283.

Reich, J. J., & Osborne, T. F. (2016). Home telehealth and the triple aim. *Telehealth and Medicine Today, 1*(4). Retrieved from http://www.telhealthandmedtoday.com/home-telehealth-and-the-triple-aim

Reynolds, A. (2013). *Age-related differences in self-efficacy and the use of e-health supports for exercise behavior in adults* (doctoral dissertation). Retrieved from http://ufdcimages.uflib.ufl.edu/UF/E0/04/54/17/00001/REYNOLDS_A.pdf

Reynolds, A., Rubens, J., King, R., & Machado, P. (2016). Technology and engagement: How digital tools are reshaping population health. *Population Health Alliance*. Retrieved from http://populationhealthalliance.org/publications/technology-and-engagement-how-digital-tools-are-reshaping-population-health.html

Rogers, E. M. (1995). *Diffusion of innovations* (4th ed.). New York, NY: Free Press.

Rogers, E. M. (2010). *Diffusion of innovations* (4th ed.). New York, NY: Simon & Schuster.

Sepah, S. C., Jiang, L., & Peters, A. L. (2015). Long-term outcomes of a web-based diabetes prevention program: 2-year results of a single-arm longitudinal study. *Journal of Medical Internet Research, 17*(4), e92. doi:10.2196/jmir.4052

Singh, R., Mathiassen, L., Stachura, M. E., & Astapova, E. V. (2011). Dynamic capabilities in home health: IT-enabled transformation of post-acute care. *Journal of the Association for Information Systems, 12*, 163–188.

Song, H., Peng, W., & Lee, K. M. (2011). Promoting exercise self-efficacy with an exergame. *Journal of Health Communication, 16*(2), 148–162. doi:10.1080/10810730.2010.535107

Svensson, M., & Lagerros, Y. T. (2010). Motivational technologies to promote weight loss, from Internet to gadgets. *Patient Education and Counseling, 79*(3), 356–360. doi:10.1016/j.pec.2010.03.004

U.S. Department of Health and Human Services, Health Resources and Services Administration. (2010). *The registered nurse population: Findings from the 2008 national sample survey of registered nurses*. Chicago, IL: Author

Wang, A., Redington, L., Steinmetz, V., & Lindeman, D. (2011). The ADOPT model: Accelerating diffusion of proven technologies for older adults. *Ageing International, 36*, 29–45.

World Health Organization. (2007). *Global age-friendly cities: A guide*. Geneva, Switzerland: Author. Retrieved from http://www.who.int/ageing/publications/Global_age_friendly_cities_Guide_English.pdf

Zickuhr, K., & Smith, A. (2012). Digital differences. Retrieved from http://www.pewinternet.org/Reports/2012/Digital-differences.aspx

3

Transitions of Care and Technology Integration

Aroop K. Pal, Diane Chau, and Jessica L. Kalender-Rich

There exist historical and current methods in which technology is used to improve transitions of care across the continuum. These programs include applications, software, and electronic tools that can improve transitions between providers in the inpatient and outpatient settings. This chapter focuses on the ways electronic health records (EHR) and cloud-based systems have thus far improved transitions, and reviews data related to readmissions, patient safety, and patient quality of care. Additionally, we explore ways in which technology is expected to be integrated into transitions into the future.

TRANSITIONS OF CARE DEFINED

Transitions of care, the movement of a patient from one setting of care or provider to another, have been identified as a focus of attention for improving patient care (Centers for Medicare & Medicaid Services [CMS], 2014; The Joint Commission, 2013). Medical care in the United States occurs across multiple sites of care, and most patients are cared for by physicians from several specialties. Each site of care, like each physician subspecialty, has a narrow scope of practice, and a patient must be in the right level of care to maximize his or her medical potential. Multiple system gaps can occur in transitions of care that technology has the potential to address; these gaps include patient safety, handoff, and risk management to improve overall patient care.

SITES OF CARE

The spectrum of care sites is wide and ranges from the highest level of acuity in an intensive care unit (ICU) in a hospital to home care with an intermittent certified nurse assistant. Patients are continuously moving between these levels of care, and at each level are cared for by an interprofessional team. Levels of care can be divided into community-based (preacute), acute, and postacute categories (see Figure 3.1).

Community-Based (Preacute) Sites of Care

Community-based (preacute) sites of care are focused on keeping patients in their current environment, maintaining their current state of health, and preventing decline of their medical conditions. This primarily includes outpatient sites of care such as the primary care physician (PCP) or subspecialists focused on prevention and treatment of chronic disease. Additionally, one can include long-term care and assisted living facilities in this category because patients are still being cared for in their site of residence. A broader perspective would expand to include pharmacies, wellness centers, ambulatory surgical centers, and diagnostic centers.

Transitions that occur in this setting are mostly related to individual providers and consultants in the community. There are also examples of care being provided by outpatient physical or occupational therapy and home health agencies with communication back to the individual referring providers.

Acute Sites of Care

Patients are typically moved to an acute hospital setting when they are being treated for an acute illness or exacerbation of a chronic illness, and when they are admitted for planned surgical intervention. There are many entry points for acute care, including the emergency department, referring clinics, outside hospitals, and the operating room. These entry points have unique workflows that impact the transition of care for patients. Regardless of entry point, the team's goal at this level of care is to treat the urgent need and then ensure a smooth transition to a less acute setting or home. Inpatient hospital care encompasses a diverse population, including both the highest levels of care available, for example, the ICU, and the lower risk elective of planned overnight stays after a procedure. In fact, this is one site where transitions of care commonly do not require a change in venue and may only include a move in location of a patient's bed.

The ICU is the site of the most critically ill patients, often requiring life-sustaining interventions on a continuous basis. These interventions may include

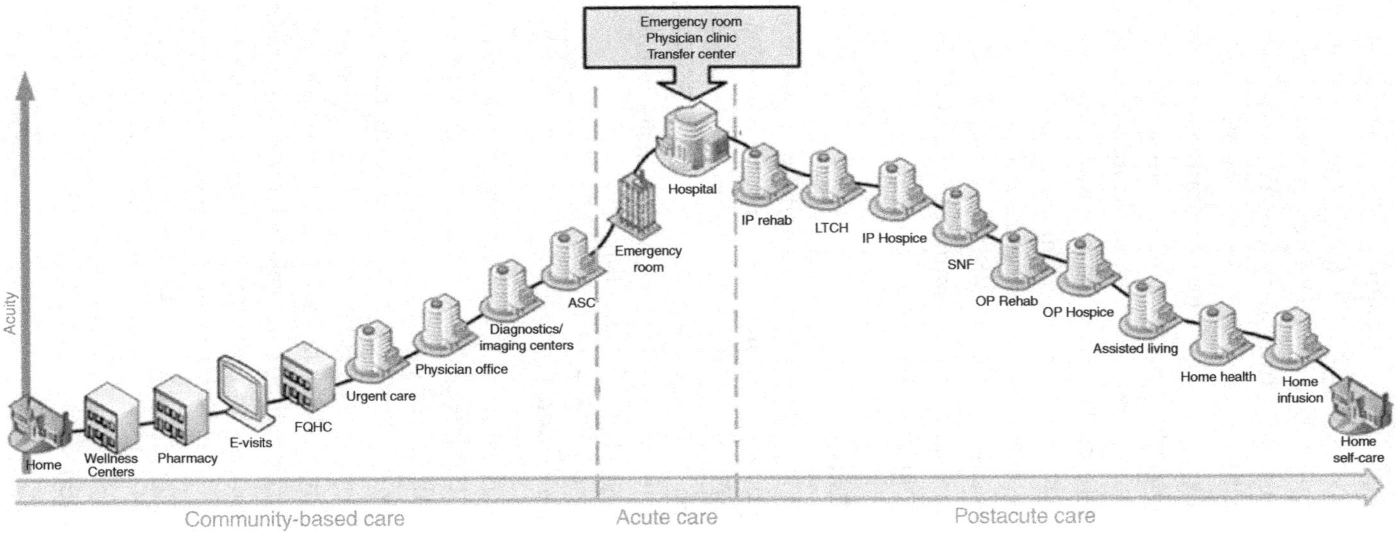

FIGURE 3.1 The continuum of care.

ASC, ambulatory surgical center; FQHC, federally qualified health center; IP, inpatient; SNF, skilled nursing facility.

Source: Modified and reprinted with permission from the University of Kansas Hospital Authority.

artificial ventilators, continuous blood pressure support with vasopressors, and invasive monitoring. The next main level of care collectively can be referred to as *floor* beds, and includes progressive care, telemetry, and medical–surgical inpatient units. The patients located on the "floor" have a variety of interventions available, including laboratory, IV treatments, blood transfusions, radiological testing, and so forth. The transition between the ICU and the "floor" bed may include a change in room, but it may also include a change in nursing staff, physicians, and therapists. Thus, there is a need for communication among providers to ensure continuity and sometimes a change in the plan of care, as driven by the new providers.

As the patient nears time for discharge from the acute setting, the inpatient team has a critical decision to make that determines how the patient's course of recovery will continue. Each level of care following the hospital is meant to focus on rehabilitation in addition to improvement in medical issues that were addressed during the hospitalization.

Postacute Sites of Care

The team's goal at each level of care after hospitalization is to help patients either return to their prior level of independence, or transition them to the next appropriate level of care to continue treatment until patients get as close to their prior level as possible. Care in these sites is comprehensive with an increased focus on activities of daily living (ADLs), including bathing, dressing, toileting, feeding oneself, and ambulating.

Long-Term Acute Care Hospital

The long-term acute care hospital (LTACH) is meant for the patient who is on a path of improvement, but is expected to have a protracted recovery requiring acute specialized nursing care. It is continuously staffed by physicians and advanced practice providers, which is unique compared to other levels of care outside of the hospital. Also, LTACHs can be independent facilities or located on a hospital campus. Each facility can provide different services, but standard available services include comprehensive wound care for advanced wounds, ventilator weaning, and care for the very complex stable patient. LTACH care is paid for by the same insurance benefit as hospital care. They are typically staffed by hospitalists, wound care physicians, infectious disease physicians, nephrologists, and pulmonary/critical care physicians.

Inpatient Rehabilitation

Inpatient rehabilitation (IPR) units can be freestanding or in a separate wing of a hospital. The hallmark of an IPR unit is that patients are medically complex, but also medically stable. Additionally, they must be able to both tolerate and benefit from 3 hours of rehabilitation daily and two different therapy areas. They are typically staffed by physical medicine and rehabilitation physicians, with consultation by internal medicine or family medicine physicians. There are also rare facilities nationwide that can comprehensively care for the pediatric patient needing IPR.

Skilled Nursing Facilities

Each community has many skilled nursing facilities (SNFs) with a wide variety of services provided. Medicare patients are required to have spent 3 midnights inpatient in the hospital in the last 30 days to qualify for SNF admission. However, some private insurance companies have begun waiving this requirement given the lower cost of an SNF stay compared to the hospital. Each SNF is required to provide therapy up to 90 minutes at least 5 days a week in addition to medical care by nursing and physicians and advanced practice providers. Medicare patients are at least partially covered for up to 100 days of care in an SNF per medical event; this number resets after 60 days that are both SNF- and hospital-free. Patients are seen by physicians and advanced practice providers on site, typically one or two times weekly.

Home Health Agencies

Home health agencies are composed primarily of nurses, aides, and therapists who come into the patient's home to provide care. Visits typically occur three to five times weekly depending on the patient's needs. Nurses may address wound care, IV antibiotic management, medication management, and a variety of other needs. Aides are often responsible for hygiene and bathing. Unlike other postacute sites of care, therapy often occurs three times weekly and most patients are given other exercises to practice between sessions. One important note about home health is that a patient must be considered homebound to qualify. This means that he or she has a significantly challenging time leaving the house, and is therefore staying home for the time being except to attend appointments with physicians and advanced practice providers or religious services. The ordering physician must certify the patient's homebound status on an ongoing basis.

Hospice

Unlike the other mentioned postacute sites of care, hospice patients have shifted their goals of care away from a treatment pathway and toward a palliative pathway. There are many hospice agencies in each community, all of which see patients in their homes and other facilities in which the patient may reside. Additionally, some hospice agencies have inpatient hospice units that are staffed continuously with nursing staff. The goal of hospice is to focus on the comfort of the patient at the end of life, administering medications and other symptom-directed treatments to patients with a life expectancy of 6 months or less.

Program of All-Inclusive Care for the Elderly and Adult Day Health Centers

Program of All-Inclusive Care for the Elderly (PACE) programs are a Medicare benefit for those aged 55 years and above who meet skilled nursing levels of care, but opt out of institutionalization. These programs are unique in addressing chronic care conditions through a day hospital concept wherein patients are provided transportation and pick up from home to attend an adult day-health center where they receive rehabilitation, wound care, medical care from a primary care provider, and medication therapy management. At the end of their day care, they are transported home and are provided home health services and caregiver services as needed, along with all durable medical equipment. Their entire cost of care is covered by the PACE organization and includes hospital care and higher levels of skilled care, if needed. Many PACE participants are palliative and under chronic disease management for conditions with life expectancies greater than 6 months. All care within PACE is performed under a comprehensive interprofessional team model. Many PACE enrollees are also under state Medicaid.

INTERPROFESSIONAL TEAMS

Successful transitions of care require a team of highly trained professionals from a wide variety of backgrounds (see Table 3.1). A varying number of these professionals are available at each site of care and their roles may be slightly varied, but they are all present to some degree. Many people do not have experience within high-functioning geriatric interprofessional teams. Clinical cases are often complex and require input from multiple disciplines to address chronic conditions and patients' psychosocial needs.

A Case Study in Transitions

Community-Based (Preacute) Care

Mr. H is a 79-year-old male who visits his PCP for a routine follow-up appointment. At this appointment, he complains of shortness of breath with exertion and new edema. His PCP sends a consult to Cardiology and orders an

TABLE 3.1 Interprofessional Team Involved in the Continuum of Care

Type of Professional	Role
Licensed independent provider (physician, nurse practitioner, physician assistant)	Management of medical illness Prescribing medications and treatments Communication with other providers and the entire interprofessional team Identification of patient's goals of care
Case manager	Coordination of care Discharge planning Coordination of postdischarge medical equipment Communication with insurance providers
Social worker	Coordination of care Discharge planning Patient and family counseling Communication with insurance providers
Registered nurse	Bedside patient care Administration of medications and treatments, including IV Venous lab draws as required
Licensed practical nurse	Bedside patient care Administration of medications and treatments
Nurse aide	Assistance with activities of daily living
Pharmacist	Provides medications as ordered Provides consultation on medication choices, dosing, administration Monitors for adverse drug events
Therapist (occupational therapist, physical therapist, speech therapist)	Functional assessment of patients Assessment for assistive devices Provide ongoing therapy to the patients and teaching to families
Respiratory therapist	Monitors oxygen usage and adjusts as needed Provides assistance with and teaching on respiratory treatments Assists in ventilator management

echocardiogram. Cardiology sees the patient after his echocardiogram and diagnoses him with congestive heart failure. The cardiologist makes recommendations, changes a few medications, and sends information back to the PCP.

Acute Care

Mr. H calls his PCP 2 weeks later with worsening shortness of breath and chest pain. He is sent to the emergency department. At the emergency department, he is evaluated for a myocardial infarction and is eventually admitted to the hospital with an exacerbation of his congestive heart failure. In the hospital, the physicians work to improve his oxygenation and optimize his medications again. Also, the physical and occupational therapists work with him to improve his functional status so he can return home. As he has been in the hospital 4 days, most of which was spent in bed, he is not strong enough to discharge home directly. Therefore, the therapy team recommends he go to an SNF. He is given a long list of options in the area and chooses one close to his home.

Postacute Care

Mr. H arrives at the SNF late in the afternoon. He is settled in a room while the nurse reviews his records. The nurse calls the on-call provider to review the patient's ordered medications and after they are approved, sends that list to the offsite pharmacy. The offsite pharmacy compiles the medications and the courier takes them to the facility. In the meantime, Mr. H has been given dinner and helped to bed. In the morning, the nursing administration reviews his hospital orders and reconciles them with the facility records. Members of the therapy team evaluate his current functional status and gather history. The physician and/or advanced practice provider come to the facility and, based on patient account and hospital records, determine treatment plan.

Over the next several weeks, the patient receives therapy on most days. He improves to very near his baseline functional status. The physician sees him several times, and both the physician and the therapy team determine he is ready for discharge. A care plan meeting occurs with nursing, therapy representatives, Mr. H, and his family to discuss discharge dates and resources needed at home.

Mr. H is discharged home with home health services. He qualified for home health services because he was considered too weak to leave his home without considerable effort. The nurse, aide, and therapy team from home health come to his house three times weekly to help with his medications, his bathing, and continue working on his independent function. He also goes back to see his PCP, who reviews the medication changes made in the hospital, and compares those with the changes made in the SNF. He also makes a few changes, which he communicates to the home health agency nurse. After a few weeks, he is considered at his functional baseline and home health discharges him.

Community-Based Care

Mr. H is now able to resume care with his PCP and cardiologist. His goal, once again, is to manage his chronic condition and stay out of the hospital.

CHALLENGES IN TRANSITION: A NEED FOR INTERVENTION

The negative outcomes associated with transitions of care include hospital readmission and adverse events. Studies have demonstrated that older adults are at risk for readmission, with as many as one in five Medicare patients being readmitted within 30 days (Forster, Murff, Peterson, Gandhi, & Bates, 2003; Jencks, Williams, & Coleman, 2009). There are many factors that have been identified to contribute to poor outcomes associated with transitions of care, including length of stay, acuity of care, comorbidities, number of medications, hemoglobin at discharge, discharge from an oncology service, sodium level at discharge, procedure during the index admission, index type of admission, number of admissions during the last 12 months, and discontinuity of care (Donze, Aujesky, Williams, & Schnipper, 2013; Taha, Pal, Mahnken, & Rigler, 2014; van Walraven et al., 2010).

One of the significant factors that has brought attention to transitions of care is the recent change in health care delivery with the advent of hospitalists. An unintended consequence of having dedicated physicians who manage patients in the hospital, different from the PCP, is discontinuity of care, and the reality of potential communication breakdown (Kripalani et al., 2007; Pham, Grossman, Cohen, & Bodenheimer, 2008). Changes in medications, pending test results, and additional workup have all been identified as contributing factors to harm (Coleman, Smith, Raha, & Min, 2005; Kripalani et al., 2007; Moore, McGinn, & Halm, 2007; Roy et al., 2005). A recent study trying to evaluate the challenges for hospitalists and outpatient physicians found similar challenges to improving communication (Solan, Sherman, DeBiasio, & Simmons, 2016).

A major driving factor for attention to the transitions of care is the costs associated with the negative outcomes. One analysis found that readmissions accounted for $15 billion annually in expenditures, and that $12 billion were potentially preventable (Medicare Payment Advisory Commission, 2007). With the reality that the elderly population is increasing, the financial impact to the United States economy is major (Administration on Aging, n.d.). The significance of the impact of readmissions and need for improvement from a cost and quality standpoint led to the creation of the Readmissions Reduction Program (RRP; Centers for Medicare & Medicaid Services, n.d.). The RRP, from the Patient Protection and Affordable Care Act, incentivized hospitals to evaluate and improve facilitation of the transition of care at hospital discharge for heart failure, pneumonia, and acute myocardial infarction, with plans to expand to other prevalent conditions.

Clearly, transitions of care became a center of attention, especially for older adults. Researchers and organizations have invested time and resources to try to optimize the outcomes of this known high-risk period. There have been many programs that have shown that multidisciplinary interventions can reduce readmission rates by improving the transition of care from the hospital to home (Boutwell, Griffin, Hwu, & Shannon, 2009; Coleman, Parry, Chalmers, & Min, 2006; Jack et al., 2009; Naylor et al., 1999). The reality is these programs are complex, and often require resources, primarily with staffing of nurse, pharmacists, and other staff. The ability to spread the work of these programs to the larger masses has been challenged by limited resources. It has been noted that up until recently, technological interventions had been very underdeveloped (Marcotte, Kirtane, Lynn, & McKethan, 2015). Factors contributing to the lack of technology at the turn of the century was primarily due to cost, lack of interoperability, and lack of availability and quality of EHR (Marcotte et al., 2015). Additionally, the state of patient engagement or involvement with their health was not high.

Two critical initiatives have sparked innovation in addressing the risks in transitions of care, and the goal of better patient engagement. The first was the RRP, which provided a financial motivation for hospitals to invest time and resources to improving the quality of transitions of care. The other was the Meaningful Use program of the Health Information Technology for Economic and Clinical Health (HITECH) Act, a part of the American Recovery and Reinvestment Act of 2009 (The Office of the National Coordinator for Health Information Technology [ONC], n.d.). These two programs are interrelated, as the funding for the HITECH Act is from the RRP. Prior to these initiatives, while a lot of work was being done to improve outcomes associated with transitions, these studies or projects were not as focused specifically on technology. The creation of the Office of the National Coordinator (ONC) for health information technology was critical to provide standards and structure for the health of the country, and to provide an emphasis on patient engagement. The Meaningful Use program has created a boom in information technology initiatives, and this chapter focuses on the state of technology and transitions of care.

CURRENT USES OF TECHNOLOGY AND TRANSITIONS OF CARE

Between Providers

Communication, consultation, clinical decision making, reference, and information gathering are just some of the ways technology has enhanced the care of elderly patients, with attention to improving the safety and quality of transitions of care (Ventola, 2014).

Communication includes automated notifications of events and ability to share information electronically. As demonstrated by the Beacon Community Awardees, these notifications are being utilized to "improve communications across care providers, improve chronic care patient management, and reduce unnecessary hospitalization" (ONC, 2013a). Sharing of all document types, including the discharge summary, has been enhanced by technology and helps support transitions. The ability to share information, including history, allergies, medications, and active problems, has helped providers be aware in a more timely manner than paper charts. This enhances consultation, or sharing one's own expert assessment and plan more easily. Telemedicine also allows providers to discuss the care of an individual patient in real time, allowing the opportunity for real-time discussion and collaboration. A good example of this type of support that can help transitions of care specifically is eReferral, developed by San Francisco General Hospital, which formalizes the "curbside consult" between primary care providers and specialists (Chen, Murphy, & Yee, 2013). Secure messaging within the electronic medical record also supports the ability for providers to communicate when a patient is transitioning care.

Sharing information on medication prescribing is a form of information sharing, and is a hot topic of interest. Electronic prescribing (also known as e-prescribing) has been a point of emphasis in Meaningful Use. The latest data show a 14-fold increased usage since 2008, with 57% new and refill scripts being sent via e-prescribing in 2013 (Gabriel & Swain, 2014). The concept of tools to keep track of what patients are and are no longer taking is termed *medication reconciliation*. Medication reconciliation has been identified as a high-risk activity impacting transitions of care (Gleason et al., 2010). Medications accounted for 66% of postdischarge errors in one study (Forster et al., 2003). Electronic medical records can help the daunting process. Additionally, health information exchange (HIE) and patient portals can help providers and patients maintain the most current list of medications (Marcotte et al., 2015).

Clinical decision-making tools can help providers identify at-risk patients and best practice interventions, including decisions on medications. The implementation of computerized provider-order entry was felt to be key to ensure accuracy of ordering, and enable clinical decision support (Agency for Healthcare Research and Quality, 2005; National Quality Forum, 2010). Common tools being utilized are order sets, best practice alerts, and hard stops to facilitate safe transitions of care (Alagiakrishnan et al., 2016).

Between Sites

At a larger scale, although still involving individual providers, some technological initiatives are being utilized to help make transitions safer. The first example is care coordination, ensuring a standard complement of important items upon discharge from the hospital. The Continuum of Care document, part of Stage 2 of Meaningful Use, is a requirement that helps provide timely and complete information, ideally in an electronic form. This includes elements critical for transition of care like medication lists, problem lists, return appointments, advance directives, among others (ONC, 2013b).

Another example is the concept of disease registries. Technology is being used to identify populations of at-risk patients and connecting interventions. Telehealth/telemonitoring for chronic disease conditions like congestive heart failure is common today, trying to provide population health strategies to control utilization (Kvedar, Coye, & Everett, 2014).

HIE with interoperability is the ultimate goal in providing seamless care from one site to another. Data support increasing use of exchanging information between sites, including over 50% of hospitals sharing radiology reports and lab results with other sites outside their system (Swain, Charles, & Furukawa, 2014).

Patient Level/Patient Engagement (Portals)

The Meaningful Use program created a standard for patient engagement, specifically in the use of patient portals. Ensuring access to their own information in a timely fashion was felt to be a pillar in increasing patients' involvement in their health. In a recent publication, the stated vision of the ONC for 2015 and beyond is "high-quality care, lower costs, healthy population and engaged people" (ONC, 2015d). According to an ONC brief, almost four in 10 Americans were offered access to their medical record in 2014 (Patel, Barker, & Siminerio, 2015). Meaningful Use specifically incentivizes communications between patients and providers. A recent report showed significant increases in text messaging and emailing from patients to providers (ONC, 2015a). Hospitals have stepped up their involvement. The percentage of hospitals providing patients the ability to view, download, or transmit their health records electronically went from 10% in 2013, to over 60% in 2014 (Charles, Gabriel, & Henry, 2015).

Other examples of current use of technology directly to patients include self-management software including wearables, patient education materials, patient-reminder applications (medication adherence), and telehealth. Telehealth is broad, and actively utilized with future direction of incorporating personal monitoring within telehealth. Personal monitoring devices allow patients to get feedback on vitals, weight, and activity to help patients track their performance. This specific industry has seen a huge increase in use, and it is projected to only increase as improvements are made (Gay & Leijdekkers, 2015). Patient education, with attention to health literacy, is another area of focus in engaging patients. The industry is recognizing that if materials are either not available, or not made in a manner that patients can comprehend, then the patient has not been well served. Medication adherence programs are popular, and include many technological options ranging from smartphone to wireless electronic–pill bottle reminders (ONC, n.d.). It is foreseeable for technology to be driven by the consumers, with integration of personal wearable data into a cloud-based medical records system and made available through portals for an on-demand telehealth visit with their providers.

Evidence of Benefit

Evidence by medical standards rests in the practice of evidence-based medicine. This requires substantial randomized and multicenter trials to validate technology and its outcomes. Although there are many new and innovative initiatives being introduced all the time, there is little statistical evidence of their benefit. This is likely because the technology is so new and constantly in flux. Technology evolves at a pace faster than the standard clinical trial practices, which include clinical trial design, submission to institutional review boards for approval, subject enrollment, data gathering, and reporting and publishing. Current evidence-based standards of medical practice are difficult to attain with many of the technology developments.

Health Information Exchange

The HIE is a promising platform to make patient information available for providers in different health systems and sites of care, but it is still in its infancy. In 2014, 42% of physicians reported electronically sharing patient health information with other providers, which is a 7% increase from 2013 (Heisey-Grove, Patel, & Searcy, 2015).

In the same year, ambulatory providers shared patient health information with other ambulatory providers outside their group in 26% of cases and with unaffiliated hospitals in only 9%. Rates of electronic sharing with home health providers, behavioral health providers, and long-term care providers were 12%, 11%, and 11%, respectively. In 2014, over one third of ambulatory physicians electronically shared laboratory results, imaging results, medication lists, medication allergies, or problem lists. However, only 26% shared at least one of those listed outside of their affiliated organization, and less than one in 10 shared all five types of information outside their affiliated organization.

Information exchange among hospitals is more advanced than in the ambulatory setting. In 2014, three quarters of hospitals exchanged information with nonaffiliated providers of care, which is a 55% increase in 1 year (Swain, Charles, Patel, & Searcy, 2015). Hospitals and outside providers exchanged information in two thirds of the hospital systems, including laboratory (63%), radiology reports (65%), clinical care summaries (64%), and medication history (58%). The exchange of clinical care summaries among hospitals has doubled since 2008.

Given the fluidity with which patients move between health care organizations, the ability to share information both within and outside the health system is crucial for care transition improvement.

Transitions Within the Hospital

Care transitions between provider teams are a source of potential medical errors. Several groups have developed computerized rounding reports to support the transition either between learners or between attending physician teams (Davis et al., 2015; Sarkar et al., 2007; van Sluisveld et al., 2015; Wohlauer, 2012). Despite the creation of these tools and published literature about their subjective benefit, outcomes measures are not widely available.

Cost Savings

It was hoped that information available in the HIE, or other electronic means, would decrease the usage and cost of unnecessarily repeated imaging and laboratory tests. Thus far, the data are mixed (Bailey, Bailey, et al., 2013; Bailey, Wan, et al., 2013; McCormick, Bor, Woolhandler, & Himmelstein, 2012; Slovis et al., 2016). Jung et al. found that the imaging cost savings per patient yearly was less than $3, and that studies that were less likely to be duplicated were also the least expensive radiological studies (Jung et al., 2015). More data are needed to fully determine cost savings.

Current Challenges

The American medical system is a series of transitions between providers, between sites, and between acute medical illnesses. Even with optimal technology in place for information sharing, there is potential for challenges (ONC, 2015b). These challenges include variation in standards across IT systems, variation in how IT stakeholders interpret government policies, and reluctance among IT stakeholders to collaborate and foster supportive business practice.

Lack of Standardization

New technology and standards of care must be adopted widely, and companies must commit significant financial resources to build systems, train their staff, and incite behavioral change (Institute of Medicine Committee on Quality of Health Care in America, 2001). Much of this change has been focused in the hospital and ambulatory settings. Additionally, although there is vast improvement even over the past year in the rates of physicians sharing information, there are key gaps in what is being shared. Bates found that standardized tools are needed for medication reconciliation, laboratory test tracking, and care plan development (Bates, 2015). The ONC for Health Information Technology has committed to developing a policy advisory on health IT by 2017 to standardize the health information exchange (ONC, 2015c).

Lack of Interoperability

Hospitals report challenges related to cumbersome workflows and systems capabilities in exchanging information electronically. An interoperable exchange includes the ability to find, send, receive, and use information. Only one in four hospitals are engaged in all four of these activities (Charles, Swain, & Patel, 2015). Seventy-eight percent of hospitals can send information, but only 56% are able to receive records from outside sources, and only 40% of hospitals can integrate the summary of care records received without manual entry. One in four hospitals report challenges in matching patients across systems, and 45% of hospitals report difficulty matching providers. Additionally, there is an associated cost in sending and receiving data outside the organization for one quarter of hospitals.

Information exchange occurs between outside hospitals and outside ambulatory care providers at a higher rate than with long-term care and postacute providers and behavioral health providers. Only 17% of hospitals reported receiving summary of care documents from long-term care providers and 16% from behavioral health providers.

Although policies such as HITECH and RRP standardize technology expectations in some settings, long-term care and postacute providers are not incentivized under the Medicare statute to implement EHR. This leaves a technological divide among sites of care even as the patient transitions across the continuum. Only 9% of hospitals send and only 7% receive summary of care documents from outside sources in electronic format alone. Paper charting must still accompany the patient to postacute settings, all appointments, and so forth. In response, long-term care and postacute facilities are implementing their own EHR systems, which lack interoperability with the systems used in the hospital and often with the HIE.

Lack of Transparency

The health IT market is known to be opaque about available products and services, which also prevents systems from integrating across multiple sites of care (ONC, 2015b). The lack of transparency prevents comparison of IT systems even related to basic information about cost, limitations, and trade-offs to lock providers into one EHR system that may not have the desired capabilities. As a result, ONC introduced new requirements for transparency of health IT in the 2015 Edition Final Rule. Some information about certified health IT is already available through a certified product list. While this new policy will increase information availability, the ONC lacks the power to require disclosure of much of the information required to thoroughly compare products.

Provider Identification

EHRs often lack the ability to identify the team taking care of the patient both within and outside of the care setting. A patient may be seeing providers from multiple medical groups and specialists without team identification in the EHR. For continuity of care, providers may not know which other specialists are involved and who to contact for collaboration (Bates, 2015).

Future Steps

Growth in health IT occurs rapidly and will likely be remarkably different even a few years from now. Since 2016, the Department of Health and Human Services has sought to further its mission for health IT adoption by using its annual congressional report to analyze the current landscape and progress toward goals (ONC, 2015c). Additionally, the ONC will update its national dashboard quarterly for review by the federal government. Success will be measured by several key factors. The ONC will review the percent of ambulatory physicians and acute care hospitals treating patients seen outside their medical organization, that have outside clinical information available at site of care and the percentage of individuals who experience gaps in health information when seeking care.

There is ongoing work to improve interoperability and remove barriers to information flow between providers and sites of care. Additionally, the Blue Button Initiative empowers individuals to access their health records online to improve patient involvement in care. One can imagine a time when health

IT enables patients to move between systems and even geographic locations, and still be able to access their personal health information.

As the medical systems move to alternative payment models, it will be crucial for IT to support the provider's ability to provide high-quality care while reducing cost. This will require collaboration with health IT companies and health care providers for optimization with clear clinical input.

The Precision Medicine Initiative is a new research initiative evaluating how we improve health and treat disease in a patient-centered manner. This is possible with the help of the HIE in addition to already commonly accessed data from Centers for Medicaid & Medicare Services.

Transitions to postacute care will benefit with this increase in electronic availability of information across health systems. Infrastructure at these sites is slowly becoming the norm and will eventually integrate into systems at both sites. Additionally, given the amount of data that can potentially be lost in this transition to postacute care from the acute care hospital, team tracking may be implemented (Bates, 2015). This would allow tracking the disease state or test result for which each provider is responsible, in addition to collaboration by providers through video conferencing or other technology.

CONCLUSION

In this chapter, we have provided the background, described the many transitions of care that patients encounter, and identified some challenges created by the transitions. We have shared the ways technology, including EHRs and cloud-based systems, have thus far improved transitions and reviewed current data related to readmissions, patient safety, and patient quality of care. We described ways in which technology is expected to be integrated into transitions into the future. Technology will play a critical role in making transitions of care as safe and efficient as possible.

REFERENCES

Administration on Aging. (n.d.). Aging stats. Retrieved from https://agingstats.gov

Agency for Healthcare Research and Quality. (2005, March). 30 safe practices for better health care. Retrieved from http://www.ahrq.gov/qual/30safe.htm

Alagiakrishnan, K., Wilson, P., Sadowski, C. A., Rolfson, D., Ballermann, M., Ausford, A., . . . Hayward, R. S. (2016, January 25). Physicians' use of computerized clinical decision supports to improve medication management in the elderly—The Seniors Medication Alert and Review Technology intervention. *Clinical Interventions in Aging, 11*, 73–81. doi:10.2147/CIA.S94126

Bailey, J. E., Pope, R. A., Elliott, E. C., Wan, J. Y., Waters, T. M., & Frisse, M. E. (2013, July). Health information exchange reduces repeated diagnostic imaging for back pain. *Annals of Emergency Medicine, 62*(1), 16–24. doi:10.1016/j.annemergmed.2013.01.006

Bailey, J. E., Wan, J. Y., Mabry, L. M., Landy, S. H., Pope, R. A., Waters, T. M., & Frisse, M. E. (2013, February). Does health information exchange reduce unnecessary neuroimaging and improve quality of headache care in the emergency department? *Journal of General Internal Medicine, 28*(2), 176–83. doi:10.1007/s11606-012-2092-7

Bates, D. W. (2015, August). Health information technology and care coordination: The next big opportunity for informatics? *Yearbook of Medical Informatics, 10*(1), 11–4. doi:10.15265/IY-2015-0020

Boutwell, A., Griffin, F., Hwu, S., & Shannon, D. (2009). *Effective interventions to reduce rehospitalizations: A compendium of 15 promising interventions.* Cambridge, MA: Institute for Healthcare Improvement. Retrieved from http://www.ihi.org/resources/Pages/Changes/EffectiveInterventionstoReduceRehospitalizationsCompendium15PromisingInterventions.aspx

Centers for Medicare & Medicaid Services. (n.d.). Readmissions Reduction Program (RRP). Retrieved from http://www.cms.gov/Medicare/Medicare-Fee-for-Service-Payment/AcuteInpatientPPS/Readmissions-Reduction-Program.html

Centers for Medicare & Medicaid Services. (2014). Transitions of care summary. Retrieved from https://www.cms.gov/Regulations-and-Guidance/Legislation/EHRIncentivePrograms/downloads/8_Transition_of_Care_Summary.pdf

Charles, D., Gabriel, M., & Henry, J. (2015). *Electronic capabilities for patients among U.S. non-federal acute care hospitals: 2008–2014.* ONC Data Brief, No. 29. Washington, DC: The Office of the National Coordinator for Health Information Technology. Retrieved from https://www.healthit.gov/sites/default/files/briefs/oncdatabrief29_patientengagement.pdf

Charles, D., Swain, M., & Patel, V. (2015, August). *Interoperability among U.S. non-federal acute care hospitals, 2014.* ONC Data Brief, No. 25. Washington, DC: The Office of the National Coordinator for Health Information Technology. Retrieved from https://www.healthit.gov/sites/default/files/briefs/onc_databrief25_interoperabilityv16final_081115.pdf

Chen, A. H., Murphy, E. J., & Yee, H. F. (2013, June 27). eReferral—A new model for integrated care. *New England Journal of Medicine, 368,* 2450–2453. doi:10.1056/NEJMp1215594

Coleman, E. A., Parry, C., Chalmers, S., & Min, S. J. (2006, September 25). The care transitions intervention: Results of a randomized controlled trial. *Archives of Internal Medicine, 166,* 1822–1828.

Coleman, E. A., Smith, J. D., Raha, D., & Min, S. J. (2005, September 12). Posthospital medication discrepancies: Prevalence and contributing factors. *Archives of Internal Medicine, 165*(16), 1842–1847. doi:10.1001/archinte.165.16.1842

Davis, J., Riesenberg, L. A., Mardis, M., Donnelly, J., Benningfield, B., Youngstrom, M., & Vetter, I. (2015, June). Evaluating outcomes of electronic tools supporting physician shift-to-shift handoffs: A systematic review. *Journal of Graduate Medical Education, 7*(2), 174–180. doi:10.4300/JGME-D-14-00205.1

Donze, J., Aujesky, D., Williams, D., & Schnipper, J. L. (2013). Potentially avoidable 30-day hospital readmissions in medical patients. *JAMA Internal Medicine, 173*(8), 632–638. doi:10.1001/jamainternmed.2013.3023

Forster, A. J., Murff, H. J., Peterson, J. F., Gandhi, T. K., & Bates, D. W. (2003, February 4). The incidence and severity of adverse events affecting patients after discharge from the hospital. *Annals of Internal Medicine, 138*(3), 161–167.

Gabriel, M. H., & Swain, M. (2014, July). *E-prescribing trends in the United States.* ONC Data Brief, No. 18. Washington, DC: The Office of the National Coordinator for Health Information Technology. Retrieved from http://healthit.gov/sites/default/files/oncdatabriefe-prescribingincreases2014.pdf

Gay, V., & Leijdekkers, P. (2015, November). Bringing health and fitness data together for connected health care: Mobile apps as enablers of interoperability. *Journal of Medical Internet Research, 17*(11), e260. doi:10.2196/jmir.5094

Gleason, K. M., McDaniel, M. R., Feinglass, J., Baker, D. W., Lindquist, L., Liss, D., & Noskin, G. A. (2010, May). Results of the Medications at Transitions and Clinical Handoffs (MATCH) study: An analysis of medication reconciliation errors and risk factors at hospital admission. *Journal of General Internal Medicine, 25*, 441–447.

Heisey-Grove, D., Patel, V., & Searcy, T. (2015, September). *Physician electronic exchange of patient health information, 2014*. ONC Data Brief, No. 31. Washington, DC: The Office of the National Coordinator for Health Information Technology. Retrieved from https://www.healthit.gov/sites/default/files/briefs/oncdatabrief31_physician_e_exchange.pdf

Institute of Medicine Committee on Quality of Health Care in America. (2001). *Crossing the quality chasm: A new health system for the 21st century*. Washington, DC: National Academies Press.

Jack, B. W., Chetty, V. K., Anthony, D., Greenwald, J. L., Sanchez, G. M., & Johnson, A. E. (2009, February 3). A reengineered hospital discharge program to decrease rehospitalization: A randomized trial. *Annals of Internal Medicine, 150*, 178–187.

Jencks, S. F., Williams, M. V., & Coleman, E. A. (2009). Rehospitalizations among patients in the Medicare fee-for-service program. *New England Journal of Medicine, 360*, 1418–1428.

The Joint Commission. (2013). Hot topics in health care, Issue #2 transitions of care: The need for collaboration across entire care continuum. Retrieved from https://www.jointcommission.org/assets/1/6/TOC_Hot_Topics.pdf

Jung, H. Y., Vest, J. R., Unruh, M. A., Kern, L. M., Kaushal, R., & The HITEC Investigators. (2015, December). Use of health information exchange and repeat imaging costs. *Journal of the American College of Radiology*, 12(12, Pt. B), 1364–1370. doi:10.1016/j.jacr.2015.09.010

Kripalani, S., LeFevre, F., Phillips, C. O., Williams, M. V., Basaviah, P., & Baker, D. W. (2007). Deficits in communication and information transfer between hospital based and primary care physicians: Implications for patient safety and continuity of care. *vJournal of the American Medical Association*, 297(8), 831–841. doi:10.1001/jama.297.8.831

Kvedar, J., Coye, M. J., & Everett, W. (2014, February). Connected health: A review of technologies and strategies to improve patient care with telemedicine and telehealth. *Health Affairs, 33*(2), 194–199.

Marcotte, L., Kirtane, J., Lynn, J., & McKethan, A. (2015, December 11). Integrating heath information technology to achieve seamless care transitions. *Journal of Patient Safety, 11*(4), 185–190. doi:10.1097/PTS.0000000000000077

McCormick, D., Bor, D. H., Woolhandler, S., & Himmelstein, D. U. (2012, March). Giving office-based physicians electronic access to patients' prior imaging and lab results did not deter ordering of tests. *Health Affairs, 31*(3), 488–496. doi:10.1377/hlthaff.2011.0876

Medicare Payment Advisory Commission. (2007, June). Payment policy for inpatient readmissions. In *Report to the Congress: Promoting greater efficiency in Medicare* (pp. 103–120). Washington, DC: Author.

Moore, C., McGinn, T., & Halm, E. (2007). Tying up loose ends: Discharging patients with unresolved medical issues. *Archives of Internal Medicine, 167*, 1305–1311.

National Quality Forum. (2010). *Safe practices for better healthcare—2010 update: A consensus report*. Washington, DC: Author. Retrieved from http://www.qualityforum.org/WorkArea/linkit.aspx?LinkIdentifier=id&ItemID=25690

Naylor, M. D., Brooten, D., Campbell, R., Jacobsen, B. S., Mezey, M. D., Pauly, M. V., & Schwartz, J. S. (1999, February 17). Comprehensive discharge planning and home follow-up of hospitalized elders: A randomized clinical trial. *Journal of the American Medical Association, 281*, 613–620.

The Office of the National Coordinator for Health Information Technology. (n.d.). Health IT legislation. Retrieved from HealthIT.gov: https://www.healthit.gov/policy-researchers-implementers/health-it-legislation

The Office of the National Coordinator for Health Information Technology. (2013a). Improving hospital transitions and care coordination using automated admission, discharge and transfer alerts. Retrieved from http://www.healthit.gov/sites/default/files/onc-beacon-lg1-adt-alerts-for-toc-and-care-coord.pdf

The Office of the National Coordinator for Health Information Technology. (2013b). Implementing Consolidated-Clinical Document Architecture (C-CDA) for meaningful use stage 2. Retrieved from https://www.healthit.gov/sites/default/files/c-cda_and_meaningfulusecertification.pdf

The Office of the National Coordinator for Health Information Technology. (2015a). Trends in individuals use of health IT: 2012–2014. Health IT Quick-Stat #46. Retrieved from http://dashboard.healthit.gov/quickstats/pages/FIG-Individuals-Health-IT-Use.php

The Office of the National Coordinator for Health Information Technology. (2015b). Health IT progress update. Retrieved from http://dashboard.healthit.gov/report-to-congress/2015-update-adoption-health-information-technology-full-text.php#progress-update

The Office of the National Coordinator for Health Information Technology. (2015c). Federal Health IT Strategic Plan: Measurement & reporting. Retrieved from http://dashboard.healthit.gov/strategic-plan/federal-health-it-strategic-plan-narrative-measurement-reporting.php

The Office of the National Coordinator for Health Information Technology. (2015d). Federal Health IT strategic plan: 2015–2020. Retrieved from https://www.healthit.gov/sites/default/files/9-5-federalhealthitstratplanfinal_0.pdf

Patel, V., Barker, W., & Siminerio, E. (2015, October). *Trends in consumer access and use of electronic health*. ONC Data Brief, No. 30. Washington, DC: Office of the National Coordinator for Health Information Technology. Retrieved from http://dashboard.healthit.gov/evaluations/data-briefs/trends-consumer-access-use-electronic-health-information.php

Pham, H. H., Grossman, J. M., Cohen, G., & Bodenheimer, T. (2008). Hospitalists and care transitions: The divorce of inpatient and outpatient care. *Health Affairs, 27*(5), 1315–1327. doi:10.1377/hlthaff.27.5.1315

Roy, C. L., Poon, E. G., Karson, A. S., Ladak-Merchant, Z, Johnson, R. E., Maviglia, S. M., & Gandhi T. K. (2005). Patient safety concerns arising from test results that return after discharge. *Annals of Internal Medicine, 143*(2), 121–128.

Sarkar, U., Carter, J. T., Omachi, T. A., Vidyarthi, A. R., Cucina, R., Bokser, S., . . . Blum M. (2007, September). SynopSIS: Integrating physician sign-out with the electronic medical record. *Journal of Hospital Medicine, 2*(5), 336–342. doi:10.1002/jhm.235

Slovis, B. H., Lowry, T., Delman, B. N., Beitia, A. O., Kuperman, G., DiMaggio, C., & Shapiro J. S. (2016, May). Patient crossover and potentially avoidable repeat computed tomography exams across a health information exchange. *Journal of American Medical Informatics Association, 25*, 30–38. doi:10.1093/jamia/ocw035

Solan, L. G., Sherman, S. N., DeBiasio, D., & Simmons, J. M. (2016, July). Communication challenges: A qualitative look at the relationship between pediatric hospitalists and primary care providers. *Academic Pediatrics, 16*(5), 453–459. doi:10.1016/j.acap.2016.03.00

Swain, M., Charles, D., & Furukawa, M. F. (2014, May). *Health information exchange among U.S. non-federal acute care hospitals: 2008–2013*. ONC Data Brief, No. 17. Washington, DC: The Office of the National Coordinator for Health Information Technology. Retrieved from http://healthit.gov/sites/default/files/oncdatabrief17_hieamonghospitals.pdf

Swain, M., Charles, D., Patel, V., & Searcy, T. (2015, April). *Health information exchange among U.S. non-federal acute care hospitals: 2008–2014*. ONC Data Brief, No. 24. Washington, DC: The Office of the National Coordinator for Health Information Technology. Retrieved from https://www.healthit.gov/sites/default/files/data-brief/ONC_DataBrief24_HIE_Final.pdf

Taha, M., Pal, A., Mahnken, J. D., & Rigler, S. K. (2014). Derivation and validation of a formula to estimate risk for 30-day readmission in medical patients. *International Journal for Quality in Health Care, 26*(3), 271–277. doi:10.1093/intqhc/mzu038

van Sluisveld, N., Hesselink, G., van der Hoeven, J. G., Westert, G., Wollersheim, H., & Zegers, M. (2015, February). Improving clinical handover between intensive care unit and general ward professionals at intensive care unit discharge. *Intensive Care Medicine, 41*(4), 589–604. doi:10.1007/s00134-015-3666-8

van Walraven, C., Dhalla, I. A., Bell, C., Etchells, E., Stiell, I. G., Zarnke, K., . . . Forster, A. J. (2010). Derivation and validation of an index to predict early death or unplanned readmission after discharge from hospital to the community. *Canadian Medical Association Journal, 182*(6), 551–557.

Ventola, C. L. (2014, May). Mobile devices and apps for health care professionals: Uses and benefits. *Pharmacy and Therapeutics, 39*(5), 356–364.

Wohlauer, M. V., Rove, K. O., Pshak, T. J., Raeburn, C. D., Moore, E. E., Chenoweth, C., & Nehler, M. R. (2012, January). The computerized rounding report: Implementation of a model system to support transitions of care. *Journal of Surgical Research, 172*(1), 11–17. doi:10.1016/j.jss.2011.04.015

4

Home Telehealth

Thomas F. Osborne, John Russo, Jr., Bryan T. Arkwright, and Joel J. Reich

Treating illness at home is a tradition that has recently been revitalized by a number of factors. Specifically, telecommunication tools, financial imperatives, quality initiatives, staffing constraints, and patient preference are among the leading drivers for this transition. Successful telehealth program outcomes depend on a number of issues, with knowledge, leadership, and management being paramount. Home telehealth programs hold the potential to improve patient outcomes with cost-effective, patient-centered care.

HISTORICAL PERSPECTIVE

Up until the early 19th century, the United States economy was primarily agricultural. In this often expansive rural landscape, most health care was provided by a household member, who was sometimes relegated to the role of full-time caregiver. Although there were limited institutions for the sick in urban areas during this period, they were primarily intended for the marginalized and poor. Around the turn of the 20th century, numerous institutional and medical advancements increased the credibility and popularity of hospitals, which dramatically grew in number from 120 hospitals in 1873 to 4,300 in 1909 (Abel, 1995; Ding,2013; Finzsch, 2003; Porter, 1994; Porter, 1999; Risse, 1999). Amid this transformation, the "house call" remained a dominant factor for a short period, accounting for 40% of encounters in 1930, but falling rapidly to 10% in the 1950s, and reaching less than 1% of older patients in the 1990s (Daschle & Dorsey, 2015).

COST PRESSURES

The unsustainable increasing costs of hospital-based care prompted numerous federal policy changes, often mirrored by private insurers. For example, in 1983, Medicare dramatically changed reimbursement policy with a newly implemented payment system of "diagnosis-related groups," which reimburses hospitals on the basis of the expected complexity of care, and not number of days. This historic change incentivized hospitals to discharge patients as soon as possible (Goldfield, 2010). However, discharging a patient too early can also lead to costly readmissions, potentially leading to unnecessary life-threatening complications. This led to the development of transitional care facilities. However, the costs for subacute care centers and long-term health care options outside of the hospital are also high, with recent U.S. estimates ranging between $210.9 billion (O'Shaughnessy, 2013) and $317.1 billion annually (Colello, Mulvey, & Talaga, 2013). Of further concern, the number of people utilizing these types of services is projected to dramatically increase from 15 million in the year 2000, to 27 million in the year 2050 (U.S. Department of Health and Human Services, 2003).

This extraordinary financial burden is a major concern for all stakeholders (Bipartisan Policy Center, 2014; Reinhard, Kassner, Houser, & Mollica, 2011; U.S. Senate Commission on Long-Term Care, 2013) and, as a result, efficient quality care is an increasingly important topic in health care reform and policy (Doty, 2010; Takahashi et al., 2012; White House Conference on Aging Staff, 2015; Wiener, 2013). Home telehealth programs offer an appealing, cost-effective alternative or extension to acute, subacute, and long-term care centers or nursing home facilities.

SHIFT BACK TO HOME HEALTH CARE

There are additional factors driving care back toward home-based care. From a clinical perspective, providing care in a patient's own residence reduces the risk of acquiring nosocomial infections, which may be antibiotic resistant. In addition, there are patients with clinical conditions ranging from Alzheimer's disease to autism, who may be more effectively treated in the home. Geographic disparities that would otherwise limit access to specialist care may also be ameliorated by home telehealth programs, and thereby make health care more equitable (Goldfield, 2010). Virtual visits and remote-accessible medical resources also improve access to basic care by overcoming transportation constraints that may otherwise limit the ability of patients to participate in routine follow-up and wellness programs. Importantly, a digitally connected home can empower independence and promote a sense of security.

It is, therefore, not surprising that there is a growing desire among many patient–consumers to shift their health care to the familiar comfort and convenience of their own residence (Cusack et al., 2008; Doty, 2010; Wiener, 2013).

SPECTRUM OF HOME HEALTH PATIENTS

Currently, the majority of home health services address the chronic needs of older patients (Gordy, & Trunkey, 2014; Harris-Kojetin et al., 2016; Haupt & Jones, 1999). The majority of diseases encountered in this setting parallel the prevalence in the geriatric population, with home telehealth services for diabetes, hypertension, heart disease, stroke, cancer, arthritis, chronic obstructive pulmonary disorder (COPD), atrial fibrillation, dementia, and depression encountered at the highest frequency (Centers for Medicare & Medicaid Services, 2013).

Although elderly long-term care is projected to be a major focus for home health services, the same basic concepts and infrastructure may be transferrable to different and/or overlapping patient populations. To this end, numerous programs are being developed for other health needs ranging from urgent care, pediatrics, rehabilitation medicine, postsurgical follow-up, and general wellness (Elias et al., 2012; Hewitt-Taylor, 2012; Patel, Park, Bonato, Chan, & Rodgers, 2012).

TECHNOLOGICAL ADVANCES

Recent technological advances in miniature sensors, low-power integrated circuits, wireless communications, and broadband data networks have enabled the development of low-cost, mobile, health data–gathering tools that can efficiently monitor many specific illnesses markers (Baig & Gholamhosseini, 2013; Milenković, Otto, & Jovanov, 2006).

In addition to technological solutions designed for individual diseases, there is also a growing need to manage more complex patients with multiple illnesses (Salive, 2013). In this situation, it is not uncommon for several different caregivers to be involved in the care of a single patient. Unfortunately, when there are different specialists working in isolation, there is a significant risk for uncoordinated care that can lead to life-threatening problems such as inappropriate polypharmacy, the incidence of which is high in older home health patients (Bao, Shao, Bishop, Schackman, & Bruce, 2012; Bronskill et al., 2012; Maher, Hanlon, & Hajjar, 2014; Scott et al., 2015). This challenge underscores the need for an integrated and interoperable enterprise health information platform that connects caregivers and facilities to help prevent medical errors.

PROVIDING VALUE AND THE TRIPLE AIM

Health care providers are being asked to do more with less, which, if not augmented by technological advancement, can result in poorer patient outcomes (Hirsbrunner, Denhaerynck, Fierz, Milisen, & Schwendimann, 2015; Dumanovsky, Rogers, Spragens, Morrison, & Meier, 2015; Kalisch, Tschannen, & Lee, 2012; Rimsza et al., 2015). At the same time, patients and payers are looking for greater value in both outcomes and overall experience. Developing effective, cost-effective, value-based, patient-centered alternatives requires a redesign of many fundamental aspects of health care delivery. Home telehealth programs hold great promise in facilitating this critical paradigm shift in health care, and success depends on interrelated factors, which are well illustrated in the context of the Triple Aim (Osborne, Reich, Arkwright, & Russo, 2016).

The Triple Aim

The *Triple Aim* is a framework developed for improved population health. This ambitious strategy was developed by the Institute for Healthcare Improvement (IHI) a decade ago in its effort to redesign the U.S. health care system. As stated by Dr. Donald Berwick, the former president and CEO of IHI, ". . . the United States will not achieve high-value healthcare unless improvement initiatives pursue a broader system of linked goals. In the aggregate, we call those goals the 'Triple Aim': improving the individual experience of care; improving the health of populations; and reducing the per capita costs of care for populations" (Berwick, Nolan, & Whittington, 2008).

Triple Aim implementation began in 2007 with a group of 15 organizations in the United States, England, and Sweden, and was quickly adopted by the Centers for Medicare & Medicaid Services (CMS) during Berwick's short tenure as administrator. The goals have subsequently become the "mantra" of health care reform, with adoption of the aims by many health care systems and accountable care organizations. As a result, in 2014, more than 150 organizations across the world participated in efforts to achieve these aims (Lewis, 2014; Osborne et al., 2016).

In recognition of the high degree of interdependence, the intent of the Triple Aim is to achieve the three linked goals simultaneously. However, the synchronized achievement of these interrelated measures is complex and challenging. The required redesign of health care financial, clinical, and operational relationships underscores that these goals will not be achieved with minor modifications to the status quo. However, for simplification of discussion, the following sections consider each component of the Triple Aim individually in relation to home telehealth.

IMPROVING THE INDIVIDUAL EXPERIENCE OF CARE

Home telehealth may improve the experience of care in various ways. For many, the familiar comfort and convenience of one's own home is much more appealing than a health care facility, and, therefore, it is not surprising that there is a growing vocal trend among seniors and Baby Boomers, soon-to-be seniors, who prefer this option (Accenture, n.d.; Family Caregiver Alliance, 2015; National Institute on Aging, n.d.). Home health care services are essential for those who are homebound and are of great value to those for whom the logistics of traveling to a provider's office is a tremendous burden. In addition, due to frailty or functional limitation, many would benefit from the added safety of digital monitoring in the home or in nonmedical residential institutions such as assisted living facilities. As a result, a technology-enabled home health system can prolong independence and a patient's control of the context of care.

User acceptance is a foundational component to achieving a positive home telehealth care experience, and begins with selecting appropriate patients who are comfortable using the specific technology (Viers et al., 2015). Many basic technological components of home telehealth, including glucometers, oximeters, and digital scales, have been available for many years as stand-alone devices. Historically, data collection and reporting has, for the most part, been manual, often in the form of patient-generated handwritten records, which are then carried to the care provider at the time of office visits. Advances in wireless device technology, increased accessibility to broadband networks, and integration, have significantly advanced the capability to report, aggregate, and share the biometric data with care provider teams to enable timely data analysis and response times.

Acceptance and endorsement from members of the care team is a sometimes neglected but critical component of success (NORC at the University of Chicago, 2012). On a similar note, engagement of appropriately designated family and friends is also a key factor for an improved health care experience. This is particularly true for friends and family of patients who are chronically ill, disabled, or frail because these caregivers are likely to be involved in home telehealth use. Therefore, measures to incorporate all of these collaborators in the enrollment, setup, management, and troubleshooting of home telehealth solutions should not be overlooked. Failure to properly address each stakeholder may result in dissatisfaction and the perception that technology has become a substitute rather than an enhancer of the team relationship (Broderick & Lindeman, 2013).

Improved acceptance and experience from each collaborator can be achieved with a thoughtful approach to the overall design of the program, and selection of the appropriate technological tools. However, balancing a technology's utility with usability can be challenging (Chau, & Hu, 2002). For example, design considerations for older patients should include providing tools and interfaces that take into account commonly encountered patient challenges such as potential vision, cognitive, and dexterity limitations, as well as potential inexperience with digital technology.

Home telehealth functions best when it is integrated into the established care process and information systems (Singh, Mathiassen, Stachura, & Astapova, 2011). Likewise, special care and attention must be given to the existing workflow and needs of care providers. Regrettably, many home telehealth programs are freestanding and not interoperable with health system electronic health records (EHRs) and population health database tools, which is a significant obstacle to success. In addition, when specific technological tools are developed without the direct consultation or understanding of a health care provider's perspectives, the results are typically suboptimal. If a home telehealth program becomes intrusive owing to poorly designed technology or workflow, the resulting decreased provider efficiency will make it virtually impossible to obtain the necessary support and participation for effective adoption. Furthermore, a well-intended tool may have negative consequences such as overly aggressive alert thresholds, resulting in disruptive false alarms that consume valuable time when staff respond to a nonevent, or, at the other extreme, delayed (or nonexistent) response, with the potential for negative outcomes due to real events missed. With either scenario, cost of care increases without obvious purpose (Murias, Sales, Garcia-Esquirol, & Blanch, 2009). Similarly, a primary care physician may derive considerable value from an organized once-per-month summary of glucose measurements; however, delivery of daily or hourly noncritical results may quickly lead to frustration. As with all other health information technology systems, privacy, data security, interoperability, data aggregation, and technical support are essential for sustainability.

Home telehealth also has the potential to significantly enhance the experience of care by facilitating communication. These benefits include, but are not limited to, creating a direct connection to care providers, friends, and family, as well as providing a sense of security via electronic safety alerts that are routed to an appropriate agency. The potential benefits of dampening the social isolation experienced by many who are chronically ill, as well as the empowerment of self-management and independence, should not be understated. The overall improved home health care experiences that can be achieved in these situations is reflected in the high patient-satisfaction scores reported by patients participating in these programs within the Veterans Health Administration system and others (Broderick & Lindeman, 2013; Jimison et al., 2008; NORC at the University of Chicago, 2012).

IMPROVING THE HEALTH OF POPULATIONS

A major goal of population health is to define the population's health needs and disparities. A key component is to identify the specific types of individuals who have these needs, and address them through care management, coordination, and clinical services.

While there are many methodologies for defining populations and their data, patients are ultimately stratified into groups to enable the most beneficial assignment of resources. Depending on the perspectives, populations may be defined by criteria such as disease type, severity scoring, source of payment, and geography. Patient stratification, often illustrated with a pyramid, is used to illustrate progressively more intense care services required. For example, beginning at the base of the pyramid, the lowest risk group is often well served by wellness programs; the moderate risk group served with coaching and self-care/management; the high-risk group with disease management; and the very high–risk group at the top of the pyramid with the addition of case management. Individuals with one or more chronic diseases in the moderate risk group, high-risk group, and noninstitutionalized very high–risk group may derive the greatest clinical value from home telehealth (Munro, 2015).

Research from the past decade has shown mixed results regarding the value, return on investment, and efficacy of home telehealth programs. There are many variables to consider, and, therefore, these studies need to be thoughtfully evaluated in the context of the specific program, patient population, and methodology. An additional challenge in the evaluation of home telehealth programs is applying research findings from studies of a single disease entity to patients in the moderate, high, and very high severity group populations who often have multiple comorbidities. As a result, the limited scope of many research studies leaves unanswered questions regarding the full potential of home telehealth for more complex patient populations (Denesen et al., 2016).

Meaningful evaluation is also confounded by the difficulty in obtaining complete follow-up data when multiple different sites of care (hospitals, physician offices, labs) are used in unrelated health systems without interoperable data systems (Goldfield, 2010). Therefore, critical considerations include factors such as the degree of network development, leadership, care provider support for home telehealth, and the extent of clinical integration at the time of the study (Ekeland, Bowes, & Flottorp, 2010; Mushcab, Kernohan, Wallace, & Martin, 2015). It is becoming clear that a successful home telehealth program needs to be well integrated into a system, which includes home health, disease management, transitional care, and primary care services (U.S. Department of Health and Human Services, 2003). Without these components, and a well-constructed response plan, its full value for populations will not be realized (Goldfield, 2010). In contrast, favorable results for home telehealth have been reported by well-organized integrated programs such as the Veterans Health Administration, Banner Health, and Geisinger Health System (Dahl, Reisetter, & Zismann, 2014; Maeng et al., 2014; NORC at the University of Chicago, 2012).

REDUCING PER CAPITA COSTS OF CARE FOR POPULATIONS

Staggering health care costs across virtually all patient populations have far-reaching implications for our economy and society as a whole. In response to this, government payers (i.e., Medicare and Medicaid) and commercial insurance companies (including employer self-funded health insurance) are shifting financial risk to health care systems and physicians through shared savings, bundled payment, and capitation programs. There are many variations in these plans; however, they all share the common goal of replacing more expensive intensive care with improved primary care, care management, preventive medicine, as well as other safe and effective alternatives (Frakt & Mayes, 2012).

The goal of efficiently lowering health care costs is particularly important for our growing senior population, who are living longer with multiple chronic conditions, functional impairment, frailty, and social stressors. This dilemma is especially problematic because this population already accounts for half of the costliest 5% of patients (Leff, Carlson, Saliba, & Ritchie, 2014). Multiple federal cost-saving measures are being initiated to meet this challenge. While there are many views on how to most effectively reduce health care spending, considerable effort is presently focused on reducing acute hospital care, and therefore home telehealth is well positioned to be an important part of the solution.

In addition, CMS rating programs, as well as those implemented by private insurance companies, use readmission as a key metric for determining rewards and penalties. This has become increasingly important because with shortened hospitalization, patients, particularly the elderly, may leave the hospital before being completely stable and without a thorough understanding of important items such as diet, medication compliance, and other follow-up discharge instructions (Nguyen et al., 2016). When combined with organized residential safety assessments, a specifically designed and technologically enabled home telehealth program can bridge this critical gap. A well-integrated system can identify early status changes for the conditions contributing the most to hospitalization and rehospitalization, such as heart failure, COPD/pneumonia, diabetes, and the myriad complications of diabetes. A common example is weight gain by a heart failure patient, which may indicate developing or worsening congestive heart failure. Early identification of this type of change in status can lead to timely intervention and management at home or at the primary care physician's office, therefore avoiding an expensive emergency department and/or hospital admission (Silow-Carroll, Edwards, & Lashbrook, 2011).

In our dynamically changing reimbursement system, calculating exactly where the cost savings occur, and to whom they accrue is challenging. In the traditional fee-for-service system, reduced hospital admissions decrease a health system's revenue, and therefore this lack of alignment has been a source of federal policy changes. On the other hand, in a physician-only shared savings program, a physician group may be financially rewarded for reducing hospital admissions. Likewise, the cost to the insurer is also reduced when hospital admissions are avoided.

In a value-based system with risk sharing, the expense to create the infrastructure that results in the savings may occur in different areas of the network. For example, a home health provider may run the home telehealth program with payment from direct monthly fees or a grant, yet the savings on reduced expenses such as acute hospitalizations may benefit a local independent accountable care organization or clinically integrated network (Davis, Bender, Smith, & Broad, 2015; Munro, 2015; Singh et al., 2011). Similarly, remote management of chronic diseases in partnership with a primary care provider may also reduce expenditures for specialist care and lab testing. Furthermore, preventive care measures provided electronically in the home, including wellness education and activity monitoring via wearable technology, may result in cost savings to multiple different entities.

While system-level cost reduction efforts have considerable importance, those accrued to individuals, families, and groups that compose the populations is an important component of system transformation's success or failure. It is difficult to place a dollar value on improved personal health and quality of life; however, there are some variables that can be calculated directly, including fewer absences from work, reduced out-of-pocket expenditures on emergency department and acute hospitalization costs, as well as the associated transportation costs.

As part of an effort to increase value, in both the fee-for-service and the value-based payment systems, CMS and private insurance programs allocate both direct financial rewards and penalties on the basis of patient experience scores. Poor patient and family experience also places considerable fee-for-service revenue at risk because of damaged institutional reputation and decreased referral rates. Because a successfully implemented home telehealth program contributes positively to patient and family experience, it therefore results in financial benefit to the care provider in many ways regardless of the payment model.

As value-based payment and accountable care arrangements mature and grow, the true benefits of home telehealth may be more fully realized. Overall, however, attainment of the Triple Aim may require substantial reallocation of health care resources from traditional fee-for-service payment arrangements to clinically integrated "value-based" payment models.

OBJECTIVE INSIGHTS

Although the promise of telehealth may seem intuitively obvious, there is also a critical need to continually and objectively evaluate assumptions. For example, a recent analysis reviewed 36 journal articles and found telehealth to be more expensive in 31% of cases. Importantly, the article authors suggested that the specific organizational model employed in the delivery of care was more important to the success of the program than the type of technology utilized (Wade, Karnon, Elshaug, & Hiller, 2010). In a separate study, the authors suggested that the lack of an effective infrastructure for case management was the pivotal factor (Takahashi et al., 2012). These examples underscore that technology by itself is not effective. Tools need to be evaluated, tested, and implemented with an understanding of existing requirements, workflows, and stakeholder insights, with the primary goal of quality patient-centered care. In the words of Jeffrey K. Liker, "Use only reliable, thoroughly tested technology that serves your people and processes" (Liker, 2004).

LEADERSHIP AND MANAGEMENT

The skills of leadership and management are critically important to success because it can take as much time, effort, and resources to implement the right solution as it does to create the wrong one. To this end, the required interplay between change and order are dependent on a number of complementary factors including clear communication, vision, empowerment, strategy, alignment, and a deep understanding of the national and local health care environment, as well as thoughtful evaluation, planning, requirements gathering, structure, and stakeholder involvement (Collins, 2001; Kearns & Sabherwal, 2006; Liker, 2004; Ploeg, Davies, Edwards, Gifford, & Miller, 2007).

Specific considerations such as potential technical limitations in broadband Internet connectivity, interoperability with critical information systems, the need for uniform standards among EHRs, cost, relevance of the proposed solutions, reliability, user acceptance, as well as legal, ethical, and facility–organizational factors need to be addressed. Understanding these types of variables and requirements will reveal valuable information about the most successful path to implementation, as well as the projected benefits and potential unintended consequences (Koch, 2006).

Planning for long-term maintenance and continual improvements based on open feedback and ongoing evaluation are also key factors to long-term achievement and sustainability (Finkbeiner, Schau, Lehmann, & Traverso, 2010; Wheelwright & Clark, 1992).

USER ACCEPTANCE

The success of any telehealth program depends on user acceptance. In the case of technologically enabled home health care, the end users are varied, and include patients, caregivers, support staff, and administrators (Cimperman, Brenčič, Trkman, & Stanonik, 2013). To be successful, the solutions must meet the needs of each major stakeholder. Thoughtfully designed user interfaces tailored to the specific audience promote an effective, intuitive, and enjoyable experience, which also decreases the need for training and elaborate change management strategies. Tools should improve upon an existing framework, and not produce an environment where people become subservient to technology (Liker, 2004).

These issues are particularly pertinent to home caregivers who may already be overworked; home health nurses work more hours than nurses in nearly any other setting (U.S. Department of Health and Human Services, Health Resources and Services Administration, 2010). Importantly, it has been shown that improved managerial support of nursing practice and better relations with physicians can translate to improved morale and better patient outcomes (Flynn, Dickson, & Moles, 2007; Lake & Friese, 2006). Therefore, technological communication tools that bridge these gaps may also provide nonlinear paths to improved patient care.

OPERATIONAL CHALLENGES OF TELEHEALTH

The intrinsic geographically isolated nature of home health care requires advanced tools for the coordinated collaboration of patients, cross-functional teams, tools, and disciplines. To this end, a successfully implemented technological infrastructure is required to provide a platform for efficient communication and engagement for everyone involved.

Therefore, the availability and reliability of Internet connections is a potential critical limitation to the deployment of specific solutions such as synchronous videoconferencing and biometrics tracking (Gindi et al., 2014; Perrin & Duggan, 2015). Nonetheless, in situations of limited Internet access, a less-desirable delayed information transfer to caregivers can still be achieved asynchronously in a "store-and-forward" process.

The connected benefits of telehealth also come with concerns regarding the security of protected health information that will be digitally transferred to offsite caregivers (Kotz, Gunter, Kumar, & Weiner, 2016; Luxton, Kayl, & Mishkind, 2012; Wilkowska & Ziefle, 2012). In addition, the various patient health metrics obtained will need to be presented to caregivers in an efficient, user-friendly format (Fleming et al., 2014; Page & Schadler, 2014).

Even with the most robust technical infrastructure, periodic in-person home visits by a caregiver are often part of a complete home health solution. However, the unstandardized home environment presents efficiency and safety challenges to visiting health care examiners, and these issues also need to be systematically addressed (Gindi et al., 2014). In addition, the use of relatively low-tech options such as railings, adjustable shower seats, and motion-activated lights provide important levels of added patient safety and independence.

FUTURE TECHNOLOGY DIRECTIONS

Iterative improvements of existing technological solutions will drive greater value and user acceptance to this disruptive home care model. However, new developments in the fields of machine learning, artificial intelligence, analytics, integrated networks, and robotics will drive a paradigm shift in how we practice medicine.

CONCLUSION

A number of interdependent factors have made home health care an attractive option for many. Leadership, management, and technology are among key factors for success. Home telehealth programs not only hold the potential to solve an escalating demand at a lower cost, but also may achieve that goal with significantly improved outcomes.

REFERENCES

Abel, E. K. (1995). A "terrible and exhausting" struggle: Family caregiving during the transformation of medicine. *Journal of the History of Medicine and Allied Sciences, 50*(4), 478–506.

Accenture. (n.d.). Tech-savvy seniors want online options to access care from home, Accenture survey shows. Retrieved from https://newsroom.accenture.com/industries/health-public-service/tech-savvy-seniors-want-online-options-to-access-care-from-home-accenture-survey-shows.htm

Baig, M. M., & Gholamhosseini, H. (2013). Smart health monitoring systems: An overview of design and modeling. *Journal of Medical Systems, 37*(2), 1–14.

Bao, Y., Shao, H., Bishop, T. F., Schackman, B. R., & Bruce, M. L. (2012). Inappropriate medication in a national sample of US elderly patients receiving home health care. *Journal of General Internal Medicine, 27*(3), 304–310.

Berwick, D. M., Nolan, T. W., & Whittington, J. (2008). The triple aim: Care, health, and cost. *Health Affairs, 27*(3), 759–769. doi:10.1377/hlthaff.27.3.759

Bipartisan Policy Center. (2014). America's long-term care crisis: Challenges in financing and delivery. Retrieved from http://bipartisanpolicy.org/wp-content/uploads/2014/03/BPC-Long-Term-Care-Initiative.pdf

Broderick, A., & Lindeman, D. (2013). Scaling telehealth programs: Lessons from early adopters. Case studies in telehealth adoption. The Commonwealth Fund. Retrieved from http://www.commonwealthfund.org/~/media/Files/Publications/Case%20Study/2013/Jan/1654_Broderick_telehealth_adoption_synthesis.pdf

Bronskill, S. E., Gill, S. S., Paterson, J. M., Bell, C. M., Anderson, G. M., & Rochon, P. A. (2012). Exploring variation in rates of polypharmacy across long term care homes. *Journal of the American Medical Directors Association, 13*(3), 309.e15–309.e21.

Centers for Medicare & Medicaid Services. (2013). *Chronic condition data warehouse*. West Des Moines, IA: Buccaneer. Retrieved from http://www.ccwdata.org/chronic-conditions/index.htm

Chau, P. Y. K., & Hu, P. J. H. (2002). Investigating healthcare professionals' decisions to accept telemedicine technology: An empirical test of competing theories. *Inform Manage, 39*, 297–311.

Cimperman, M., Brenčič, M. M., Trkman, P., & Stanonik, M. D. L. (2013). Older adults' perceptions of home telehealth services. *Telemedicine and e-Health, 19*(10), 786–790.

Colello, K. J., Mulvey, J., & Talaga, S. R. (2013, April). *Long-term services and supports: Overview and financing*. In Congressional Research Service Report for Congress. Retrieved from http://digital.library.unt.edu/ark:/67531/metadc462393/m1/1/high_res_d/R42345_2013Apr04.pdf

Collins, J. C. (2001). *Good to great: Why some companies make the leap . . . and others don't*. New York, NY: Random House.

Cusack, C. M., Pan, E., Hook, J. M., Vincent, A., Kaelber, D. C., & Middleton, B. (2008). The value proposition in the widespread use of telehealth. *Journal of Telemedicine and Telecare, 14*(4), 167–168.

Dahl, D., Reisetter, J. A., & Zismann, N. (2014). People, technology, and process meet the triple aim. *Nursing Administration Quarterly, 38*(1), 13–21.

Daschle, T., & Dorsey, E. R. (2015). The return of the house call. *Annals of Internal Medicine, 162*(8), 587–588.

Davis, C., Bender, M., Smith, T., & Broad, J. (2015). Feasibility and acute care utilization outcomes of a post-acute transitional telemonitoring program for underserved chronic disease patients. *International Encyclopedia of Public Health, 21*(9), 705–713.

Denesen, B., Nonnecke, B., Lindeman, D., Toft, E., Kidholm, K., & Jethwani, K. (2016). Personalized health in the future: A global research agenda. *Journal of Medical Internet Research, 18*(3), e53.

Ding, A. (2013). The history of health care in the United States pre-1965. In M. K. Sethi & W. H. Frist (Eds.), *An introduction to health policy* (pp. 3–13). New York, NY: Springer.

Doty, P. (2010). The evolving balance of formal and informal, institutional and non-institutional long-term care for older Americans: A thirty-year perspective. *Public Policy & Aging Report, 20*(1), 3–9.

Dumanovsky, T., Rogers, M., Spragens, L. H., Morrison, R. S., & Meier, D. E. (2015). Impact of staffing on access to palliative care in US hospitals. *Journal of Palliative Medicine, 18*(12), 998–999.

Ekeland, A. G., Bowes, A., & Flottorp, S. (2010). Effectiveness of telemedicine: A systematic review of reviews. *International Journal of Medical Informatics, 79*(11), 736–771.

Elias, E. R., Murphy, N. A., Liptak, G. S., Adams, R. C., Burke, R., Friedman, S. L., . . . Norwood, K. W. (2012). Home care of children and youth with complex health care needs and technology dependencies. *Pediatrics, 129*(5), 996–1005.

Family Caregiver Alliance. (2015). Selected long-term care statistics. Retrieved from https://www.caregiver.org/selected-long-term-care-statistics

Finkbeiner, M., Schau, E. M., Lehmann, A., & Traverso, M. (2010). Towards life cycle sustainability assessment. *Sustainability, 2*(10), 3309–3322.

Finzsch, N., & Jütte, R. (2003). *Institutions of confinement: Hospitals, asylums, and prisons in Western Europe and North America, 1500–1950*. New York, NY: Cambridge University Press.

Fleming, N. S., Becker, E. R., Culler, S. D., Cheng, D., McCorkle, R., Graca, B. D., & Ballard, D. J. (2014). The impact of electronic health records on workflow and financial measures in primary care practices. *Health Services Research, 49*(1, Pt. 2), 405–420.

Flynn, L., Dickson, G., & Moles, D. J. (2007). Focus on caregiving. Enhancing the nursing workplace: In a recent study of long term care nurses, key organizational factors emerge as most important in supporting a productive work environment. *Provider, 33*(1), 35–39.

Frakt, A. B., & Mayes, R. (2012). Beyond capitation: How new payment experiments seek to find the 'sweet spot' in amount of risk providers and payers bear. *Health Affairs, 31*(9), 1951–1958. doi:10.1377/hlthaff.2012.0344

Gindi, R. M., Zipf, G., Galinsky, A. M., Miller, I. M., Nwankwo, T., & Terry, A. L. (2014). Comparison of in-home collection of physical measurements and biospecimens with collection in a standardized setting: The health measures at home study. *Vital and Health Statistics. Series 2, Data Evaluation and Methods Research*, (164), 1–16.

Goldfield, N. (2010). The evolution of diagnosis-related groups (DRGs): From its beginnings in case-mix and resource use theory, to its implementation for payment and now for its current utilization for quality within and outside the hospital. *Quality Management in Healthcare, 19*(1), 3–16.

Gordy, S., & Trunkey, D. (2014). Changing demographics of the American population. In J. A. Yelon & F. A. Luchette (Eds.), *Geriatric trauma and critical care* (pp. 3–9). New York, NY: Springer.

Harris-Kojetin, L., Sengupta, M., Park-Lee, E., Valverde, R., Caffrey, C., Rome, V., & Lendon, J. (2016). Long-term care providers and services users in the United States: Data from the National Study of Long-Term Care Providers, 2013–2014. National Center for Health Statistics. *Vital & Health Statistics, 3*(38), 1–118.

Haupt, B. J., & Jones, A. (1999). The national home and hospice care survey: 1996 summary. *Vital and Health Statistics. Series 13, Data from the National Health Survey,* (141), 1–238.

Hewitt-Taylor, J. (2012). Planning the transition of children with complex needs from hospital to home. *Nursing Children and Young People, 24*(10), 28.

Hirsbrunner, T., Denhaerynck, K., Fierz, K., Milisen, K., & Schwendimann, R. (2015). Nurse staffing, patient turnover and safety climate and their association with in-patient falls and injurious falls on medical acute care units: A cross-sectional study. *Journal of Hospital Administration, 4*(3), 54.

Jimison, H., Gorman, P., Woods, S., Nygren, P., Walker, M., Norris, S., & Hersh, W. (2008). *Barriers and drivers of health information technology use by the elderly chronically ill and underserved*. AHRQ Publication No. 09-E004. Retrieved from http://www.ahrq.gov/downloads/pub/evidence/pdf/hitbarriers/hitbar.pdf

Kalisch, B. J., Tschannen, D., & Lee, K. H. (2012). Missed nursing care, staffing, and patient falls. *Journal of Nursing Care Quality, 27*(1), 6–12.

Kearns, G. S., & Sabherwal, R. (2006). Strategic alignment between business and information technology: A knowledge-based view of behaviors, outcome, and consequences. *Journal of Management Information Systems, 23*(3), 129–162.

Koch, S. (2006). Home telehealth—Current state and future trends. *International Journal of Medical Informatics, 75*(8), 565–576.

Kotz, D., Gunter, C. A., Kumar, S., & Weiner, J. P. (2016). Privacy and Security in Mobile Health: A Research Agenda. *Computer, 49*(6), 22–30.

Lake, E. T., & Friese, C. R. (2006). Variations in nursing practice environments: Relation to staffing and hospital characteristics. *Nursing Research, 55*(1), 1–9.

Leff, B., Carlson, C. M., Saliba, D., & Ritchie, C. (2014). The invisible homebound: Setting quality-of-care standards for home-bound primary and palliative care. *Health Affairs, 34*(1), 21–29.

Lewis, N. (2014). A primer on defining the Triple Aim. Retrieved from http://www.ihi.org/communities/blogs/_layouts/ihi/community/blog/itemview.aspx?List=81ca4a47-4ccd-4e9e-89d9-14d88ec59e8d&ID=63

Liker, J. K. (2004). *The Toyota way*. New York, NY: McGraw-Hill.

Luxton, D. D., Kayl, R. A., & Mishkind, M. C. (2012). mHealth data security: The need for HIPAA-compliant standardization. *Telemedicine and e-Health,18*(4), 284–288.

Maeng, D. D., Starr, A. E., Tomcavage, J. F., Sciandra, J., Salek, D., & Griffith, D. (2014). Can telemonitoring reduce hospitalization and cost of care? A health plan's experience in managing patients with heart failure. *Population Health Management, 17*(6), 340–344.

Maher, R. L., Hanlon, J., & Hajjar, E. R. (2014). Clinical consequences of polypharmacy in elderly. *Expert Opinion on Drug Safety, 13*(1), 57–65.

Milenković, A., Otto, C., & Jovanov, E. (2006). Wireless sensor networks for personal health monitoring: Issues and an implementation. *Computer Communications, 29*(13), 2521–2533.

Munro, D. (2015). Targeting the 'superusers' of healthcare with telehealth. *Forbes*. Retrieved from http://www.forbes.com/sites/danmunro/2015/05/03/targeting-the-superusers-of-healthcare-with-telehealth/#3296cb6d5dd3

Murias, G., Sales, B., Garcia-Esquirol, O., & Blanch, L. (2009). Telemedicine in critical care. *The Open Respiratory Medicine Journal, 3*, 10–16. doi:10.2174/1874306400903010010

Mushcab, H., Kernohan, W. G., Wallace, J., & Martin, S. (2015). Web-based remote monitoring systems for self-managing type 2 diabetes: A systematic review. *Diabetes Technology & Therapeutics, 17*(7), 498–509.

National Institute on Aging. (n.d.). There's no place like home—for growing old. Retrieved from https://www.nia.nih.gov/health/publication/theres-no-place-home-growing-old

Nguyen, O. K., Makam, A. N., Clark, C., Zhang, S., Xie, B., Velasco, F., & Halm, E. A. (2016). Vital signs are still vital: Instability on discharge and the risk of post-discharge adverse outcomes. *Journal of General Internal Medicine, 32*, 42–48. doi:10.1007/s11606-016-3826-8

NORC at the University of Chicago. (2012). Health IT and health disparities: Patient provider telehealth network—using telehealth to improve chronic disease management. Retrieved from https://www.healthit.gov/sites/default/files/pdf/RCCHCandPHS_CaseStudy.pdf

O'Shaughnessy, C. V. (2013). *The basics: National spending for long-term services and supports, 2012*. Washington, DC: National Health Policy Forum, George Washington University. Retrieved from http://www.nhpf.org/library/the-basics/Basics_LTSS_03-27-14.pdf

Osborne, T. F., Reich, J. J., Arkwright, M. H. A., & Russo, J., Jr. (2016). On the digital road to home healthcare. *Telehealth and Medicine Today*. Retrieved from http://www.telhealthandmedtoday.com/on-the-digital-road-to-improved-home-healthcare

Page, C. A. K., & Schadler, A. (2014). A nursing focus on EMR usability enhancing documentation of patient outcomes. *Nursing Clinics of North America, 49*(1), 81–90.

Patel, S., Park, H., Bonato, P., Chan, L., & Rodgers, M. (2012). A review of wearable sensors and systems with application in rehabilitation. *Journal of Neuroengineering and Rehabilitation, 9*(1), 1.

Perrin, A., & Duggan, M. (2015). Americans' internet access: 2000–2015. Retrieved from http://www.pewinternet.org/2015/06/26/americans-internet-access-2000-2015

Ploeg, J., Davies, B., Edwards, N., Gifford, W., & Miller, P. E. (2007). Factors influencing best-practice guideline implementation: Lessons learned from administrators, nursing staff, and project leaders. *Worldviews on Evidence-Based Nursing, 4*(4), 210–219.

Porter, D. (Ed.). (1994). *The history of public health and the modern state* (Vol. 26). Amsterdam, The Netherlands: Rodopi.

Porter, R. (1999). *The greatest benefit to mankind: A medical history of humanity (The Norton History of Science)*. New York, NY: W. W. Norton.

Reinhard, S. C., Kassner, E., Houser, A., & Mollica, R. (2011). *Raising expectations: A state scorecard on long-term services and supports for older adults, people with physical disabilities, and family caregivers*. Washington, DC: AARP. Retrieved from http://www.longtermscorecard.org

Rimsza, M. E., Hotaling, A. J., Keown, M. E., Marcin, J. P., Moskowitz, W. B., Sigrest, T. D., & Simon, H. K. (2015). The use of telemedicine to address access and physician workforce shortages. *Pediatrics, 136*(1), 202–209.

Risse, G. B. (1999). Health care in hospitals: the past 1000 years. *The Lancet, 354*, SIV25.

Salive, M. E. (2013). Multimorbidity in older adults. *Epidemiologic Reviews, 35*(1), 75–83.

Scott, I. A., Hilmer, S. N., Reeve, E., Potter, K., Le Couteur, D., Rigby, D., . . . Jansen, J. (2015). Reducing inappropriate polypharmacy: The process of deprescribing. *JAMA Internal Medicine, 175*(5), 827–834.

Silow-Carroll, S., Edwards, J. N., & Lashbrook, A. (2011). Reducing hospital readmissions: Lessons from top-performing hospitals. *The Commonwealth Fund*. Retrieved from http://www.commonwealthfund.org/publications/case-studies/2011/apr/reducing-hospital-readmissions

Singh, R., Mathiassen, L., Stachura, M. E., & Astapova, E. V. (2011). Dynamic capabilities in home health: IT-enabled transformation of post-acute care. *Journal of the Association for Information Systems, 12*, 163–188.

Takahashi, P. Y., Pecina, J. L., Upatising, B., Chaudhry, R., Shah, N. D., Van Houten, H., . . . Hanson, G. J. (2012). A randomized controlled trial of telemonitoring in older adults with multiple health issues to prevent hospitalizations and emergency department visits. *Archives of Internal Medicine, 172*(10), 773–779.

U.S. Department of Health and Human Services, Health Resources and Services Administration. (2010). *The registered nurse population: Findings from the 2008 national sample survey of registered nurses.* Chicago, IL: Author.

U.S. Department of Health and Human Services. (2003). *The future supply of long-term care workers in relation to the aging baby boom generation: Report to Congress*. Washington, DC: Author. Retrieved from https://aspe.hhs.gov/pdf-report/future-supply-long-term-care-workers-relation-aging-baby-boom-generation

U.S. Senate Commission on Long-Term Care. (2013). *Report to the Congress.* Retrieved from http://www.gpo.gov/fdsys/pkg/GPO-LTCCOMMISSION/pdf/GPO-LTCCOMMISSION.pdf

Viers, B. R., Pruthi, S., Rivera, M. E., O'Neil, D. A., Gardner, M. A., Jenkins, S. M., . . . Gettman, M. T. (2015). Are patients willing to engage in telemedicine for their care: A survey of preuse perceptions and acceptance of remote video visits in a urological patient population. *Urology, 85*(6), 1233–1240. doi:10.1016/j.urology.2014.12.064

Wade, V. A., Karnon, J., Elshaug, A. G., & Hiller, J. E. (2010). A systematic review of economic analyses of telehealth services using real time video communication. *BMC Health Services Research, 10*(1), 1.

Wheelwright, S. C., & Clark, K. B. (1992). Creating project plans to focus product development. *Harvard Business Review, 70*(2), 70–82.

White House Conference on Aging Staff. (2015). Long-term services and supports policy brief. In *2015 White House Conference on Aging*. Washington, DC: U.S. Department of Health and Human Services.

Wiener, J. M. (2013). After CLASS: The long-term care commission's search for a solution. *Health Affairs, 32*(5), 831–834.

Wilkowska, W., & Ziefle, M. (2012). Privacy and data security in E-health: Requirements from the user's perspective. *Health Informatics Journal, 18*(3), 191–201.

5

Telemedicine and Its Effects on Elder Care in Rural Areas

Roxana Aminbakhsh

The American Telemedicine Association defines telemedicine as "use of medical information exchanged from one site to another via electronic communications to improve a patient's clinical health status. Telemedicine includes a growing variety of applications and services using two-way video, email, smartphones, wireless tools, and other forms of telecommunications technology" (What is Telemedicine, American Telemedicine Association, n.d.).

BRIEF HISTORY OF TELEMEDICINE

Clinicians, health providers, and others have always tried to use the latest and most advanced telecommunication and information technologies to improve health care. Historically, concerns about distance and availability of medical expertise in remote regions was the driving force for use of telecommunication devices; technology costs were the prohibitive factor.

1959

In 1959, Cecil Whittson established the first functional telemedicine program. This program focused on psychiatric patient care and medical education. For patient care, telemedicine was used in group therapy. The system was also used to train medical students by connecting the clinics and classrooms (Kiel, 2001).

1968

In April 1968, Logan Airport Medical Station and Massachusetts General Hospital established a microwave video link between the hospital and the airport. This program intended to provide immediate access to a physician without assigning one permanently to the airport. The program proved to be useful in avoiding medical delays due to patient/physician travel (Kiel, 2001).

New telecommunication devices were, at first, expensive and out of reach for many health care providers. Telemedicine in its early days made sense only when the patients were on a remote island, in arctic regions, or other sparsely populated areas.

1970s

In the 1970s, Kaiser Foundation International and Lockheed Missiles and Space Company teamed up to create a remote monitoring system at Papago Indian Reservation in southwestern Arizona for health care delivery. This area was a rural location without many medical services. Physician assistants in this program were able to send patient information using remote monitoring tools to another hospital or medical facility many miles away. It was hoped that this program would allow remote rural areas around the world to receive better health care services. This remote monitoring project lasted until 1977 and results uncovered typical challenges such as equipment malfunction and the time needed for video consultations ("The History of Remote Monitoring, Telemedicine Technology," 2015).

2010s

Due to advances in technology, National Aeronautics and Space Administration (NASA) is looking to ensure that remote monitoring capabilities would lead to stronger medical care possibilities for long-duration space missions ("The History of Remote Monitoring, Telemedicine Technology," 2015).

Telemedicine is rapidly advancing technologically, and costs have been reduced drastically. However, telemedicine still faces numerous challenges including reimbursement, physician licensure, legal/bureaucratic barriers, and high infrastructure costs.

These challenges, however, have not stopped many hospitals and health care systems from implementing various telemedicine programs. Serving as virtual health coaches, web consults with specialists, and cloud-based physicians are becoming daily tasks for some physicians in government and the private sector.

Presently, telemedicine and its applications have two main forms: real-time direct communication (synchronous) and store-and-forward (asynchronous). Real-time communications are mainly used to consult with a distant specialist. However, they can also be used for interpretive and educational purposes such as conferences and training.

Alternatively, store-and-forward refers to transmitting digital data and images between various locations to obtain additional input for a diagnosis. Data can be used instantaneously or be stored for future use by specialists. Currently, this is commonly done in the fields of radiology and dermatology. Home health care and monitoring can also be considered in this category.

More advanced remote control and surgical robotics are being performed at an experimental level, which require advanced devices and great teamwork among many experts working together at various sites. These applications are new and were not possible even a few years ago.

TECHNOLOGICAL ADVANCES

Telemedicine started with limited use of basic telephone, faxing echocardiograms and other investigation results, mailing digital images on a CD, and videoconferencing technology to connect local providers with distant specialists for consultation. This type of real-time communication is still used today. However, advances in communication technology such as more affordable wireless broadband and advanced communication devices make it more efficient and less expensive. Videoconferencing can create a closer relationship between the consulting doctor and a patient in another location. These systems can be utilized to provide patients with better counseling or other mental health care that may be unavailable if they live in a remote location, or simply are not able to go to the specialists.

In addition to improved videoconferencing technology, the ability to measure and transfer diagnostic information almost instantaneously is advancing synchronous telemedicine. Devices that can measure, track, and report a patient's vital signs and condition are being used to provide vital information to remote specialists by facilitating an almost interactive physical examination. Bluetooth-enabled devices can monitor patients' conditions and generate alerts based on threshold breaches in vital sign readings. These innovations are allowing doctors to monitor patients with chronic medical conditions, improve safety, and decrease medical costs by reducing unnecessary doctor visits or hospital admissions.

Physicians have started using cloud technology to share high-quality medical photographs, x-rays, CT scans, MRI scans, PET scans, and other images among specialists in various locations who can provide assistance with a patient's diagnosis. Services such as teleradiology and telestroke have also become standards of care.

Home health monitoring and care is another area that has tremendously benefited from improved technology. The desire to reduce length of hospital stay and lower costs by patients and providers has increased utilization of telemedicine. Data exchange between hospital and home by Internet is now simple and inexpensive. Automated monitoring and measurement devices for blood pressure, blood glucose, peak respiratory flow rate data collection, and transfer of data between home and hospital are less expensive with new technology. Cardiac arrhythmia monitoring with Cardio Memo, diabetic patients' data collection and exchange on glucose control, asthmatic controls with peak flow meter connected to miniaturized computers and palm devices, and control of fluid balance with data from patients with heart failure are just few examples of home monitoring and care applications. Some telemedicine practitioners believe that virtualization of health care is the future of medicine. Many hospital and private practice services may be outsourced by telemedicine.

FACTORS ADVANCING TELEMEDICINE

Technological advances are transforming health care. Patients and providers are forcing politicians and other decision makers to implement new health care policies to take advantage of advanced technology to reduce costs and provide a more efficient health care system.

Other forces are at work as well. According to an article by Nathaniel M. Lacktman, five trends will drive telemedicine's continued growth and transformation of health care delivery (Five Telemedicine Trends Transforming Health Care in 2016, 2015):

Expanding Reimbursement and Payment Opportunities

Reimbursement has been the primary obstacle to telemedicine implementation. However, new laws requiring coverage of telemedicine-based services have been implemented at the state level. Providers are also becoming increasingly receptive to exploring payment models beyond fee-for-service reimbursement. Examples include institution-to-institution contracts and greater willingness by patients to pay out of pocket for telemedicine services.

Uptick in International Arrangements

Increasingly, U.S. hospitals and health care providers will work with overseas medical institutions. These international partnerships will provide access to more patients and create additional revenues. According to the American Telemedicine Association, more than 200 academic medical centers in the United States already offer video-based consulting in other parts of the world (Five Telemedicine Trends Transforming Health Care in 2016, 2015).

Continued Momentum at the State Level

In the United States, state governments are leading the way in telemedicine expansion. While state law makers are trying to incorporate telemedicine into the health care system, two recent developments point to attempts at the federal level to expand telemedicine. The Centers for Medicare & Medicaid Services (CMS) is considering expansion of Medicare coverage for telemedicine, and a bill working its way through the U.S. House of Representatives would pay physicians for delivering telemedicine services to Medicare beneficiaries in any location.

Retail Clinics and Employer Onsite Health Centers Are on the Rise

Some studies suggest that nearly 70% of employers will offer telemedicine services as an employee benefit by 2017. Additionally, consumers have shown willingness to visit retail medical clinics and pay out of pocket even when telemedicine is not covered by their insurance plans.

More Accountable Care Organizations Are Using Technology to Improve Care and Cut Costs

Since the introduction of Medicare Accountable Care Organizations (ACOs), the number of Medicare beneficiaries served has grown consistently. These organizations can qualify for CMS cost-reduction incentives if they can reduce costs. However, only 27% of ACOs achieved enough savings to qualify for those incentives in 2015. Only 20% of ACOs use telemedicine services, according to a recent study. Telemedicine can provide the savings that these organizations need (Five Telemedicine Trends Transforming Health Care in 2016, 2015).

TELEMEDICINE AT THE STATE AND FEDERAL LEVELS

Lack of coverage and reimbursement has also been another important barrier to telemedicine access. Therefore, improving coverage and reimbursement are considered among the most important factors for expanding telemedicine.

Medicare reimburses for telemedicine services when the originating site (patient location) is a health professional shortage area (HPSA) or in a county that is outside of any metropolitan statistical area (MSA). Telemedicine services provided at the patient's home cannot qualify for reimbursement. There is no restriction on the distant site (i.e., the location of eligible health care provider). However, the originating site (location of the Medicare patient) has to meet the following conditions (Your Medicare Coverage—Telehealth, n.d.):

- A doctor's office
- A hospital
- A critical access hospital (CAH)
- A rural health clinic
- A federally qualified health center
- A hospital-based or critical access hospital-based dialysis facility
- A skilled nursing facility (SNF)
- A community mental health center (CMHC)

A study by Harvard Medical School researchers, published in *JAMA*, describes trends in telemedicine utilization in Medicare from 2003 to 2013. According to this study, examination of Medicare claims data revealed that the number of telemedicine visits provided to Medicare beneficiaries has increased by 28% per year from 2004 to 2013 with 107,000 visits provided in 2013 (Mehrotra et al., 2016).

On July 7, 2015, the Medicare Telehealth Parity Act of 2015 (House—Energy and Commerce; Ways and Means, 2015) was introduced to modernize the way Medicare pays for telehealth services. Amendments to title XVIII (Medicare) of the Social Security Act will expand telemedicine coverage in three implementation phases over a 4-year period. The Act will change the Medicare telemedicine payment methodologies and expand coverage to residents of both rural and urban areas. The three implementation phases are listed in an article by Nathaniel M. Lacktman (2015).

In April 2016, the state of Indiana passed legislation regarding the expanded use of telemedicine ("New Indiana Law Expands Use of Telemedicine," 2016). The new law, which became effective on July 1, 2016, defines telemedicine as either the use of secure videoconferencing or the monitoring of a patient by a physician, via technology, who is located elsewhere geographically.

This Indiana law is designed to streamline the telemedicine process by expanding a physician's ability to treat a patient using the technology from any location. The most significant feature of the law is that physicians, physician assistants, optometrists, and nurse practitioners will now be able to prescribe certain kinds of medication after a video-call consultation. Previously, a patient had to be introduced to the care provider at least once in person before medication could be prescribed. The revised law requires that an initial authentic physician–patient relationship be established before medication can be prescribed via videoconferencing. At a minimum, physician–patient relationship includes the following ("New Indiana Law Expands Use of Telemedicine," 2016):

- Obtaining the patient's name and contact information and (a) a verbal statement or other data from the patient identifying the patient's location, and (b) to the extent reasonably possible, the identity of the requesting patient;
- Disclosing the provider's name and whether the provider is a physician, physician assistant, advanced practice nurse, or optometrist;
- Obtaining informed consent from the patient;
- Obtaining the patient's medical history and other information necessary to establish a diagnosis;
- Discussing with the patient the (a) diagnosis, (b) evidence for the diagnosis, and (c) risks and benefits of various treatment options, including when it is advisable to seek in-person care;
- Creating and maintaining a medical record for the patient and, subject to the consent of the patient, notifying the patient's primary care provider of any prescriptions the provider has written for the patient, if the primary care provider's contact information is provided by the patient. This requirement is not applicable when the provider is using an electronic health record system that the patient's primary care provider is authorized to access;
- Issuing proper instructions for appropriate follow-up care;
- Providing a telemedicine visit summary to the patient, including information that indicates any prescription that is being prescribed.

If these procedures are not performed, the relationship is deemed unauthentic and telemedicine prescriptions are considered illegal.

The new law also contains a provision regarding the kinds of medication that cannot be prescribed. For example, it is illegal to give patients abortion-inducing drugs, controlled substances, and vision enhancing aids, such as glasses, via telemedicine ("New Indiana Law Expands Use of Telemedicine," 2016).

Congress has also been introducing a number of telemedicine-related bills such as Tele-Med Act of 2015, which allows some Medicare providers licensed in a state to provide telemedicine services to Medicare beneficiaries in other states without having to be licensed in the other states.

Nurses (registered nurses and licensed practical nurse/vocational nurses) have long had a Licensure Compact. Nurses who declare a "compact state" as their primary state of residence can practice physically and remotely in other compact states without having to obtain another license. There are 25 states that are members of the nurse compact (National Council of State Boards of Nursing, n.d.).

Licensure Compact for physicians is also being developed. The Interstate Medical Licensure Compact for physicians offers a new, voluntary expedited pathway to licensure for qualified physicians who wish to practice in multiple states. Telemedicine supporters believe physician licensure compacts will increase access to health care for patients in underserved or rural areas, and allow them to more easily connect with medical experts through the use of new technologies. Presently, the compact is being implemented in 17 states (Interstate Medical Licensure Compact, n.d.).

On June 17, 2016, the U.S. Health Resources and Services Administration (HRSA), an agency of the U.S. Department of Health and Human Services, announced that it will provide funding to support state medical and osteopathic boards as they implement the administrative and technical infrastructure of the new Interstate Medical Licensure Compact. The grant from HRSA of $250,000 annually for 3 years is intended to help the compact become operational and provide support for educational outreach to help expand participation in the compact by other states. Grant funding began on July 1, 2016:

> The Compact is expected to expand access to health care, especially to those in rural and underserved areas of the country, and facilitate the use of telemedicine technologies in the delivery of health care. (Federation of State Medical Boards, n.d.)

OPPOSITION TO TELEMEDICINE

Telemedicine has the potential to drastically reshape health care and fundamentally change medical care. Proponents of telemedicine claim that with advance in technology, telemedicine will continue to produce the following benefits:

- Increase access to health care to those who may, for whatever reason, be unable to visit with a physician;
- Cut health care costs;
- Generate revenue.

On the other hand, critics worry that such services will sacrifice quality care for convenience and cost reductions. Opponents believe that unchecked growth of telemedicine can break down and damage the relationship between health care providers and patients, and also may cause a breakdown in relationships among health professionals themselves, which will lower the quality of care.

Consulting a random doctor who patients will never meet may create more problems. Opponents point out that even minor issues such as upper respiratory infections cannot be carefully evaluated by a doctor who cannot listen to a patient's heart, culture a patient's throat, or feel the patient's swollen glands.

In a dermatology study in *JAMA*, researchers posing as patients with skin problems submitted a series of dermatological cases with photographs, including neoplastic, inflammatory, and infectious conditions, using regional and national telemedicine websites and smartphone applications offering services to California residents. In 62 cases from 16 websites, none asked for identification or raised concerns about pseudonym use or false photographs. Less than one third disclosed clinicians' credentials or let patients choose; only 32% discussed potential side effects of prescribed medications. According to this research, several sites misdiagnosed serious conditions and failed to ask basic follow-up questions (Resneck et al., 2016).

In February 2016, "the Mississippi State Medical Association and more than 60 state physicians and medical students opposed a bill in the state House that would allow out-of-state physicians to treat patients by telephone" (Hall, 2016b). These doctors and medical students believed that high-quality care is impossible without a physician visit.

There are many skeptical health care providers, doctors, and nurses who are not eager to use telemedicine. The resistance is not usually because of the new technology; the issue is maintaining and complying with the existing standards of care. Traditional health care providers must comply with care standards that telemedicine physicians want to modify to perform their job efficiently across regional, national, and international boundaries.

Credentialing and licensing issues add another layer of difficulty when implementing a telemedicine program. Opponents of telemedicine do not want a physician licensed in other states to be permitted to diagnose a patient in their state without ever visiting the patient.

Telemedicine providers must be able to ensure high-quality service remotely, and comply with the Health Insurance Portability and Accountability Act's (HIPAA) privacy and security requirements; these requirements are the same for telemedicine practitioners and traditional hospitals and providers.

Telemedicine providers want to make deployment of telemedicine less challenging and decrease costs by modifying security and HIPAA requirements. Opponents of telemedicine view these efforts by telemedicine providers as an attack on patient security and privacy.

Opponents believe that telemedicine encounters are still susceptible to third-party interferences, hacker attacks, signal errors, or transmission outages. These cases can result in loss of data, interrupted communications, identity theft, or the alteration of important clinical information. These and other liability risks could lead to HIPAA privacy and security violations. For example, third-party interference with transmission may be considered a security breach under the HIPAA security regulations; transmission outages or hacker attacks may result in loss of important clinical data during transmission. These issues could be viewed as a failure to adequately maintain the integrity of protected information, as required under the HIPAA security and privacy regulations.

Professional organizations are concerned that unchecked and rapid growth of telemedicine will adversely impact patient care and may also have adverse effects on their members, including employment of physicians and their income. National politics and legislative processes affect how medical licensing and credentialing vary from state to state and country to country. In the United States, each of the 50 states and the District of Columbia administer their own regional medical licensure with their own state medical boards. Each board has separate fees and requirements. Multistate licensure can become very expensive. The paperwork involved and the cost of maintaining multistate licensure have been some of the biggest impediments to telemedicine.

Many state medical boards are cautious about telemedicine applications in their state. For example, the State Medical Board of Ohio is changing its administrative code to define an "active patient" as one who a provider has visited in person during the past 24 months, or performed an evaluation via an approved video platform. The rule also clarifies the standards for establishing a physician–patient relationship for prescription of drugs when the physician is not at the same location as a patient (Wicklund, 2016a).

In April 2016, the Texas Medical Board also required face-to-face patient visits before doctors could issue a prescription. According to the board, the care must be provided at an appropriate location and also requires the presence of qualified staff to assist in the evaluation of the patient. Thus, treatment and consultation recommendations made via telemedicine are held to the same standards of acceptable medical practices as those made in the traditional in-person clinical settings (Texas Medical Board, n.d.).

FUTURE OF TELEMEDICINE

Opponents and proponents of telemedicine will continue their efforts to ensure that the best technology and procedures are used for safer and better patient care. Marketplace, law makers, and other stakeholders will also increasingly integrate telemedicine into health care.

New technologies, if they are efficient, convenient, and cost-effective, have always forced social and legal changes to satisfy consumer demand and social needs. Increasing acceptance of telemedicine as a standard of care is quickly being established.

Progress in international data transmission networks will make it possible to provide medical care and education internationally. There are still many issues to overcome, such as licensure, certifications, and regulations.

As radiology, stroke care, mental health, and dermatology have proven to be very effective fields for outsourcing via telemedicine, some hospitals and care providers like Spectrum Health will start offering their own telemedicine services and building their own platforms.

In November 2015, Spectrum Health, with a 12-hospital and 184-site network, based in western Michigan, launched its own platform, bringing a three-pronged virtual care program in-house and under its own control. The service offers on-demand and specialty care, as well as home-monitoring tools (Wicklund, 2016b).

Spectrum Health is part of a large number of providers who are progressively moving into telemedicine. These providers had started working with a vendor to establish a virtual platform and then, after gaining experience, gradually moved to their own platform and internal system.

Experts estimate that 40% of health providers who have virtual care networks have followed this direction before starting their own in-house telemedicine platform, and they expect the number of providers following this route to grow as the technology becomes more universal (Wicklund, 2016b).

GROWING ELDERLY POPULATION IN RURAL AREAS

The population of persons 65 years and older is projected to double over the next 25 years across the country (Rural Health Information Hub, 2016). This population of elderly in each county is directly related to the level of rurality of that county. Nearly one fourth of the population of the United States lives in rural areas. The more rural and less populated areas have a larger percentage of older populations. Figure 5.1 is a map, based on 2010 census data, that illustrates the percentage of the population over 65 years by each county (Rural Health Foundation Hub, n.d.). Two thirds of the 3,142 counties in the United States are considered rural (Freeman, Thompson, Howard, Randolph, & Holmes, 2015).

DISPARITIES BETWEEN RURAL AND URBAN AREAS

In general, population in the rural areas of the United States has lower income, fewer employment opportunities, and lesser services than the urban

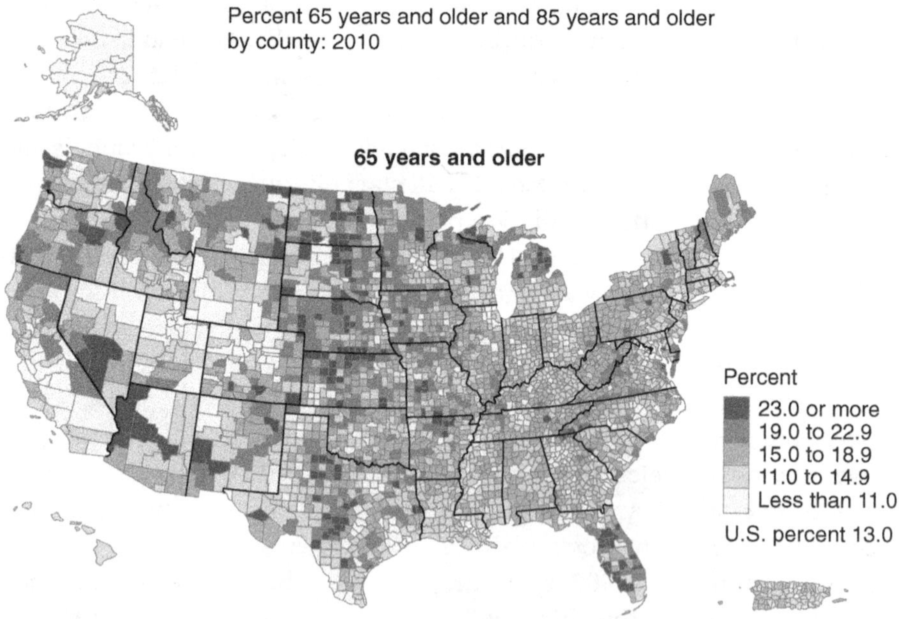

FIGURE 5.1 Percentage of population 65 years and older by county.

Source: Werner (2011).

areas. Rural areas also have lower numbers of health care professionals, hospitals, and clinics than the urban areas. According to the National Rural Health Association, only 10% of physicians practice in rural areas (Rural Health Foundation Hub, n.d.).

The health care infrastructure in much of rural areas consists of small hospitals, clinics, and nursing homes. These facilities generally do not have large patient populations and sufficient capital to invest in most advanced technologies. Therefore, it is increasingly difficult for rural residents to gain access to top medical care, and for health care providers to provide highest quality services in many rural areas. According to the North Carolina Rural Health Research Program, the typical rural hospitals are critical access hospitals (53.5% of all rural hospitals; Freeman et al., 2015). These hospitals have less than 25 inpatient beds, and maintain an annual average length of stay of less than 96 hours for acute inpatient care.

Many rural hospitals are struggling to survive. The National Health Association has identified that more than 10% of all rural hospitals across the country are in danger of closing (Demko, 2015). Therefore, rural hospitals are being forced to shift from inpatient to outpatient care, as prevalent technology and practice patterns have concentrated specialized inpatient care services in urban areas (American Hospital Association, 2011).

When a rural hospital shuts down, the community is not losing only a hospital, but also additional services such as hospice, home health services, skilled nursing, adult day care, and assisted living, as rural hospitals are usually the only facilities in rural areas that provide these services. Therefore, it is vital for the elderly population to have access to good rural hospitals that are financially sustainable.

TRANSFORMING RURAL SPECIALTY CARE WITH NEW TECHNOLOGIES

While the nation struggles with health care reform and government programs that intend to increase access for rural populations to good medical care, many rural health providers are investing in innovative communication and telemedicine technologies to provide viable services and remain financially sustainable.

New technologies that can enhance communication between the patients and providers in a rural community with specialists in other regions of the country can overcome many of the traditional problems of rural health care providers. Rural primary care providers often do not have close connection to specialists who are usually based in larger academic medical centers (AMCs). Virtual learning, electronic consultation, and telemedicine are three approaches that have shown promising results for delivering quality care to areas that have limited availability of specialist physicians.

Virtual Learning

A good example of virtual learning and consultation technology is Project ECHO in New Mexico (University of New Mexico School of Medicine, n.d.). ECHO is the abbreviation for Extension for Community Healthcare Outcomes. Since 2003, this project, which is funded by the Agency for Healthcare Research and Quality (AHRQ), has been delivering care via the Internet to rural, low-income, and often uninsured patients (Arora, n.d.). This program is designed to address the access needs of rural communities to specialty care. Project ECHO trains rural primary care clinicians to provide specialty care services in their own community, which usually improves patient outcome and reduces costs. It acts as a "performance optimizer." It also provides professional growth and job satisfaction for health care professionals who might feel isolated in remote rural areas, and provides a forum in which primary care providers and specialists can learn from each other.

The expert specialists are located in an AMC or other specialty care site that are called "hubs." Primary care clinicians located in rural communities are the "spokes." These clinicians become a learning community where they receive training and provide feedback to each other and to the hub specialists. Under ECHO, primary care providers use communication technologies to participate in "guided practice" with specialists who are mentors and trainers. This will assist primary care clinicians to learn new skills that would allow them to treat rural patients in their own community, rather than refer them to urban areas. ECHO increases access to specialty care by sharing knowledge.

When a rural care provider or clinic joins ECHO, its staff would receive initial training from University of New Mexico in Albuquerque (UNM). UNM's information technology (IT) experts help the care providers install and use site-appropriate software that would help them with care management and data reporting. In this way, the clinic or rural provider joins a disease-specific "knowledge network" that meets online each week for case presentations and discussions (Arora, n.d.).

Because of its success, Project ECHO has become the model for the Department of Veteran Affairs Specialty Care Access Network–Extension for Community Healthcare Outcomes (SCAN-ECHO) program (Hall, 2016a). Also, in April 28, 2016, a bill was introduced in the senate by Senators Hatch and Schatz (S.2873-ECHO Act) "to require studies and reports examining the use of, and opportunities to use, technology-enabled collaborative learning and capacity building models to improve programs of the Department of Health and Human Services, and for other purposes" (S.2873-ECHO Act, 114th Congress, 2015–2016). In an announcement related to the introduction of this bill, Ms. Barbara McAneny, past chair of the American Medical Association, said that ECHO is "an exemplary model for using new technologies to improve patient care, Project ECHO has potential to bolster access to specialists, reduce incidences of chronic disease, and rein in costs through reduced travel and fewer ER visits" (Hall, 2016a).

Online Medical Consultation

Presently, many online medical services and websites offer a virtual doctor visit 24 hours a day, 365 days a year, by phone, by web, or by smartphone. These websites offer to match a patient with a board-certified physician, counselor, therapist, or psychologist who is licensed in the patient's state. These experts can review medical records, diagnose, and prescribe medication to treat patients.

The advantages of online medical consultations (OMCs) are apparent for elderly populations who are restricted to home or are at remote rural locations with limited health care provider access. Some patients would like to have a second opinion from another doctor.

A study called ECHO-Age was conducted to assess the effects of remote video consultation program that connected specialists in management of behavioral disorders to patients with dementia in nursing homes in 11 sites in Massachusetts and Maine. The results indicated that a case-based videoconferencing program (telepsychiatry) can improve the care of geriatric patients with dementia and/or delirium in nursing homes (Catic et al., 2014).

On the individual and personal level, many older people in rural areas suffer from higher levels of social isolation and loneliness due to distance and insufficient affordable transportation. Isolation, loneliness, and anxiety can have mental and physical impacts on the elderly population.

The OMC services are best suited to alleviate the feelings of isolation, loneliness, and anxiety by connecting the counselors or specialists with patients. Also, if the problems do not require a physical examination, virtual or phone visits are convenient and effective.

These services must comply with privacy requirements and cyber security standards such as HIPAA requirements in the United States and cyber security standards of ISO 27002 internationally (International Organization for Standards; ISO 27002, n.d.; Who is required to Comply with HIPAA Requirements, HRSA Health Information Technology, n.d.).

Telemedicine for Rural Health

In this section, we review the services that telemedicine can provide to rural communities, such as

- Teleradiology
- Telepsychiatry
- Teleophthalmology
- Teledermatology
- Teledentistry
- Telepharmacy

Telemedicine's functions and capabilities are expanding exponentially with advances in communication technology and innovation in medical devices. Videoconferencing, consultation and interviews, assessment and monitoring of patients, access and review of patient data and records, and education for patients and physicians are becoming routine tasks in telemedicine.

Telemedicine inventions are continuously introducing monitoring devices that allow a physician to monitor and analyze the patient from a remote location. The patient wears a device at one location to transfer temperature readings, heart rate and respiration rate or pulse oximetry to the physician in another location. Special cameras can be used to examine the eyes or a special stethoscope can be used to allow the remote physician to auscultate. Touchless temporal smartphone-connected thermometers, smartphone glucometer devices, telestroke robots, and a whole array of new devices are being continuously introduced to allow delivery of medical information from a distance.

In an experiment cofunded by the Korean and New Zealand governments, and conducted by University of Auckland researchers, a robot was used to measure blood pressure, heart rate, and temperature of four elderly patients. These touchscreen robots also had videoconferencing and gaming capabilities. The researchers found that basic companionship from the robots was important for the elderly subjects. The robots reminded the patients when to take their medications and helped the patients connect to the Internet (Plumb, 2015).

Telemedicine services have improved geriatrics care in rural health. In rural areas, more hospitals and clinics are using telemedicine to improve access and increase their connections with other health care providers. In Arkansas, for example, all of the centers on aging are presently receiving monetary, connectivity, and equipment support to start their own clinics and geriatrics educational programs across the state. The Center for Distance Health (CDH) within the College of Medicine at University of Arkansas is also working on connecting nursing homes with physicians and emergency departments to reduce the need to transport their patients from the rural areas (UAMS Centre for Distance Health, n.d.).

In North Carolina, in-home monitoring using telemedicine has decreased hospitalization rates for elderly patients enrolled in the First Health Home Care Chronic Disease model. Patients previously diagnosed with heart failure, diabetes, or chronic obstructive pulmonary disease (COPD), and who experience frequent hospitalizations are monitored by telemedicine devices at home between periodic visits from nursing staff. Response and intervention times have improved considerably, according to the program (Ripton & Winkler, 2016).

A study by The Commonwealth Fund concluded that nursing homes that use telemedicine to provide after-hour care can reduce hospitalization rates for their residents. This study showed that enabling patients to simply visit with physicians by video or other telecommunications devices can lower the hospitalization rates and save money for Medicare (The Commonwealth Fund, n.d.).

Telegeriatrics for Rural Areas

Using telemedicine in geriatrics care is expanding in rural areas. Most of the current uses are for monitoring, virtual consultation, and providing support and companionship.

Increasingly, providers are trying to develop telemedicine approaches that can perform traditional geriatric diagnoses and treat illnesses from distant locations. In general, and more so for rural areas, barriers to early diagnosis of geriatric problems include lack of routine screening and access to specialty consultative services. Therefore, if telegeriatrics can be proven to be safe and reliable, it can contribute greatly to geriatrics care in rural areas.

Extensive studies are still needed to demonstrate that geriatrics diagnoses and treatment can be effective. These efforts are underway and will continue. Daily advances in technology and new approaches to diagnosing and treating illness are replacing the traditional face-to-face specialist visits. For many rural patients, this is a necessity, not a preferred choice. According to AARP, "a shortage of geriatricians is leading to a major public health concern" (Peterson, 2016).The shortage of geriatricians in rural areas will be even more significant. Therefore, more research and funding could be channeled toward new development in telegeriatrics to provide viable approaches to elderly care.

A study to determine the diagnostic accuracy of telegeriatrics for the diagnosis of dementia by videoconferencing indicated that videoconferencing was not inferior to face-to-face assessment (Martin-Khan et al., 2012). In a subsequent study (Martin-Khan, Salih, Rowland, Wootton, & Gray, 2015), it was shown that general practitioners, patients, and caregivers support using telegeriatric memory disorder consultation for elderly diagnosis. This study claims that diagnosis of dementia is reliable when videoconferencing is used. Research also showed that a telegeriatric memory disorder consultation is only feasible when the general practitioners in the remote area have confidence in the assessment process (Martin-Khan et al., 2015).

Telehomecare in Rural Areas

Telehomecare refers to telemedicine and communication approaches that are used to connect the patient at home and the formal caregiver such as a nurse or physician at a distant location (Day, n.d.). These electronic virtual visits may also require some means for the distance care provider to access patient vital signs and receive patient-initiated medical tests. The patient or, if applicable, the in-home informal caregiver must be trained to use appropriate telemedical monitoring or test equipment that sends the relevant video images or data using various communication devices to the distant health provider.

For many elderly patients in rural areas who prefer to stay in their homes rather than going to a distant nursing home away from their families and community, telehomecare is a great choice. They can get some of the required assistance at home. Therefore, insurances and Medicare need to investigate how to make telehomecare more available and affordable for the elderly rural population to ensure delivery of better home care.

Medicare reimburses for limited telehomecare services. The following paragraph presents how Medicare considers the payment for telehomecare services (Day, n.d.).

> 201.13 Telehealth—An HHA [home health agency] may adopt telehealth technologies that it believes promote efficiencies or improve quality of care. Telehomecare encounters do not meet the definition of a visit set forth in regulations at 42 CFR 409.48(c) and the telehealth services may not be counted as Medicare covered home health visits or used as qualifying services for home health eligibility. An HHA may not substitute telehealth services for Medicare-covered services ordered by a physician. However, if an HHA has telehealth services available to its clients, a doctor may take their availability into account when he or she prepares a plan of treatment (i.e., may write requirements for telehealth services into the POT). Medicare eligibility and payment would be determined based on the patient's characteristics and the need for and receipt of the Medicare-covered

services ordered by the physician. If a physician intends that telehealth services be furnished while a patient is under a home health plan of care, the services should be recorded in the plan of care along with the Medicare covered home health services to be furnished.

Geriatricians and other providers must consider appropriate telehomecare while preparing the patient's home health plan.

DIFFICULTIES OF USING NEW TECHNOLOGIES FOR RURAL HEALTH CARE

As technologies develop to improve delivery of health care to elderly patients in remote rural locations, many complex legal, ethical, and sociopolitical issues must be carefully debated and resolved to ensure safe and reliable implementation of procedures designed to deliver remote services to all patients.

Major legal concerns surrounding telemedicine include cross-state licensure of health providers, compliance with fraud and abuse laws, informed consent issues, and internal/external review policies and procedures such as adverse situations that may arise from administrating telemedicine services.

State laws for telemedicine vary significantly from state to state. Some insurance companies exclude telemedicine as a part of the professional liability policy. Companies must add malpractice insurance as a rider.

Privacy and security considerations are always cited as other major issues. While patients and their physicians may be eager to use the innovative technologies such as smartphones, these devices are not always secure. While new self-monitoring devices and applications are becoming easier to use, it is critical that medical consults be delivered by a secure HIPAA-compliant system.

Also, it is important to understand and consider the social barriers to telemedicine. Some vulnerable patients are from communities that are economically disadvantaged or are homeless and lack access to an Internet connection and videoconferencing equipment. According to National Alliance to End Homelessness, about 7% of the homeless population lives in rural areas (National Alliance to End Homelessness, n.d.).

Rural health care providers, caregivers to the homeless population, and those who provide care in underserved areas cannot provide the best telemedicine technologies without government policies and health care providers who would fund and support these innovative technologies.

On April 18, 2016, the U.S. Department of Agriculture (USDA) announced its plans to award $11.7 million in grants through the Community Connect grant program. The grant funds development of broadband infrastructures for underserved areas. Since 2002, USDA has invested $160 million to bring broadband to underserved rural communities (USDA, 2016). Telemedicine companies and private health care providers should contribute and fund such projects to assist the rural communities.

CONCLUSION

Historically, concerns about distance and availability of medical expertise in remote regions were the driving force for the use of new and innovative telecommunication devices. Health care providers and health care systems always try to use the latest and the most advanced telecommunication and information technologies to improve health care delivered to patients.

Telemedicine has the potential to significantly reshape health care, and fundamentally change medical care. Proponents of telemedicine claim that with advances in technology, telemedicine will continue to increase access to physicians, decrease health care costs, and generate revenue. On the other hand, critics are concerned that such services might sacrifice quality of care. Opponents believe that uncontrolled growth of telemedicine has a potential to break down the relationship between health care providers and patients, and the relationship among health professional themselves, which will result in lowering the quality of care. Opponents also believe that telemedicine encounters are still susceptible to third-party interferences, hacker attacks, and technical problems such as signal errors or transmission outages. However, it is important to realize and consider that barriers to telemedicine, in general, can also be applied to rural health care systems.

Licensing and regulations are part of the challenges that telemedicine is facing. National politics and legislative processes affect how medical licensing and credentialing vary from state to state and country to country. In the United States, each of the 50 states and the District of Columbia administer their own regional medical licensure with their own state medical boards. State governments are leading the way in telemedicine expansion. Law makers are trying to incorporate telemedicine into the health care system, and the CMS is considering expansion of Medicare coverage for telemedicine.

Looking at rural health care infrastructure and telemedicine's ability to improve care in remote areas makes telemedicine a favorable modality to overcome some of the challenges that health care systems are facing in rural areas. Populations in the rural areas of the United States has lower income and fewer services than the urban areas. There are also fewer health care professionals, hospitals, and clinics in rural areas compared with urban regions. Only 10% of physicians practice in rural areas. Small hospitals, clinics, and nursing homes in rural areas with small patient populations do not have sufficient funds to invest in the most advanced technologies. As a result, rural residents have difficulty gaining access to top medical care, and it is challenging for health care providers to provide highest quality of services to rural residents. Many rural hospitals are struggling to survive and are forced to shift from inpatient to outpatient services. Therefore, new technologies that can enhance communication between the patients and providers in rural communities with specialists in other regions can overcome many of these struggles.

Virtual learning, electronic consultations, and telemedicine are three modalities that have shown promising results in improving quality of care provided to rural residents. Telemedicine can provide teleradiology, telepsychiatry, teleophthalmology, teledermatology, teledentistry, and telepharmacy services at remote areas and improve health care for millions.

REFERENCES

American Hospital Association. (2011). The opportunities and challenges for rural hospitals in an era of health reform. Retrieved from http://www.aha.org/research/reports/tw/11apr-tw-rural.pdf

Arora, S. (n.d.). Project ECHO: Bringing specialty care to rural New Mexico. Retrieved from https://healthit.ahrq.gov/ahrq-funded-projects/transforming-healthcare-quality-through-health-it/project-echo-bringing

Catic, A. G., Mattison, M. L. P., Bakaev, I., Morgan, M., Monti, S. M., & Lipsitz, L. (2014). ECHO-AGE: An innovative model of geriatric care for long-term care residents with dementia and behavioral issues. *Journal of the American Medical Directors Association, 15*(12), 938–942. doi:10.1016/j.jamda.2014.08.014

Day, T. (n.d.). Guide to long term care planning—About medical care for elderly. Retrieved from https://www.longtermcarelink.net/eldercare/medical_care_issues.htm

Demko, P. (2015). Modern health care, as rural hospitals struggle, solution sought to preserve healthcare access. Retrieved from http://www.modernhealthcare.com/article/20150516/MAGAZINE/305169959

Federation of State Medical Boards. (n.d.). Federal grant awarded to support state medical boards in implementing Interstate Medical Licensure Compact. Retrieved from http://licenseportability.org/wp-content/uploads/2016/06/Compact-HRSA-Grant_June-2016_FINAL.pdf

Five telemedicine trends transforming health care in 2016. (2015). *National Law Review*. Retrieved from http://www.natlawreview.com/article/five-telemedicine-trends-transforming-health-care-2016

Freeman, V. A., Thompson, K., Howard, H. A., Randolph, R., & Holmes, G. (2015). *The 21st century rural hospital—A chart book* (p. 5). Retrieved from http://www.shepscenter.unc.edu/wp-content/uploads/2015/02/21stCenturyRuralHospitalsChartBook.pdf

Grabowski, D. C., & O'Malley, A. J. (2014). Use of telemedicine can reduce hospitalization of nursing home residents and generate savings for Medicare. *Health Affairs, 33*(2), 244–250.

Hall, S. D. (2016a). Bill recommends project ECHO as national model. Retrieved from http://www.fiercehealthcare.com/it/bill-recommends-project-echo-as-national-model

Hall, S. D. (2016b). Mississippi docs oppose telephone-based telemedicine bill, cite need for visual component. *Fierce Healthcare*. Retrieved from http://www.fiercehealthcare.com/it/mississippi-docs-oppose-telephone-based-telemedicine-bill-cite-need-for-visual-component

House-Energy and Commerce; Ways and Means. (2015). Summary: H.R.2948—114th Congress (2015-2016) Medicare Telehealth Parity Act of 2015. Retrieved from https://www.congress.gov/bill/114th-congress/house-bill/2948

Interstate Medical Licensure Compact. (n.d.). The IMLC. Retrieved from http://www.licenseportability.org

ISO 27002. (n.d.). ISO 27002 (International Organization for Standardization 27002). Retrieved from http://searchcompliance.techtarget.com/definition/ISO-27002-International-Organization-for-Standardization-27002

Kiel, J. M. (2001). *Information technology for the practicing physician* (p. 228). New York, NY: Springer-Verlag.

Lacktman, N. M. (2015). Congress wows with Medicare Telehealth Parity Act of 2015, but will it succeed? *Health Care Law Today*. Retrieved from https://www.healthcarelawtoday.com/2015/07/15/congress-wows-with-medicare-telehealth-parity-act-of-2015-but-will-it-succeed

Martin-Khan, M., Flicker, L., Wootton, R., Loh, P.-K., Edwards, H., Varghese, P., . . . Gray, L. C. (2012). The diagnostic accuracy of telegeriatrics for the diagnosis of dementia via video conferencing. *Journal of the American Medical Directors Association, 13*(5), 487. doi:10.1016/j.jamda.2012.03.004

Martin-Khan, M., Salih, S. A., Rowland, J., Wootton, R., & Gray, L. C. (2015). General practitioners, patients, and care givers support the use of a telegeriatric memory disorder consultation for older adults. *Advances in Alzheimer's Disease, 4*(01), 1–9. doi:10.4236/aad.2015.41001

Mehrotra, A., Jena, A. B., Busch, A. B., Souza, J., Uscher-Pines, L., & Landon, B. E. (2016). Utilization of telemedicine among rural Medicare beneficiaries. *Journal of the American Medical Association, 315*(18), 2015–2016. doi:10.1001/jama.2016.2186

National Alliance to End Homelessness. (n.d.). Rural homelessness. Retrieved from http://www.endhomelessness.org/pages/rural

National Council of State Boards of Nursing. (n.d.). Nurse licensure compact. Retrieved from https://www.ncsbn.org/nurse-licensure-compact.htm

New Indiana law expands use of telemedicine. (2016). *The National Law Review*. Retrieved from http://www.natlawreview.com/article/new-indiana-law-expands-use-telemedicine

Peterson, J. (2016). Where are the doctors you'll need? Retrieved from http://www.aarp.org/health/conditions-treatments/info-2016/geriatrician-geriatric-doctor-physician.html

Plumb, S. (2015, November 1). Who needs docs? Meet iRobot. *New Zealand Herald*. Retrieved from http://www.nzherald.co.nz/technology/news/article.cfm?c_id=5&objectid=11538191

Resneck, J. S., Abrouk, M., Steuer, M., Tam, A., Yen, A., Lee, I., . . . Edison, K. E. (2016). Choice, transparency, coordination, and quality among direct-to-consumer telemedicine websites and apps treating skin disease. *JAMA Dermatology, 152*(7), 768. doi:10.1001/jamadermatol.2016.1774

Ripton, J. T., & Winkler, C. S. (2016). How telemedicine is transforming treatment in rural communities. *Becker's Health IT & CIO Review*. Retrieved from http://www.beckershospitalreview.com/healthcare-information-technology/how-telemedicine-is-transforming-treatment-in-rural-communities.html

Rural Health Foundation Hub. (n.d.). About rural health care. Retrieved from http://www.ruralhealthweb.org/go/left/about-rural-health/what-s-different-about-rural-health-care

Rural Health Information Hub. (2016). Rural aging. Retrieved from https://www.ruralhealthinfo.org/topics/aging

S.2873-ECHO Act, 114th Congress. (2015–2016). Retrieved from http://assets.fiercemarkets.net/public/004-Healthcare/internal/echo.pdf

Texas Medical Board. (n.d.). Telemedicine FAQs. Retrieved from http://www.tmb.state.tx.us/page/laws-gc-faqs-telemedicine

The Commonwealth Fund. (n.d.). Use of telemedicine can reduce hospitalizations of nursing home residents and generate savings for Medicare. Retrieved from http://www.commonwealthfund.org/publications/in-the-literature/2014/feb/use-of-telemedicine

The history of remote monitoring, telemedicine technology. (2015, November 09). *mHealth Intelligence*. Retrieved from http://mhealthintelligence.com/news/the-history-of-remote-monitoring-telemedicine-technology

UAMS Centre for Distance Health. (n.d.). Geriatrics. Retrieved from http://cdh.uams.edu/providers/programs/geriatrics

U.S. Department of Agriculture. (2016, April 18). USDA seeks applications for nearly $12 million in broadband grants for rural communities. Retrieved from http://www.usda.gov/wps/portal/usda/usdahome?contentidonly=true&contentid=2016/04/0092.xml

University of New Mexico School of Medicine. (n.d.). Project ECHO. Retrieved from http://echo.unm.edu

Werner, C. A. (2011). *The older population: 2010 census briefs*. United States Census Bureau. Retrieved from https://www.census.gov/prod/cen2010/briefs/c2010br-09.pdf

What is telemedicine, American Telemedicine Association. (n.d.). Retrieved from http://www.americantelemed.org/about-telemedicine/what-is-telemedicine#.V33bjLgrJ2R

Who is required to comply with HIPAA requirements, HRSA Health Information Technology. (n.d.). Retrieved from http://www.hrsa.gov/healthit/toolbox/HIVAIDSCaretoolbox/SecurityAndPrivacyIssues/whoisreq2comply.html

Wicklund, E. (2016a). Ohio moves to limit telehealth in cross-coverage situations. Retrieved from https://www.pharmacist.com/ohio-moves-limit-telehealth-cross-coverage-situations

Wicklund, E. (2016b). Spectrum health takes its telehealth platform in-house. Retrieved from http://mhealthintelligence.com/news/spectrum-health-takes-its-telehealth-platform-in-house

Your Medicare coverage—Telehealth. (n.d.). Retrieved from https://www.medicare.gov/coverage/telehealth.html#1368

6

Technology Design for Frailty

Adriana J. Salas, Ashley Reynolds, and Colin M. Thomas

As of 2013, the average life expectancy in the United States was 84.3 years, with a continued upward trend ("Deaths: Final Data for 2013, table 7," 2013). As technology and medical advancements continue to improve, so does the proportion of older adults compared to those less than 65 years of age. According to the 2015 U.S. Census Bureau report, 14.88% of the populations is currently 65 years and older, and it is estimated to reach 23.55% by the year 2060 (Percent Distribution of the Projected Population by Sex and Selected Age Groups for the United States: 2015 to 2060 [NP2014-T6], 2014). Despite technological advancements in medical care, a portion of those aged 65 years and older will become frail. However, depending on the criteria used to operationalize the definition of frailty, the incidence will vary.

Frailty has been defined as either a physical phenotype, or as an index that quantifies the accumulation of a large number of deficits across multiple systems, and is reported as a ratio of abnormal systems to total systems measured (Clegg, Young, Iliff, Rikkert, & Rockwood, 2013). Fried et al. (2001) operationalized a physical phenotype of frailty as five physical attributes: weight loss, exhaustion, weakness, slowness, and low physical activity. Both phenotype and cumulative deficit models effectively identify elderly patients who are at risk for increased disability, hospitalization, nursing home admission, and mortality. Phenotype models are more amenable to implementation in busy clinical settings. In contrast, frailty indices incorporate a larger number of systems and variables that are more challenging to implement, but may capture a broader spectrum of frailty that is not captured completely by phenotype models. For instance, frailty indices may capture combinations and interactions of cognitive, immune, nutritional, psychosocial, and physiological deficits that are not measured directly in frailty phenotype models.

Regardless of the model used, frailty is a syndrome with multiple deficits across numerous body systems that predict poor health outcomes for the elderly population (Xue, 2011). Frailty has impacts beyond specific measures of physical function, such as diminished cognitive function, decreased muscle mass, depressive disorders, and social isolation—all contributing to greater levels of dependence, inability to tolerate stressors, and poor quality of life. Frailty is a state of vulnerability where small stressors result in a significant decline in functional status, followed by a slow and incomplete recovery to a new functional baseline (see Figure 6.1). According to the National Health and Aging Trend Study on 7,439 older noninstitutionalized participants, 15% were found to be frail and 45% prefrail (Badeen-Roche et al., 2015). Higher rates of frailty were also observed among women, Hispanic, and Black persons in residential care facilities, and persons with lower socioeconomic status (Badeen-Roche et al., 2015). For those residing in nursing homes, about half met the criteria of frailty (Kojima, 2015). Although the prevalence of frailty is high in some populations, some aspects of frailty can be managed, slowed, or reversed with interventions (P.-H Lee, Y.-S. Lee, & Chan, 2012).

In this chapter, we examine technologies that can assist with screening, assessment, and delay or prevention of the physical, cognitive, nutritional, and psychosocial aspects of frailty. A minority of these technologies have strong evidence for use in frailty. Consequently, we also explore technologies that are in use or have potential applications to frailty, but have not been rigorously evaluated for this purpose.

TECHNOLOGY TO ASSIST WITH SCREENING AND ASSESSMENT OF FRAILTY

Screening is a process by which healthy people who may be at risk for a disease or condition are identified (Morrison, 1998). Prior to beginning a screening program for any condition, it is important to assess whether the condition is appropriate for screening. Screening programs involve a systematic application of tests or instruments that have the ability to discriminate between those at average and those at high risk for the outcome of interest. Screening tests are not designed to diagnose a disease or condition. Screening programs can be rendered ineffective by either an excess of false-negative or false-positive results. False-negative results fail to identify those with the condition of interest and false-positive results can cause unnecessary anxiety over a condition that is not present and/or incur additional cost for unnecessary diagnostic testing. When disease prevalence is low,

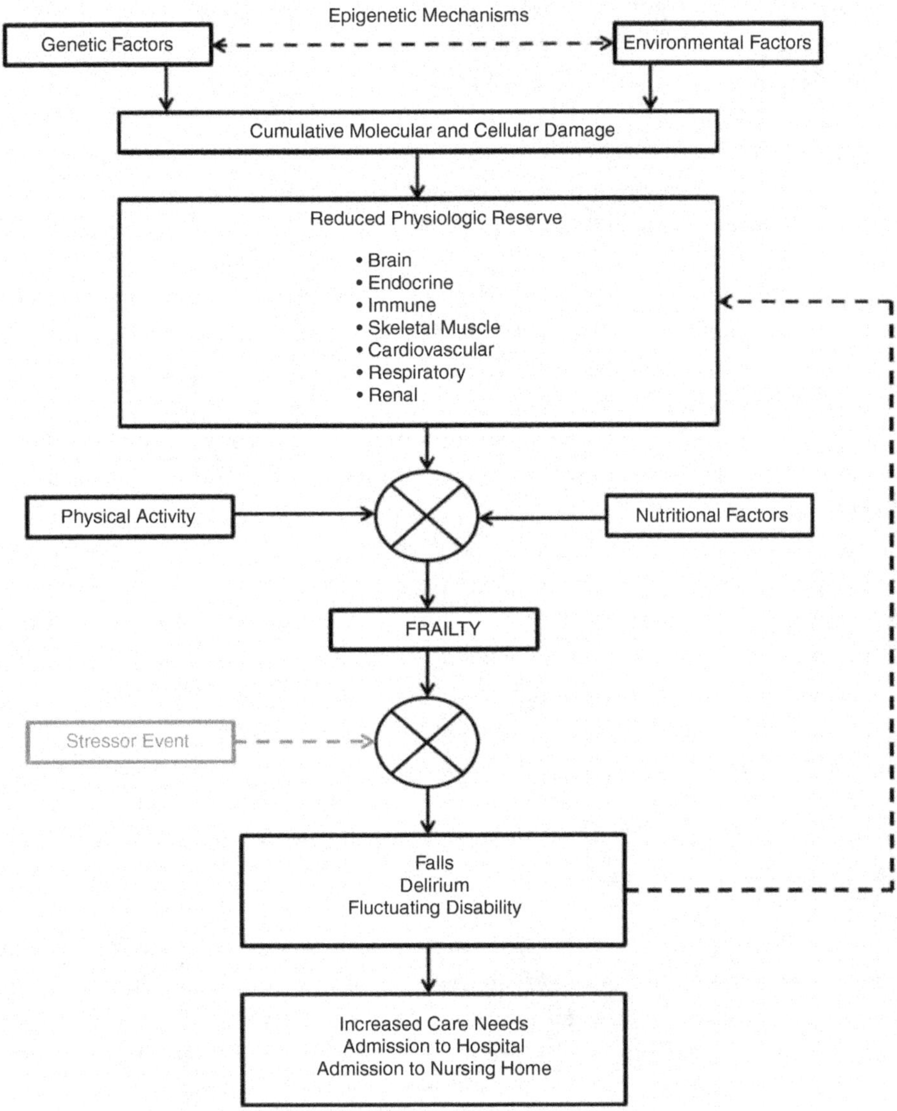

FIGURE 6.1 Pathophysiology of frailty.

the proportion of false-positive results increases (Fletcher, 2014). Screening tests are often developed by the selection of a small number of key elements from a more detailed diagnostic assessment battery. Alternatively, a subset of variables from a diagnostic instrument may be adapted to elements of an existing data set that was gathered for other purposes to retrospectively or concurrently screen a population. Another important element of screening programs is to target conditions for which interventions can positively impact the progression, course, and outcomes of the disease (Lee et al., 2012).

Frailty is a condition that has potential for screening because it has a definable clinical syndrome and targets for intervention to prevent or manage negative outcomes. An ideal frailty screening program would target a population of older, healthy individuals attempting to identify those who are at risk for developing frailty. Frailty is sufficiently common in adults over the age of 65 years (Collard, Boter, Schoevers, & Oude Voshaar, 2012) to warrant consideration as a target population for screening. Frailty screening can be abbreviated into brief instruments that can be performed in the context of a routine clinical visit (Oubaya et al., 2014).

Several large clinical trials have successfully incorporated frailty screening instruments into their protocols with acceptable accuracy. Some of these have included the Cardiovascular Health Study, the Canadian Study of Health and Aging, and the Study of Osteoporotic Fractures (Orlando Frailty Conference Group, 2013). Instruments used in these trials have options for self-reported or informant-reported brief questionnaires that can be completed in less than 5 minutes, which ideally would be tailored to a larger scale screening effort. Other screens focus on physical aspects of frailty and incorporate tests such as the Timed Up and Go (TUG; Podsiadlo & Richardson, 1991) test or a gait speed test (Bohannon, 1997). The TUG test can be reliably applied by following a simple set of instructions to measure the number of seconds it takes a subject to rise from a chair, walk three meters, turn around, walk back, and sit again (Lin et al., 2004). For gait speed, a fixed distance in meters is marked on the floor, and the clinician simply times a normal walking speed across the known distance.

Some individuals will require further diagnostic assessments either because of a positive frailty screen or for medical evaluation of symptoms that may indicate frailty. However, diagnostic assessments for complex geriatric syndromes like frailty are more extensive than screening tests and generally require a skilled clinician. The assessment usually includes documentation of the time course of the frailty symptoms along with comorbid medical conditions, medication review, and a physical examination of the pertinent body systems affected. In addition to this general assessment, a validated diagnostic instrument such as the Fried Frailty Criteria (Fried et al., 2001) or a Frailty Index (Jones, Song, & Rockwood, 2004) should also be completed to fully describe the extent and severity of frailty. Screening tools generally need to be brief and easy to execute. However, in a clinical diagnostic setting, instruments that are more accurate, expensive, difficult to interpret, or time consuming may be used to precisely quantify deficits and identify effective interventions.

Technological solutions are currently available that can facilitate implementation of screening through dissemination of tools to clinicians, patients, and/or their caregivers. Several self-report instruments have been validated for the purpose of screening for frailty (Metzelthin et al., 2010). Existing screening and assessment instruments can be implemented as web-based interfaces, or as tablet or smartphone applications. One example, the Edmonton Frail Scale (Rolfson, Majumdar, Tsuyuki, Tahir, & Rockwood, 2006) is available as a free application for android devices, iPhones, and iPads.

Modern smartphones also contain inertial sensors, which can be utilized to quantify many types of physical motion. For example, inertial sensors can be used to measure the TUG test (Galán-Mercant, Barón-López, Labajos-Manzanares, & Cuesta-Vargas, 2014). Inertial sensors can also be used to measure a more integrated, overall level of physical activity (Galán-Mercant & Cuesta-Vargas, 2015). Although this technology has not been validated against prior frailty assessment scales, it has the potential to provide a much more accurate way of quantifying the concept of low physical activity compared with self-report tools.

Capitalizing on the functionality of smartphones has several advantages. Application software for these measurements can be easily distributed to end users through existing application stores. Many people already own smartphones equipped with these types of sensors, which would allow initiation of monitoring with minimal or no additional cost for application software. Wearable wrist inertial sensors are also available for general public use and have capabilities to monitor activity levels and sleep (Tulley, McBride, Heron, & Hunter, 2014). Pedometers and wearable or smartphone global positioning system (GPS) tracking also offer alternatives to assess total activity levels and gait speed. Both are available in existing platforms and are accurate in healthy populations (Cyarto, Myers, & Tudor-Locke, 2004). However, pedometers can be less sensitive for detecting steps in low gait speeds that are frequently present in frail elderly people (Le Masurier & Tudor-Locke, 2003). All of these technologies are available in existing consumer-based platforms, and can be used in either a clinic or home setting by caregivers or cognitively intact patients.

Strength measurement is also included in many assessments of frailty, most commonly grip strength. This is traditionally measured using a spring-based, analog hand dynamometer. An alternative to this instrument has been developed that makes use of sophisticated pressure and temperature sensors within an inflated ball to measure hand-grip force. Sensors connect via Bluetooth and deliver grip-strength data, which can be used for both assessment and tracking of improvement during a rehabilitation program (Jaber, Hewson, & Duchêne, 2012).

Visual technology used in gaming, and other applications such as Microsoft Kinect, have also successfully been applied to elements of frailty assessment. The five times sit-to-stand (5STS) is one test used to assess fall risk and physical function, which has been specifically adapted to analysis by optical and inertial sensor technology (Ejupi et al., 2016). The testing protocol and equipment are simple and inexpensive enough to use in either a clinic or home setting. Similar technologies have been tested for use with the TUG test. In addition to measuring the primary time measurement of the TUG test, the visual technology has the capability to measure many other elements of gait that are predictive of frailty such as trunk angle, time from sit to stand, and back-to-sit movements (Hassani, Kubicki, Brost, & Mourey, 2015). Kinematic technology also has the potential to assess and quantify numerous specific components of gait analysis that were previously reserved for highly skilled technicians in research settings or qualitative assessment by experienced clinicians with specific training and expertise in gait analysis. Screening tests like the TUG are attractive primarily for their simplicity to perform and interpret. They reliably identify risk, but they do not elucidate any specific underlying causes, tailor interventions to reduce fall risk, or improve gait. The use of technology to assess specific elements of gait that are failing may also lead to more targeted and successful interventions in the future.

TECHNOLOGY AND FRAILTY-ASSOCIATED CHANGES

In addition to the changes previously described, frailty may also be associated with cognitive changes that may impact which tools or how technology should be designed when considering use in frail elderly patients. In this section, we explore these changes and how they may impact technology use.

Cognitive Changes

Changes in cognition associated with aging results in decreased ability to perform mental operations such as simultaneously remembering and incorporating new information, multitasking, and comprehending text (Schneider & Pichora-Fuller, 2000). These cognitive changes can actually begin in early adulthood (Salthouse, 2004). According to Salthouse (2004), vocabulary scores remain stable until age 55 years, then decline slightly over time. Even more compelling, Salthouse found large negative correlations between advancing age and pattern comparison speed (−.47), reasoning (−.48), and memory (−.43). Other evidence points to a typical linear cognitive decline in how new information is stored (encoding), how quickly information is processed, and spatial awareness (Hedden & Gabrieli, 2004). Other age-related physiological changes impacting cognition include reduced cerebral gray matter and neural demyelination, which results in slowed motor response and reaction time (Kochunov et al., 2007). Keeping the user interface without extraneous details and with clear, simple, and concise instructions will aid usability for frail older adults. These changes should be considered when designing user interfaces for older adults.

Physical Changes

Electronic exercise games may be a useful tool to increase physical activity in older adults (Dunning, 2008a; Gerling, Schild, & Masuch, 2010). However, physical decline normally associated with the aging process can raise challenges for older game players who wish to use movement-based interfaces to exercise (Gerling et al., 2010). Game players who are not successful owing to their physical limitations may not find the experience enjoyable, thereby decreasing the likelihood of continued interaction. Therefore, the physical limitations in frailty should be taken into account when designing and providing alternatives such as exertive video games (Reynolds, 2013). For instance, alternatives should be flexible enough to allow various styles of game play that accommodate the physical limitations such as difficulty standing or maintaining balance. As an added benefit, some dance games with team-based play facilitate social interaction and teamwork, which many older adults find enjoyable (Boschman, 2010; Dunning, 2008b).

Older adults prefer games with simplicity, adjustable displays, immediate performance feedback, and fewer required steps (Gerling, Schulte, & Masuch, 2011). As a result, including these design features may also improve older adults' enjoyment of exercise games. However, exertive game controls should avoid complicated interfaces that require balance and coordination that frail patients may not possess. Consider using physical activity or alternative controls that allow exertion while stable, such as seated in a wheelchair or on a couch.

Visual Changes

Age-related changes in vision impact how older adults interact with their environment. These changes are of great importance to e-Health research as many of these tools are visually based. As we age, the lens of the eye loses its ability to accommodate or change shape, so that moving a focal point from far to near or vice versa takes longer, or requires corrective lenses (Ham, Sloane, Warshaw, Potter, & Flaherty, 2007). Age-related ocular structural changes (changes in lens shape and size of the iris) limit the amount of light entering the eye, thereby decreasing visual acuity. In addition, retinal neural attrition decreases the amount of visual information received and processed by the brain (Morrell, 2001). These changes, including the loss of ability to discern details or contrast (Crassini, Brown, & Bowman, 1988) and color discrimination (Haegerstrom-Portnoy, Schneck, & Brabyn, 1999), coupled with increased sensitivity to glare, makes it difficult for older adults to read and visualize certain types of information (Echt, Morrell, & Park, 1998). Design features suiting visual changes in frailty should include larger font sizes (National Institute on Aging, 2008), leveraging larger displays such as tablet computers (Smith, 2014), and high-contrast displays.

Motor Skill Changes

Designing digital health tools for frail patients should include consideration of the users' age and tool preferences. Digital health device interfaces for frail users must also account for associated age-related motor skill changes, so that the experience can be less overwhelming and more enjoyable (Reynolds, 2013). In addition, older adults' physical limitations such as mobility and balance may make digital health tools, which require stability to operate, difficult or uncomfortable to use. Having ergonomically designed controllers, or games in which the player is able to set the difficulty or controller characteristics to suit their physical limitations, would be beneficial. Designers should avoid complicated gesture controls or those that require accurate pointing or hand gestures as frail adults may not be able to perform these actions and become frustrated with the experience (Reynolds, 2013).

Fitness Applications and Activity Monitors

Self-monitoring tools can support self-regulatory mechanisms such as feedback and goal setting. Using instruments that track data, contextual activities, or feedback on data points provides the user with information regarding health behaviors. This self-monitoring information can be exceptionally powerful at influencing health behaviors. Pedometers or other self-monitoring devices have been found to have significant effects, such as increased adherence with various health behaviors and as disease self-management and exercise (Heesch, Mâsse, Dunn, Frankowski, & Mullen, 2003; Hollis et al., 2008). Although little evidence exists about how different age groups use these devices, increasing numbers of adults are adopting self-monitoring health tools, especially with the introduction of mobile technology. Older adults are using self-monitoring tools for health maintenance more frequently than their younger counterparts. However, this is due, in part, to the increased illness burden (Reynolds, 2013).

Physical and cognitive changes in frailty represent unique challenges and opportunities for digital health tools to support healthy activities. Providers should contemplate these changes when considering a particular digital health intervention with frail elderly patients. When appropriately applied, these digital tools can aid patients and their caregivers in managing an often difficult and complex stage of life. However, when inappropriately applied, it may cause harm.

TECHNOLOGY TO PREVENT OR DELAY PROGRESSION OF NUTRITIONAL FRAILTY

Weight loss, muscle wasting, and malnutrition are core components of the frailty syndrome. Adequate nutritional intake is required for maintaining a normal body weight and muscle mass. However, nutritional supplementation alone has not been effective in counteracting the muscle weakness associated with frailty (Fiatarone et al., 1994). In addition, a growing body of literature is suggesting that inflammation and proinflammatory cytokines may be playing a role in the development of frailty (Chen, Mao, & Leng, 2014). This concept is supported by evidence that inflammatory cytokines such as IL-6 and neopterin are elevated in frail elderly individuals, and are associated with anorexia and weight loss (Mantovani, 2006).

Smartphone applications, with or without peripheral devices, can be used to measure and track body weight and caloric intake and expenditure. When these measurements are integrated, it is possible to track the total caloric balance. Currently available fitness applications are largely designed and marketed for overweight individuals. However, they also have great potential for use in the management of undernutrition and frailty. Unfortunately, manual entry of food calories is both labor and cognitively intensive, and therefore less applicable to frail and prefrail elders in the absence of a healthy caregiver. Smart kitchen scales improve on the automation of calorie counting and upload intake to an integrated application, but still require a high level of interaction with the user. There is one wearable device on the market that can perform automatic calorie counts without the usual intensive data input. However, significant validation of the accuracy of smart and wearable devices in thin and frail elderly individuals will be required before they can be used with confidence. Smart bathroom scales can automatically record and track weight, but require some skill to set up. On the other hand, smart bathroom scales can also include body composition analysis by bioelectrical impedance. A low-voltage current is used to measure electrical impedance across the patient as they stand on the scale, and the impedance measurement is used to estimate percentage of body fat. This method has been validated in healthy adult subjects (Lukask, Johnson, Bolonchuk, & Lykken, 1985). Clinical trials with either prefrail or frail older adults supported by caregivers will also be required to demonstrate whether these device-based interventions are effectively maintaining or improving weight and strength in prefrail and frail older individuals.

TECHNOLOGY TO IMPROVE SOCIAL FUNCTION IN PREFRAIL AND FRAIL ELDERS

Although social isolation and loneliness are not included in frailty indices and scales, they are core components of the frailty syndrome that have a major impact on quality of life. As with other aspects of comprehensive geriatric care, focusing exclusively on a medical model but ignoring socioeconomic variables often fails. It is, therefore, necessary to evaluate and enhance socialization of the frail elderly population. Technological advancements have the potential to impact the social elements of frailty, particularly social isolation and loneliness. However, technology can be intimidating, complicated, and costly. In this part of the chapter we review risk factors for social isolation, differences between social isolation and loneliness, consequences of social isolation, and tools available for assessment, interventions to relieve social isolation and loneliness in the prefrail and frail elderly populations.

Risk Factors for Social Isolation and Loneliness

Older adults find themselves in a shrinking social network immediately after retirement, losing contact with coworkers of many years. This may be followed by eventual loss of spouse, family, or other close friends of similar age as they outlive those around them. Living in a highly mobile society, many of their children are residing out of state with limited contact or involvement in their well-being. Consequently, an estimated 29% of elderly individuals will end up living alone, with a limited number of social interactions outside of the home, often relying on long-distance relationships with family (Administration for Community Living, 2015). Another 5% of elderly individuals will ultimately require nursing home placement, going up as high as 50% for those greater than 95 years of age, with further decreased levels of socialization compared to those living at home alone (Demko, 2016).

With retirement, there is also a significant drop in income, likely affecting the degree to which older adults can participate in activities outside of the home. In 2013, the median family income of older adult homeowners in the United States was $34,452 versus $17,268 for renters (Administration for Community Living, 2015), compared to $52,250 for all adults (Noss, 2014). In addition, the communities they live in can become impoverished over time and perceived as having poor safety, therefore causing elders to avoid leaving the home.

With advancing age, older adults are also faced with physical changes that may include sensory loss, altered mobility, and altered bowel or bladder continence. Impaired vision will interfere with the ability to walk safely outside of the home without falling. They may start to avoid social situations where their diminished hearing is impeding two-way conversations with others. Even telephone conversations can become difficult resulting in fewer telephone interactions with friends and family. As their vision, hearing, dexterity, and reflexes diminish, their ability to drive safely is also affected. Both the frequency and driving distance reduces and sometimes ceases all together. According to the U.S. Department of Transportation, 29% of older adults continue to hold a driver's license, although it is unclear the percentage that are actually driving (U.S. Department of Transportation: Federal highway statistics 2014, n.d.). Altered mobility may also make it difficult for elders to take public transportation, or even walk outside their homes, becoming dependent on family, friends, or community organizations for door-to-door transportation.

If the older adult is having difficulties with continence, they start to feel self-conscious of their appearance and smell, especially if having to wear protective garments. Proximity and feasibility of restroom facilities becomes the focus, sometimes deterring them from leaving the home (Fultz & Herzog, 2001).

Cognitive decline affects the functional status of the elderly individuals in many different areas of their lives. It is estimated that 5% of those 65 to 69 years of age, and 32% of those greater than 85 years of age will suffer from moderate to severe memory impairment (Federal Interagency Forum on Aging-Related Statistics, 2004), placing them at higher risk for getting lost as their memory declines. As a result, older adults and their families may start to avoid activities outside of the home.

Depending on their socioeconomic resources, physical status, and cognition, they will have different degrees of social isolation and loneliness. The higher the number of chronic illnesses, the higher the risk of social isolation (Hall, Havens, & Jivan, 2004).

Social Isolation Versus Loneliness

Social isolation has been simply defined as the objective absence or contact with people (Cornwell & Waite, 2009), while loneliness is the subjective feeling of limited or lost companionship or social support (Cattan, White, Bond, & Learmouth, 1999). Loneliness is further broken down into social or emotional loneliness. Social loneliness is the absence of meaningful relationships, while emotional loneliness is the lack of attachment, intimate bond, or a confidant (DiTommaso & Spinner, 1997). Most of the components of social isolation and loneliness have been studied with different scales available to try and quantify degrees of social isolation and loneliness. Depending on the definition being utilized, the scale being applied, and the location where the older adult is residing, social isolation can range drastically from 21% to 54% (Nicholas & Nicholson, 2010).

Effects of Social Isolation in the Elderly Population

Social isolation is a risk factor for numerous negative health outcomes that are core components of frailty, such as malnutrition (Lucie, 2014), physical weakness, falls (Cauley, Faulkner, Griffin, Nevitt, & Zmuda, n.d.), or other outcomes indirectly associated with frailty, such as mood disorders, self-harming behavior, decreased quality of life, and dementia (Fratiglioni, Paillard-Borg, & Winblad, 2004), with resultant increased morbidity and mortality (Demakakos, Shankar, & Steptoe, 2013). Self-harming behaviors include personal neglect and substance use disorders (Hanson, 1994), while mood disorders include anxiety and depression, sometimes leading to suicide. Quality of life can also be affected by social isolation from decreased life satisfaction, decreased sense of self-control and self-esteem. Figure 6.2 illustrates the interaction between social isolation, morbidity, mortality, quality of life, frailty, and the inherent biopsychosocial interactions.

Technology for Screening and Assessment of Social Isolation and Loneliness

Several attempts have been made to measure the degree of social isolation and loneliness in the elderly population. But like frailty, social isolation and loneliness are multidimensional concepts with a broad range of definitions in the academic literature, making them difficult to operationalize and measure. The two terms are also used interchangeably, making it difficult, if not impossible, to compare research findings. No scale to date has been determined to be comprehensive in its evaluation of social isolation or loneliness,

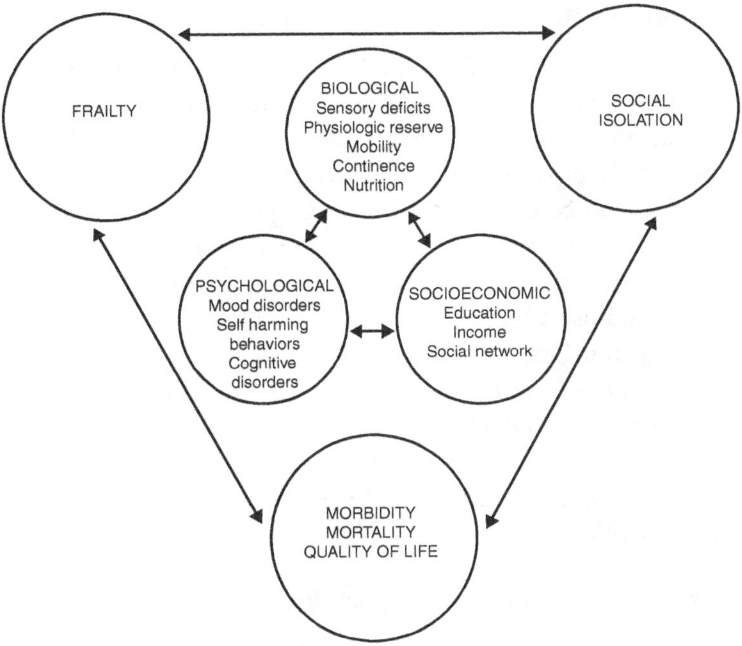

FIGURE 6.2 Biopsychosocial model of frailty.

only measuring components at any given time. Most scales also tend to be lengthy and cumbersome to apply, and therefore used in a research rather than a clinical setting.

However, there have been several instruments used to screen and measure subcomponents of social isolation and loneliness that have shown adequate validity and reliability within the subgroups being tested. For example, the Lubben Social Network Scale measures the size, closeness, and frequency of contact of a respondent's social network (Lubben, 2006). It is a 12-item questionnaire that gives the option of performing a short 6-item version, which can easily be implemented in the clinic setting. There is also the University of California Los Angeles (UCLA) loneliness scale (Russell, 1996), a 20-item scale designed to measure a person's feeling of social isolation and loneliness. Because these instruments are short, it is reasonable to implement them in the clinical setting. However, most instruments remain in paper form and not readily available. The digitalization of these instruments, specifically into a mobile application that can automatically sum up and transfer results into the medical record, would be ideal and of great benefit to the clinician. It would expedite and further encourage their use.

Interventions to Reduce Social Isolation

Reducing social isolation in the elderly population is of great importance, given the detrimental health effects. Literature has shown a 50% reduction in mortality rates for all individuals with strong social support (Dickens, Richards, Greaves, & Campbell, 2011). However, it is not clear the types of interventions that would be effective in improving social isolation in the elderly population. Numerous studies have attempted to evaluate this construct; however, many of them had design flaws such as a small sample size, no control group, and use of different instruments measuring different domains with conflicting findings. Nevertheless, the following paragraphs discuss current interventions in place to help reduce social isolation and loneliness in the elderly population that may or may not have strong evidence to support their application. Interventions for the community-dwelling and homebound adult are discussed, including the use of technology to improve social isolation and loneliness.

Community Group Resources for Socialization

For the more functional older adult, a limited amount of community resources already exists that provide group activities among seniors and improve socialization. However, participants must be mobile enough to leave their homes with established means of transportation, making group activities more appropriate for those who are not homebound and have not yet advanced to frailty. For that reason, most studies implementing group-type interventions were found in adult day care centers, senior centers, rehabilitation centers, community centers, or on-site if it involved voluntary work by the senior, such as a mentoring program or reading to children.

The overall type of gathering can be categorized into four different groups: support, educational, social, and physical activity groups. Support groups covered areas such as bereavement (Constantino, 1988) or open discussion groups (Lokk, 1990). There was also group-based reminiscence therapy that looked at depression, loneliness, and psychological well-being, finding significant improvements (Chiang, 2010). An educational support group was composed of a gardening program that included lectures on how to garden, giving them responsibility for their own plants, having significant improvement in loneliness, life satisfaction, and social network (Tse, 2010). In the social activities group, people got together to participate in diverse group activities, such as art, exercise, discussions, and writing with improved structural social support, though no other areas of social or mental health were measured (Routasalo, Tilvis, Kautiainen, & Pitkala, 2009). Religious engagement was also associated with decreased rates of social isolation

(Nicholas & Nicholson, 2010). Although the physical activity groups usually aim for improved physical functioning, they also offered consequent social interaction with one study improving depression, but had no effect on loneliness (Aaltonen, Pohjolainen, Puukka, Hinkka, & Pöntinen, 2008).

Family and Friends as a Resource for Socialization

The frail elderly population frequently develops physical disabilities that preclude them from leaving the home, sometimes dependent on their family and friends for any type of social interaction. Family may play a major role in the amount of socialization the older adult receives, yet they are limited by their own constraints of child care and job responsibilities. Friends also help with socialization, but most elders' friends are of similar age with similar health problems, and/or disabilities limiting their own ability to socialize. Unfortunately, telephone conversations with family and friends end up replacing physical visitations. Telephone conversations can improve social isolation and loneliness, but face-to-face social interactions continue to be superior to telephone interactions, reducing the incidence of depression (Teo et al., 2015).

Community Resources for the Homebound to Improve Socialization

For the older adults who are homebound with limited or no access to family or friends, there are community resources targeting social isolation and loneliness by sending people to the home for such things as visitations, music, and animal-assisted therapy (AAT). There are also radio programs targeting social isolation and loneliness such as KPBS, a San Diego, California–based Radio Reading Service broadcasting the readings of newspapers, books, and magazines to those with low vision, blindness, and other impairments 24 hours a day over a private audio channel. Similarly, a radio program in Australia for the elderly population addressed social isolation and loneliness by focusing on music and other programs relevant to those who grew up in the 1920s to 1950s, showing statistical improvement in depressive symptoms and quality of life (Travers & Bartlett, 2010).

Information Communication Technology to Reduce Social Isolation and Loneliness

Social isolation and loneliness can lead to severe depression and functional decline. Family, friends, and community resources can be limited, and sometimes unsuccessful, in alleviating social isolation for elderly individuals who are homebound, frail, or live in a rural area where access to family, friends, or community resources is limited. Despite people's beliefs that the older adult does not or cannot use information communication technology (ICT), the data show otherwise. Information and communication technology might then be the bridge for this marginalized group of people to stay connected with society. Information and communication technology can be the key to reaching those at risk for social isolation and improve health outcomes, where standard interventions have proven to be minimally to moderately effective at best.

Use of ICT in the Elderly Population Compared to the General Population

One source of communication technology that has partially filled this gap is the cell phone, with 92% of adult Americans owning a cell phone and 67% owning a smartphone (Rainie & Zickuhr, 2015). The smartphone is portable, wireless, with the same capabilities of a personal computer at similar or less cost (without the maintenance), exchangeable, and upgradable. Cell phone use in the 65 years and older group has increased over time, trailing behind those who are younger with an estimated use of 74% in 2014 (Pew Research Center: Internet, Science and Technology, 2014), with 48% using mobile applications (Rainie & Zickuhr, 2015). The elderly population today is more likely to own a smartphone than a personal computer.

Computer or Internet use in the elderly population has not increased at the same rate as cell phone use, creating a digital divide based on differences in physical, social, economic, or regional conditions. Regardless, computer and Internet use is now rapidly increasing, with 75% of Americans using the Internet, 56% being greater than 65 years old (Morris, 2016). A survey of Internet users found the elderly population to be using email 86% of the time, with 27% searching the Internet for health/medical information, and 34% using it for social networking (Madden & Zickuhr, 2012). The elderly population is also using different social network platforms such as Facebook 48%, Pinterest 16%, LinkedIn 12%, Twitter 6%, and Instagram 4% of the time (Duggan, 2015). The proportional use of these social networks by those greater than 65 years has also been sequentially increasing over time. For example, Facebook use in older adults increased from 35% in 2012 and 45% in 2013, to 56% in 2014 (Duggan, Ellison, Lampe, Lenhart, & Madden, 2015). Overall Internet use has further increased with the introduction of smartphones, mobile broadband, and Wi-Fi, making them highly mobile and accessible for all age groups. However, the elderly population continues to have problems with program design and interface, lack of training and support, and high cost in relation to their income. It can also be stressful and challenging for the elderly population to adopt new technology.

The tablet computer is a hybrid between the smartphone and the personal computer, being lightweight and only measuring 12 inches. The tablet has, therefore, improved computer use in the elderly population who lack strength and ability to sit in front of a desktop computer. Touch screen technology allows older adults with dexterity problems to avoid using the keyboard altogether. In 2014, 42% of Americans owned a tablet computer (Pew Research Center: Internet, Science and Technology, 2014), allowing them to access the same or similar social networks as with their personal computer, yet with easier feasibility than with their cell phones.

Effects of ICT on Socialization/Loneliness in the Elderly Population

Evidence shows that a significant number of elderly individuals are using ICT. However, it is still to be determined if ICT can improve social isolation and loneliness. A systematic review evaluating the effectiveness of various interventions designed to alleviate social isolation and loneliness in older adults was performed by others reviewing 4,940 studies between the years 1978 and 2009. Thirty-two studies met their selection criteria (Dickens et al., 2011). From the 32 studies, four involved the implementation of ICT in the form of computer/Internet training (Fokkema & Knipscheer, 2007; Slegers, van Boxtel, & Jolles, 2008; White et al., 1999; White et al., 2002), and one involved telephone support to an older adult population (Heller, Thompson, Trueba, Hogg, & Vlachos-Weber, 1991). All five studies were found to have a moderate to high degree of bias and only one study showed overall reduction in loneliness at 3 years (Fokkema & Knipscheer, 2007).

Another systematic review looked at interventions to alleviate loneliness in adults greater than 55 years of age between the years 1996 and 2011, with 34 studies meeting inclusion criteria (Jiska Cohen-Mansfield & Rotem Perach, 2015). This review included the five already mentioned studies reviewed by Dickens et al. (2011), plus eight additional studies implementing interventions in computer training (Bickmore, Caruso, Clough-Gorr, & Heeren, 2005; Moses, 2003; Shapira, Barak, & Gal, 2007), videoconferencing (Tsai, Tsai, Wang, Chang, & Chu, 2010; Tsai & Tsai, 2011), teleconferencing (Swindell & Mayhew, 1996), a telephone support group (Stewart et al., 2001), and a radio program (Travers & Bartlett, 2010). Of the eight new studies, three significantly reduced loneliness, which included emailing with friends and family (Moses, 2003), videoconferencing with family (Tsai & Tsai, 2011), and Internet browsing (Shapira, Barak, & Gal, 2007).

A third systematic review looked at interventions to alleviate social isolation and depression in adults 77 to 86 years, reviewing 403 articles between the years of 2009 and 2013, with five studies meeting inclusion criteria (Franck, Molyneux, & Parkinson, 2016). The review included one already mentioned study on the first two reviews. Out of the four remaining studies, only one implemented the use of a home video gaming console with significant improvement in loneliness (Kalbaugh, 2011).

A more recent systematic review looked at ICT interventions to reduce social isolation in adults greater than 55 years, reviewing a total of 424 publications between the years 2002 and 2015, with a total of 25 articles meeting the inclusion criteria (Chen, 2016). Interventions included email, online chat rooms, videoconferencing, social networking, telehealth systems, telephone befriending, smartphone, iPad, Nintendo Wii, and virtual pet companion application for a pet avatar. Of the studies that looked at the effects of ICT on social isolation, four were found to significantly reduce social isolation (Cattan, Kime, & Bagnall, 2011; Cotten, Anderson, & McCullough, 2013; Karimi & Neustaedter, 2012; Khvorostianov, Elias, & Nimrod, 2011). Out of the 18 studies that looked at the effects of ICT on loneliness, 15 had a significant reduction (Chen, 2016). However, most of the studies did convenience sampling, posing a high risk for selection bias, some had a small sample size, while others had a high attrition rate.

Challenges Faced by the Elderly Population When Using ICT

The challenges the elderly population faces in attempting to adopt social networking include a decline in vision, hearing, fine motor skills, coordination, cognition, self-efficacy, and frequently a low socioeconomic status. A study conducted by Wright found that older adults with disabilities in vision, hearing, physical mobility, dexterity, or a homebound status had significantly less use of technology (Hill & Wright, 2009). According to the Unified Theory of Acceptance and Use of Technology (UTAUT), the adoption of computer and Internet use in the elderly population will be determined mainly by their ability to see usefulness for it, ease of use, and the influence of society around them, in addition to inherent moderators such as age, gender, experience, and voluntariness of use (Demiris, Gell, LaCroix, Patel, & Rosenberg, 2015). The digital divide, regardless of current support systems or interventions in place, is anticipated to improve over time as the younger generations that have been exposed to this technology most of their lives get older. However, a gap in use between the young and old will always be expected, given that people will always suffer from physical or cognitive disability that will interfere with the use of ICT.

ICT-Adaptive Equipment

To reduce the digital divide for those with disabilities and improve accessibility, there are three widely used guidelines for website development, which include the U.S. Federal Government section 508 guidelines of the Rehabilitation Act, the National Institute on Aging (NIA)/National Library of Medicine (NLM) guidelines, and the World Wide Web Consortium's Web Accessibility Initiative (WAI) guidelines, which require that all web browsers be adapted for people with disabilities (Jaeger & Xie, 2009). Because of these guidelines, the visually impaired older adult can now zoom in or magnify text in both smartphones and personal computers. However, a windows mobile magnifier application may need to be downloaded to have the feature on the phone. If the phone has too small a screen despite the magnifier, a tablet or personal computer may be the answer. There is also Microsoft Reader's Frutiger Linotype and ClearType, a setting that smooths the edges of screen fonts to make text more readable.

For the hearing impaired, there are light alerts for both mobile phones and personal computers. According to Demiris et al. (2015), "Technology use did not vary by the presence of hearing impairment or balance or coordination impairments. However, impairments in vision and memory were associated with decreased usage of email and text messaging and the Internet." However, if proper adaptations are made for the visually impaired, it is expected that they will utilize ICT with greater ease.

For older adults lacking dexterity, sensation, coordination, or fine motor skills, there are touch screen features on both tablets and personal computers. Although touch screen technology can improve ease of use, it can still be a problem for older adults with tremors. For this reason, mobile phone and computer manufacturers have developed bigger and more prominent keys, word predictors, larger text, yes/no menu, text-to-speech tools or voice commands, to minimize or avoid typing altogether.

For the older adult with cognitive problems, there are simpler-to-use interfaces such as IBM Easy Web Browsing, layouts and designs with easier-to-use applications, and no time limitations when completing forms, site registration, or answering messages. The cognitively impaired older adult may require added time for learning, in addition to individualized learning. Then again, no amount of training will compensate for progressive cognitive impairment.

Self-efficacy is the extent or strength of one's belief in one's own ability to complete tasks and reach goals (Ormrod, 2006), sometimes viewed as the same concept as self-esteem (Judge, Erez, Bono, & Thoresen, 2002). If the individual does not believe that he or she can learn to use technology and is not willing to try, it will be difficult to utilize any type of ICT. Introduction of ICT may need to take place gradually for these individuals.

Overcoming Socioeconomic Barriers to ICT

Educational level, income, profession, gender, race, and age have all been associated with rates of computer/Internet use (Werner, Carlson, Jordan-Marsh, & Clark, 2011). The U.S. government and nonprofit organizations are attuned to this problem, and have implemented programs to reduce this digital divide by improving access to computers and cell phones. For example, "Computers for Learning" is a U.S. government program that provides computers for low-income families by redistributing federal and corporation surplus computers. There is also access to free computers from local, county, state, or national corporate-sponsored programs, and nonprofit agencies that take computer donations to turn around and give to others in need. For example, "Share the Technology" allows seniors with disabilities to request a computer from a pool of donated resources (Share the Technology Computer Recycling Project, 2016). Some programs may require proof of family income or a referral by a government assistance program.

Government programs such as "Link Up" help pay for the cost of basic local telephone services. There is also "Lifeline," which provides a smartphone to low-income individuals, popularly referred to as the "Obama phone." The Lifeline program is sponsored by the federal government, but regulated at the state level with similar eligibility requirements, but different state-to-state services, with some offering 250, 1,000, or even unlimited monthly minutes and texts (Lifeline, 2016).

Social isolation is an important component of the frailty syndrome. Family, friends, and community resources can help improve social isolation, but a large gap remains. Despite popular belief, the elderly population has adopted the use of ICT at greater rates than expected, contributing to increased social interactions. However, further updated research studies are needed to support the belief that ICT improves social isolation and loneliness in the pre-frail and frail elderly populations.

A CASE STUDY IN USE OF ICT FOR FRAIL ELDERS

A 74-year-old male presents to clinic for follow-up after a hospitalization and rehabilitation period for injuries sustained from a fall. He has a history of dementia, hypertension, degenerative disc disease, lumbar spinal stenosis, a left leg radiculopathy, and a 15-lb weight loss in the past 6 months. He reports falling forward and striking directly on his face. In the fall, he fractured his right facial bone and sustained a laceration to his right arm. The head injury caused bleeding inside his skull, or subdural hematoma. He is unable to recall how the fall occurred, but denies losing consciousness. He did not require surgery for his subdural hematoma or his facial fractures, but he did require stitches to repair the forearm laceration. He was sent to a rehabilitation unit for physical and occupational therapy for 4 weeks and was discharged home. During the visit, it is noted that the patient entered the exam room propelling himself very slowly in a wheelchair. He had difficulty rising from the wheelchair, even using both arms, still requiring extensive assistance from the nurse to reach the exam table. He explains that he was provided with a walker upon discharge from the rehabilitation center, but does not use it. He prefers to use the wheelchair and braces on the furniture inside his home for transfers. He also uses the wheelchair for longer distances, but usually stays home because his endurance is poor.

During the exam, he is noticeably slim with food particles and stains on his shirt, and poor foot hygiene. His blood pressure is low when he is standing upright. Physical exam is without new head or facial trauma, and right arm laceration is well healed. He answers all questions, but some of the information he provides is contradictory with information in the medical record. He can state his full name and location, but is not able to remember the date. Since discharge from the rehabilitation unit, he has not gone out of his home. A neighbor brought food from the market once, but is not able to do this consistently. He describes eating one meal a day, which is not unusual for him. He states that he can do everything for himself, but on the basis of observed functional status in clinic, he does not appear capable of personal hygiene, cooking, cleaning, or shopping for food.

He was married and divorced three times and has no children. He lives in a low-income apartment with an elevator to enter. He reports having one niece across the country, whom he talks to on the phone once a month, but has not seen her in 20 years. He states that his care team recommended he remain in a nursing home for custodial care, but he refused and signed himself out as he knows he can take care of himself. He has not designated a power of attorney for health care or completed a living will, requesting full resuscitative measures if he should experience a cardiac or respiratory arrest. He has both Medicare Part A and Part B, but does not have Medicaid or any other private insurance. His only source of income is social security. His ability to care for himself safely at home is questionable.

Given the complexity of the patient's presentation, a multicomponent treatment plan was developed addressing assessment and management of frailty elements, including cognitive impairment, weight loss, nutrition, strength, fall risk, community mobility, and social isolation.

Because the patient was noted to have memory problems, a Saint Louis University Mental Status (SLUMS) exam was performed using a smartphone application with a score of 15 out of 30, indicative of dementia (Tariq, Tumosa, Chibnall, Perry, & Morley, 2006). Once the patient obtained a government-subsidized cell phone, he had his home address entered in Google Maps for him to be able to return home using this application, if he ever became disoriented. His niece was also able to log on to the Internet and monitor his cell phone location in case he ever got lost. The niece was also considering in-home cameras for further monitoring.

The patient's malnutrition was attributed to his lack of access to food. The social worker was consulted to initiate Meals On Wheels, a home food delivery program for older adults. The nutritionist was also consulted to formally evaluate caloric and protein intake. A prescription for supplemental drinks was provided. He was also provided with a bathroom scale to help monitor his weight. The patient was then scheduled for an outpatient follow-up with the nutritionist. An appetite stimulant would be considered if he failed to gain weight once he had access to nutrition.

He was then referred for home physical and occupational therapy to improve his strength, endurance, balance, and to evaluate the home for environmental hazards. The occupational therapist was also consulted to perform a Kohlman Evaluation of Living Skills (KELS) to assess performance of instrumental and basic activities of daily living (IADLs and ADLs), and the capacity to live independently (Sabrina Pickens, 2007). His new government-issued cell phone would also be able to estimate daily activity by counting his steps and intensity of activity by measuring his heart rate.

Because it is no longer safe for the patient to drive, the social worker also assisted the patient to apply for subsidized metropolitan transit system (MTS) services that can drive him to future medical appointments without taking the risk of him driving or getting lost. MTS services would also be able to transport him to community group meetings/gatherings to increase his socialization. A Department of Motor Vehicles form was filled out for a disabled placard, so when he receives rides from his neighbor, he can park in the reserved parking spaces for disabled individuals.

The patient's income was limited, making it difficult for him to have a cell phone. However, he was referred to Lifeline to obtain a federally subsidized cell phone, which allowed him to contact his niece or call for emergency services as needed. In the future, he would be assisted to apply for a subsidized computer to videoconference with his niece, enhancing his communication connection to his only relative.

It was found unsafe for the patient to return home to independent living, but he refused placement. Risks and benefits of staying home in his current condition were discussed with the patient. Because the patient was able to describe a plan for how he would secure food and shelter, and repeat the risks and benefits of going back home, he was deemed as having decision-making capacity. However, adult protective services were still contacted. He also lacked the resources for placement in a skilled nursing facility for long-term custodial care. He was referred to the social worker who initiated an application for Medicaid, as this would help fund a home health aide, and potentially fund placement in a skilled nursing facility for custodial care in the future. The niece was to discuss finances with her uncle to make sure that his bills continued to get paid.

His goals and preferences for medical care were discussed in detail, and he expressed preferences to at least pursue trials of aggressive therapy, but he clarified that he would want to have care withdrawn if his initial trials of therapy were unsuccessful. He also agreed to have his niece named as his power of attorney for health care. His preferences were documented in a living will, which was placed in his medical record.

After 6 months at home, the patient suffered another fall. He was unable to get up, but was able to call his neighbor using his cell phone who activated emergency medical services. He was taken to a local hospital for care where he was found to have no significant injuries. However, by this time, his Medicaid application had been processed and approved. After this fall, the patient realized that it was no longer safe for him to remain home alone, and agreed to placement in a skilled nursing facility.

CONCLUSION

As the overall life expectancy, number, and proportion of elderly people increases, we can only expect that the number of frail elderly people will also increase. It is, therefore, imperative that the proper resources to care for the prefrail and frail elderly people are in place. Currently, a large portion of prefrail and frail elderly individuals remains marginalized, impoverished, with lack of medical and long-term care as they age. The economics and family structure in the United States is such that it makes it difficult for family and friends to supplement their care, and community resources are limited owing to lack of financial incentives.

We then turned to technology to help bridge this gap in the care of the prefrail and frail elderly population. Technology can assist providers, the elderly population, and their caretakers by facilitating early identification of frailty, quantification and measurement of deficits associated with frailty, interventions to delay progression, and improvement in social isolation via ICT. However, as previously mentioned, a minority of these technologies have strong evidence to support their use. This is partially attributed to the lack of up-to-date studies, the biased belief that older adults are unwilling or incapable of adopting technology, and the rapid turnover in technology.

Improved technology geared toward the elderly, plus research to support its use, is desperately needed. For now, providers, prefrail and frail elderly populations, and their caretakers will have to continue to improvise with the resources currently available to them.

REFERENCES

Aaltonen, T., Pohjolainen, T., Puukka, P., Hinkka, K., & Pöntinen, S. (2008). Alleviating loneliness among frail older people—Findings from a randomised controlled trial. *International Journal of Mental Health Promotion, 10*, 26–34.

Administration for Community Living. (2015). Profile of older Americans: Housing. Retrieved from http://www.aoa.acl.gov/Aging_Statistics/Profile/2015/11.aspx

Badeen-Roche, K., Seplaki, C. L., Huang, J., Buta, B., Kalyani R. R., & Varadhan R. (2015, July 14). Frailty in older adults: A nationally representative profile in the United States. *Journals of Gerontology, Series A: Biological Sciences and Medical Sciences, 70*(11), 1427–1434. doi:10.1093/gerona/glv133

Bickmore, T. W., Caruso, L., Clough-Gorr, K., & Heeren, T. (2005). It's just like you talk to a friend: Relational agents for older adults. *Interact Comput, 17*, 711–735.

Bohannon, R. W. (1997). Comfortable and maximum walking speed of adults aged 20–79 years: Reference values and determinants. *Age and Ageing, 26*(1), 15–19.

Boschman, L. R. (2010). *Exergames for adult users: A preliminary pilot study.* Proceedings of the International Academic Conference on the Future of Game Design and Technology (pp. 235–238). New York, NY: Association for Computing Machinery.

Cattan, M., Kime, N., & Bagnall, A.-M. (2011, March). The use of telephone befriending in low level support for socially isolated older people—An evaluation. *Health and Social Care Community, 19*(2), 198–206. doi:10.1111/j.1365-2524.2010.00967.x

Cattan, M., White, M., Bond, J., & Learmouth, A. (1999). Preventing social isolation and loneliness among older people: A systematic review of health promotion interventions. *Aging and Society, 25*(1), 41–67. doi:10.1017/S0144686X04002594

Cauley, J., Faulkner, K., Griffin, J., Nevitt, M., & Zmuda, J. (n.d.). Is social integration associated with the risk of falling in older community-dwelling women? *Journals of Gerontology, Series A: Biological Sciences and Medical Sciences, 58*, M954–M959. Retrieved from http://biomed.geronologyjournals.org/cgi/content/full/58/10/M954

Chen, X., Mao, G., & Leng, S. (2014). Frailty syndrome: An overview. *Clinical Interventions in Aging, 9*, 433–441.

Chen, Y. S. (2016, January). The effect of information communication technology interventions on reducing social isolation in the elderly: A systematic review (G. Eysenbach, N. Diviani, & J. Clemensen, Eds.). *Journal of Medical Internet Research, 18*(1), e18. doi:10.2196/jmir.4596

Chiang, K. (2010). The effects of reminiscence therapy on psychological well-being, depression, and loneliness among institutionalized aged. *International Journal of Geriatric Psychiatry, 2*, 380–388.

Clegg, A., Young, J., Iliff, S., Rikkert, M. O., & Rockwood, K. (2013). Frailty in elderly people. *The Lancet, 381*, 752–762. doi:10.1016/S0140-6736(12)62167-9

Collard, R. M., Boter, H., Schoevers, R. A., & Oude Voshaar, R. C. (2012). Prevalence of frailty in community-dwelling older persons: A systematic review. *Journal of the American Geriatrics Society, 60*, 1487–1492. doi:10.1111/j.1532-5415.2012.04054.x

Constantino, R. (1988). Comparison of two group interventions for the bereaved. *Journal of Nursing Scholarship, 20*, 83–88.

Cornwell, E. Y., & Waite, E. J. (2009, March). Social disconnectedness, Perceived isolation and health among older adults. *Journal of Health and Social Behavior, 50*(1), 31–48.

Cotten, S. R., Anderson, W. A., & McCullough, B. M. (2013). Impact of internet use on loneliness and contact with others among older adults: Cross-sectional analysis. *Journal of Medical Internet Research, 15*(2), 39. doi:10.2196/jmir.2306

Crassini, B., Brown, B., & Bowman, K. (1988). Age-related changes in contrast sensitivity in central and peripheral retina. *Perception, 17*(3), 315–332.

Cyarto, E. V., Myers, A. M., & Tudor-Locke, C. (2004). Pedometer accuracy in nursing home and community-dwelling older adults. *Medicine & Science in Sports & Exercise, 36*(2), 205–209. doi:10.1249/01.MSS.0000113476.62469.98

Deaths: Final data for 2013, table 7. (2013). Retrieved from http://www.cdc.gov/nchs/fastats/older-american-health.htm

Demiris, G., Gell, N., LaCroix, A., Patel, K., & Rosenberg, D. (2015). Patterns of technology use among older adults with and without disabilities. *The Gerontologist, 55*(3), 412–421. doi:10.1093/geront/gnt166

Demko, D. (2016). How many seniors really end up in nursing homes? *Nursing Home Diaries: Information, stories and articles about nursing homes*. Retrieved from http://nursinghomediaries.com/howmany

Dickens, A. P., Richards, S. H., Greaves, C. J., & Campbell, J. L. (2011). Interventions targeting social isolation in older people: A systematic review. *Biomedical Central, 11*, 647–669. Retrieved from http://www.biomedcentral.com/1471-2458/11/647

DiTommaso, E., & Spinner, B. (1997, March). Social and emotional loneliness: A re-examination of Weiss' typology of loneliness. *Personality and Individual Differences, 22*(3), 417–427. doi:10.1016/S0191-8869(96)00204-8

Duggan, M. (2015, August 19). The demographics of social media users. Retrieved from http://www.pewinternet.org/2015/08/19/the-demographics-of-social-media-users

Duggan, M., Ellison, N., Lampe, C., Lenhart, A., & Madden, M. (2015, January 9). Demographics of key social network platforms: Social media update 2014. Retrieved from http://www.pewinternet.org/2015/01/09/demographics-of-key-social-networking-platforms-2

Dunning, T. (2008a). Aging, activities, and the internet. *Activities, Adaptation and Aging, 32*(1), 59–60.

Dunning, T. (2008b). Dance, dance revolution (DDR). *Activities, Adaptation & Aging, 32,* 238–239.

Echt, K. V., Morrell, R. W., & Park, D. C. (1998). Effects of age and training formats on basic computer skill acquisition in older adults. *Educational Gerontology: An International Quarterly, 24*(1), 3–25.

Ejupi, A., Brodie, M., Gschwind, Y. J., Lord, S. R., Zagler, W. L., & Delbaere, K. (2016). Test for clinical and in-home assessment of fall risk in older people. *Gerontology, 62,* 118–124. doi:10.1159/000381804

Federal Interagency Forum on Aging-Related Statistics. (2004). *Older Americans 2004: Key indicators of well-being.* Washington, DC: U.S. Government Printing Office.

Fiatarone, M., O'Neill, E., Ryan, N., Clements, K., Solares, G., Nelson, M., . . . Evans, W. (1994). Exercise training and nutritional supplementation for physical frailty in very elderly people. *New England Journal of Medicine, 330*(25), 1769–1775. doi:10.1056/NEJM199406233302501

Fletcher, R. H. (2014). Prevention. In R. H. Fletcher, S. W. Fletcher, & G. S. Fletcher (Eds.), *Clinical epidemiology: The essentials* (pp. 152–163). Philadelphia, PA: Lippincott Williams & Wilkins.

Fokkema, T., & Knipscheer, K. (2007). Escape loneliness by going digital: A quantitative and qualitative evaluation of a Dutch experiment in using ECT to overcome loneliness among older adults. *Aging and Mental Health, 11,* 496–504.

Franck, L., Molyneux, N., & Parkinson, L. (2016). Systematic review of interventions addressing social isolation and depression in aged care clients. *Quality of Life Research, 25,* 1395–1407. doi:10.1007/s11136-015-1197-y

Fratiglioni, L., Paillard-Borg, S., & Winblad, B. (2004). An active and socially integrated lifestyle in late life might protect against dementia. *Lancet Neurology, 3,* 343–353. doi:10.1016/S1474-4422(04)00767-7

Fried, L. P., Tangen, C. M., Walston, J., Newman, A. B., Hirsch, C., Gottdiener, J. . . . McBurnie, M. A. (2001, March). Frailty in older adults: Evidence for a phenotype. *Journal of Gerontology Series A: Biological Sciences and Medical Sciences, 56*(3), M146–M156.

Fultz, N., & Herzog, A. (2001). Self-reported social and emotional impact of urinary incontinence. *Journal of the American Geriatrics Society, 49,* 892–899. doi:10.1046/j.1532-5415.2001.49179.x

Galán-Mercant, A., Barón-López, F. J., Labajos-Manzanares, M. T., & Cuesta-Vargas, A. I. (2014). Reliability and criterion-related validity with a smartphone used in timed-up-and-go test. *BioMedical Engineering OnLine, 13,* 156–167.

Galán-Mercant, A., & Cuesta-Vargas, A. I. (2015). Clinical frailty syndrome assessment using inertial sensors embedded in smartphones. *Physiological Measurement, 36,* 1929–1942.

Gerling, K. M., Schild, J., & Masuch, M. (2010). *Exergame design for elderly users: The case study of SilverBalance.* Proceedings of the 7th International Conference on Advances in Computer Entertainment Technology (pp. 66–69). New York, NY: Association for Computing Machinery.

Gerling, K. M., Schulte, F. P., & Masuch, M. (2011). *Designing and evaluating digital games for frail elderly persons.* Proceedings of the 8th International Conference on Advances in Computer Entertainment Technology (p. 62). New York, NY: Association for Computing Machinery.

Haegerstrom-Portnoy, G., Schneck, M. E., & Brabyn, J. A. (1999). Seeing into old age: Vision function beyond acuity. *Optometry & Vision Science, 76*(3), 141–158.

Hall, M., Havens, B., & Jivan, T. (2004). Social isolation and loneliness: Differences between older rural and urban Manitobans. *Canadian Journal on Aging, 23*, 129–140. doi:10.1353/cja.2004.0022

Ham, R. J., Sloane, P. D., Warshaw, G. A., Potter, J. F., & Flaherty, E. (2007). *Ham's primary care geriatrics: A case-based approach*. Philadelphia, PA: Mosby.

Hanson, B. (1994). Social network, social support and heavy drinking in elderly men: A population study of men born in 1914, Malmo, Sweden. *Addiction, 89*, 725–732. doi:10.1111/j.1360-0443.1994.tb00958.x

Hassani, A., Kubicki, A., Brost, V., & Mourey, F. (2015). Kinematic analysis of motor strategies in frail aged adults during the Timed Up and Go: How to spot the motor frailty? *Clinical Interventions in Aging, 10*, 505–513.

Hedden, T., & Gabrieli, J. D. (2004). Insights into the ageing mind: A view from cognitive neuroscience. *Nature Reviews Neuroscience, 5*(2), 87–96.

Heesch, K. C., Mâsse, L. L., Dunn, A. L., Frankowski, R. F., & Mullen, P. D. (2003). Does adherence to a lifestyle physical activity intervention predict changes in physical activity? *Journal of Behavioral Medicine, 26*(4), 333–348.

Heller, K., Thompson, M. G., Trueba, P. E., Hogg, J. R., & Vlachos-Weber, I. (1991). Peer support telephone dyads for elderly women: Was this the wrong intervention? *American Journal of Community Psychology, 19*, 53–74.

Hill, T., & Wright, D. (2009). Prescription for trouble: Medicare part D and patterns of computer and internet access among the elderly. *Journal of Aging and Social Policy, 21*, 172–186. doi:10.1080/08959420902732514

Hollis, J, F., Gullion, C. M., Stevens, V. J., Brantley, P. J., Appel, L. J., Ard, J., . . . Laferriere, D. (2008). Weight loss during the intensive intervention phase of the weight-loss maintenance trial. *American Journal of Preventive Medicine, 35*(2), 118–126.

Jaber, R., Hewson, D. J., & Duchêne, J. (2012). Design and validation of the Grip-ball for measurement of hand grip strength. *Medical Engineering and Physics, 34*(9), 1356–1361. doi:10.1016/j.medengphy.2012.07.001

Jaeger, P. T., & Xie, B. (2009, June). Developing online community accessibility guidelines for persons with disabilities and older adults. *Journal of Disability Policy Studies, 20*(1), 55–63. doi:10.1177/1044207308325997

Jiska Cohen-Mansfield, P. A., & Rotem Perach, M. (2015, February). Interventions for alleviating loneliness among older persons: A critical review. *American Journal of Health Promotion, 29*(3), 109-125.

Jones, D. M., Song, X., & Rockwood, K. (2004). Operationalizing a frailty index from a standardized comprehensive geriatric assessment. *Journal of the American Geriatrics Society, 52*(11), 1929–1933.

Judge, T. A., Erez, A., Bono, J. E., & Thoresen, C. J. (2002). Are measures of self-esteem, neuroticism, locus of control, and generalized self-efficacy indicators of a common core construct? *Journal of Personality and Social Psychology, 83*(3), 693–710. doi:10.1037/0022-3514.83.3.693

Kalbaugh, E. S. (2011). Effects of playing Wii on well-being in the elderly: Physical activity, loneliness, and mood. *Activities, Adaptation, and Aging, 35*, 331–344.

Karimi, A., & Neustaedter, C. (2012, February). *From high connectivity to social isolation: Communication practices of older adults in the digital age*. Proceedings of the ACM 2012 conference on Computer Supported Cooperative Work Companion (pp. 127–130). New York, NY: Association for Computing Machinery. doi:10.1145/2141512.2141559

Khvorostianov, N., Elias, N., & Nimrod, G. (2011, November 11). Without it I am nothing: The internet in the lives of older immigrants. *New Media and Society, 14*(4), 583–599. doi:10.1177/1461444811421599

Kochunov, P., Thompson, P. M., Lancaster, J. L., Bartzokis, G., Smith, S., Coyle, T., . . . Fox, P. T. (2007). Relationship between white matter fractional anisotropy and other indices of cerebral health in normal aging: Tract-based spatial statistics study of aging. *Neuroimage, 35*(2), 478–487.

Kojima, G. (2015, November 1). Prevalence of frailty in nursing homes: A systematic review and meta-analysis. *Journal of American Medical Directors Association, 16*(11), 940–945. doi:10.1016/j.jamada.2015.06.025

Le Masurier, G. C., & Tudor-Locke, C. (2003, Mar). Comparison of pedometer and accelerometer accuracy under controlled conditions. *Medicine & Science in Sports & Exercise, 35*(5), 867–871. doi:10.1249/01.MSS.0000064996.63632.10

Lee, P.-H., Lee, Y.-S., & Chan, D.-C. (2012). Interventions targeting geriatric frailty: A systemic review. *Journal of Clinical Gerontology & Geriatrics, 3*(2), 47–52. doi:10.1016/j.jcgg.2012.04.001

Lifeline. (2016, November 28). Retrieved from http://www.obamaphone.com/obama-phone-eligibility

Lin, M.-R., Hwang, H.-F., Hu, M.-H., Wu, H.-D. I., Wang, Y.-W., & Huang, F.-C. (2004). Psychometric comparisons of the timed up and go, one-leg stand, functional reach, and Tinetti balance measures in community-dwelling older people. *Journal of the American Geriatrics Society, 52*(8), 1343–1348.

Lokk, J. (1990). Emotional and social effects of a controlled intervention study in day-care unit for elderly patients. *Scandinavian Journal of Primary Health Care, 8*, 165–172.

Lubben, J. B. (2006). Performance of an abbreviated version of the Lubben Social Network Scale among three European community–dwelling older adult populations. The *Gerontologist, 46*(4), 503–513. Retrieved from http://www.brandeis.edu/roybal/docs/LSNS_website_PDF.pdf

Lucie, K. (2014). Social isolation as a risk factor for inadequate diet of older Eastern Europeans. *International Journal of Public Health, 59*, 707–714. doi:10.1007/s00038-014-0582-6

Lukask, H. C., Johnson, P. E., Bolonchuk, W. W., & Lykken, G. I. (1985, April). Assessment of fat-free mass using bioelectrical impedance measurements of the human body. *The American Journal of Clinical Nutrition, 41*(4), 810–17.

Madden, M., & Zickuhr, K. (2012). Older adults and internet use. Retrieved from http://www.pewinternet.org/reports/2012/older-adults-and-internet-use.aspx

Mantovani, G. (2006). Cytokines in cachexia. In P. Matthys & A. Biliau (Eds.), *Cachexia and wasting: A modern approach* (pp. 205–207). Milan, Italy: Springer-Verlag.

Metzelthin, S. F., Daniëls, R., van Rossum, E., de Witte, L., van den Heuvel, W. J., & Kempen, G. I. (2010). The psychometric properties of three self-report screening instruments for identifying frail older people in the community. *BioMed Central Public Health, 10*, 176–184. doi:10.1186/1471-2458-10-176

Morrell, R. W. (2001). *Older adults, health information, and the World Wide Web.* Mahwah, NJ: Psychology Press.

Morris, J. (2016, March 21). First look: Internet use in 2015. Retrieved from https://www.ntia.doc.gov/blog/2016/first-look-internet-use-2015

Morrison, A. S. (1998). Screening. In K. J. Rothman & S. Greenland (Eds.), *Modern epidemiology* (2nd ed., p. 499). Philadelphia, PA: Lippincott-Raven Publishers.

Moses, B. (2003). *Technology as a means of reducing loneliness in the elderly* (PhD dissertation). Walden University, Minneapolis, MN.

National Institute on Aging. (2008, May). Making your printed health materials senior friendly. Retrieved from https://www.nia.nih.gov/sites/default/files/making_your_printed_health_materials_senior_friendly_1.pdf

Nicholas, R., & Nicholson, J. (2010). *Predictors of social isolation in community dwelling older adults* (dissertation) (p. 223). Retrieved from http://gradworks.umi.com/34/15/3415135.html

Noss, A. (2014, September). Household income: 2013. *American Community Survey Briefs*. Retrieved from https://www.census.gov/content/dam/Census/library/publications/2014/acs/acsbr13-02.pdf

Orlando Frailty Conference Group. (2013). Raising awareness of the urgent need to implement frailty into clinical practice. *Journal of Frailty and Aging*, *2*(3), 121–124.

Ormrod, J. (2006). *Educational psychology: Developing learners*. Upper Saddle River, NJ: Pearson/Merrill Prentice Hall.

Oubaya, N., Mahmoudi, R., Jolly, D., Zulfiqar, A., Quignard, E., Cunin, C., . . . Drame, M. (2014). Screening for frailty in elderly subjects living at home: Validation of the modified short emergency geriatric assessment (SEGAm) instrument. *Journal of Nutrition, Health & Aging*, *18*(8), 757–763.

Percent distribution of the projected population by sex and selected age groups for the United States: 2015 to 2060 (NP2014-T6). (2014, December). Retrieved from http://www.census.gov

Pew Research Center: Internet, Science and Technology. (2014, January). Mobile fact sheet. Retrieved from http://www.pewinternet.org/fact-sheet/mobile

Podsiadlo, D., & Richardson, S. (1991). The timed "Up & Go": A test of basic functional mobility for frail elderly persons. *Journal of the American Geriatrics Society*, *39*, 142–148.

Rainie, L., & Zickuhr, K. (2015, August 26). Chapter 1: Always on connectivity: Americans' view on mobile etiquette. Retrieved from http://www.pewinternet.org/2015/08/26/chapter-1-always-on-connectivity

Reynolds, A. (2013). *Age-related differences in self-efficacy and the use of e-health supports for exercise behavior in adults* (dissertation). University of Florida, Gainesville, FL.

Rolfson, D. B., Majumdar, S. R., Tsuyuki, R. T., Tahir, A., & Rockwood, K. (2006). Validity and reliability of the Edmonton Frail Scale. *Age and Ageing*, *35*, 526–529.

Routasalo, P. E., Tilvis, R. S., Kautiainen, H., & Pitkala, K. H. (2009). Effects of psychosocial group rehabilitation on social functioning, loneliness and well-being of lonely, older people: Randomized controlled trial. *Journal of Advanced Nursing*, *65*, 297–306.

Russell, D. (1996). UCLA Loneliness Scale (Version 3): Reliability, validity, and factor. *Journal of Personality Assessment*, *66*, 20–40. Retrieved from http://fetzer.org/sites/default/files/images/stories/pdf/selfmeasures/Self_Measures_for_Loneliness_and_Interpersonal_Problems_VERSION_3_UCLA_LONELINESS.pdf

Sabrina Pickens, M. A.-B. (2007, March). The utility of the KELS test in substantiated cases of elder self-neglect. *Journal of the American Academy of Nurse Practitioners*, *19*(3), 137–142. doi:10.1111/j.1745-7599.2007.00205.x

Salthouse, T. A. (2004). What and when of cognitive aging. *Current Directions in Psychological Science*, *13*(4), 140–144.

Schneider, B., & Pichora-Fuller, M. (2000). Implications of perceptual deterioration for cognitive aging research. In F. Craik & T. Salthouse (Eds.), *Handbook of aging and cognition* (2nd ed.). Hillsdale, NJ: Erlbaum.

Shapira, N., Barak, A., & Gal, I. (2007). Promoting older adults' well-being through Internet training and use. *Aging and Mental Health*, *11*, 477–484.

Share the technology computer recycling project. (2016, November 28). Retrieved from http://www.envirolink.org/resource.html?itemid=200211211049020.236091&catid=5

Slegers, K., van Boxtel, M. P. J., & Jolles, J. (2008). Effects of computer training and internet usage on the well-being and quality of life of older adults: A randomized control study. *Journals of Gerontology, Series B: Psychological Sciences and Social Sciences, 63*, P176–P184.

Smith, A. (2014, April 3). *Older adults and technology use*. Retrieved from http://www.pewinternet.org/2014/04/03/older-adults-and-technology-use

Steptoe, A., Shankar, A., Demakakos, P., & Wardle, J. (2013). Social isolation, loneliness, and all-cause mortality in older men and women. *Proceedings of the National Academy of Sciences of the United States of America, 110*(15), 5797–5801. doi:10.1073/pnas.1219686110

Stewart, M., Mann, K., Jackson, S., Downe-Wamboldt, B., Bayers, L., Slater, M., & Turner, L. (2001). Telephone support groups for seniors with disabilities. *Canadian Journal on Aging, 20*, 47–72.

Swindell, R., & Mayhew, C. (1996). Educating the isolated ageing: Improving the quality of life of the housebound elderly through educational teleconferencing. *International Journal of Lifelong Education, 15*, 85–93.

Tariq, S. H., Tumosa, N., Chibnall, J. T., Perry, M. H., & Morley, J. E. (2006, November). Comparison of the Saint Louis University Mental Status examination and the Mini-Mental State Examination for detecting dementia and mild neurocognitive disorder—A pilot study. *Journal of American Geriatric Psychiatry, 14*(11), 900–910. doi:10.1097/01.JGP.0000221510.33817.86

Teo, A. R., Choi, H. J., Andrea, S. B., Valenstein, M., Newsom, J. T., Dobscha, S. K., & Zivin, K. (2015). Does mode of contact with different types of social relationships predict depression in older adults? Evidence from a nationally representative survey. *Journal of the American Geriatrics Society, 63*(10), 2014–2022.

Travers, C., & Bartlett, H. B. (2010). Silver Memories: Implementation and evaluation of a unique radio program for older people. *Aging and Mental Health, 15*, 169–177.

Tsai, H.-H., & Tsai, Y.-F. (2011). Changes in depressive symptoms, social support, and loneliness over 1 year after a minimum 3-month videoconference program for older nursing home residents. *Journal of Medical Internet Research, 13*, e93.

Tsai, H.-H., Tsai, Y.-F., Wang, H.-H., Chang, Y.-C., & Chu, H. H. (2010). Videoconferencing program enhances social support, loneliness, and depressive status of elderly nursing home residents. *Aging and Mental Health, 14*, 947–954.

Tse, M. (2010). Therapeutic effects of an indoor gardening programme for older people living in nursing homes. *Journal of Clinical Nursing, 19*, 949–958.

Tulley, M. A., McBride, C., Heron, L., & Hunter, R. F. (2014, December 23). The validation of Fitbit Zip™ physical activity monitor as a measure of free-living physical activity. *BioMed Central Research Notes, 7*, 952.

U.S. Department of Transportation: Federal highway statistics 2014. (n.d.). Distribution of licensed drivers—2014 by sex and percent in each age group and relation to population. Retrieved from http://www.fhwa.dot.gov/policyinformation/statistics/2014/dl20.cfm

Werner, J. M., Carlson, M., Jordan-Marsh, M., & Clark, F. (2011, October). Predictors of computer use in community dwelling, ethnically diverse older adult. *Human Factors and Ergonomics Society, 53*(5), 431–447. doi:10.1177/0018720811420840

White, H., McConnell, E., Clipp, E., Branch, L. G., Sloane, R., Pieper, C., & Box, T. L. (2002). A randomized control trial of the psychological impact of providing internet training and access to older adults. *Aging and Mental Health, 6*, 213–221.

White, H., McConnell, E., Clipp, E., Bynum, L., Teague, C., Navas, l., . . . Halbrecht, H. (1999). Surfing the net in later life. *Journal of Applied Gerontology, 18*, 358–378.

Xue, Q.-L. (2011). The frailty syndrome: Definition and natural history. *Clinics in Geriatric Medicine, 27*(1), 1–15. doi:10.1016/j.cger.2010.08.009

7

Technology and Cognitive Impairment

Ian C. Neel, Roxana Aminbakhsh, Lauren Cook, and T. J. McCallum

OVERVIEW OF COGNITIVE IMPAIRMENT

The term *cognitive impairment* refers to a collection of disorders that affect a person's ability to process the world. Specifically, cognitive function is not a single action, but rather a collection of abilities that enables the processing and problem solving necessary to interact with the world. Cognition itself is broken down into several domains including visuospatial reasoning, executive functioning, naming, memory, attention, language, abstraction, and orientation. The impairment of these domains of cognition, therefore, is the strict definition of cognitive impairment, and when identified, must be explored to determine the underlying cause.

The *Diagnostic and Statistical Manual of Mental Disorders* (5th ed.; *DSM-5;* American Psychiatric Association, 2013) helps clinicians in the process of diagnosing the cause of cognitive impairment. In the *DSM-5*, cognitive disorders are broken down into major neurocognitive disorders and minor neurocognitive disorders, as well as delirium.

Mild Neurocognitive Disorder

Mild neurocognitive disorder is defined as having impairment in cognitive performance, as evidenced by clinical assessment of cognitive function, preferably via standardized neuropsychiatric testing. The definition also necessitates concern on behalf of the patient or clinician that there has been a decline in cognitive function. As to what differentiates mild and major neurocognitive disorders, it is that the deficits of mild neurocognitive disorder do not interfere with one's ability to function in the world. Specifically, one should not have an impairment in activities of daily living (ADLs) or instrumental activities of daily (IADL; American Psychiatric Association, 2013).

ADLs are the standard activities persons need to perform to be able to function in everyday society. The six ADLs are eating, bathing, dressing, toileting, transferring, and bowel/bladder continence. IADLs, meanwhile, are more complex tasks that enable one to live independently. The IADLs include tasks such as shopping, housekeeping, food preparation, medication management, managing finances, using a telephone, and navigating transportation. IADLs are typically the first functions to become impaired in cognitive disorders; it is rare to see ADLs impaired at the onset of a cognitive disorder.

Major Neurocognitive Disorder

In contrast to mild neurocognitive disorder, major neurocognitive disorder, by definition, interferes with one's ability to function in the world. The criteria for defining a patient as having a major neurocognitive disorder include, first and foremost, that there is evidence of impairment of at least one domain of cognition in the realm of learning and memory, language, executive function, attention, visuospatial planning, or social cognition. Further, the deficits must interfere with one's performance of everyday activities, either via a decline in social functioning or ADLs/IADLs. Further, the impairment must be an acquired disorder, to differentiate it from genetic disorders, which are beyond the scope of this overview. The disorder itself also must be of insidious onset and have evidence of a progressive decline. Importantly, the disorder cannot be accounted for by another underlying psychiatric disorder such as schizophrenia or depression. Most importantly, the disorder must not occur only during a period of delirium.

Delirium

Delirium is an entity that is important to distinguish from the preceding major and minor neurocognitive disorders. Delirium is marked by an acute change in cognition brought on by an underlying medical disturbance. The causes of delirium are vast, and hence it is important when performing a diagnostic assessment of someone with a cognitive impairment to rule out delirium before diagnosing them with a cognitive disorder. Typical etiologies of delirium include constipation, infection, pain, hepatic or renal disease, electrolyte disturbance, dehydration, and often polypharmacy. Medications are a common, and often unrecognized, cause of delirium, most notably medications that have anticholinergic action. It is important to recognize delirium and treat or reverse the underlying cause, as there is a mortality risk associated with the presence of delirium. Delirium itself is defined as a waxing and waning cognitive impairment, most notably with impaired attention, compared to other domains of cognition.

Dementia

Within the domain of major neurocognitive disorder lie the dementia disorders, most typically known by their individual definitions in the *DSM-IV*. The *DSM-5* revised the diagnosis to the more generalized major neurocognitive disorder with the caveat that the clinician should also specify the likely underlying etiology. For example, a diagnosis of a person with cognitive deficits in the domains primarily of memory and executive function, who has had a slow, progressive decline without underlying alternate psychiatric or medical explanation for the decline, with significant impairment on cognitive testing and impaired functional ability in everyday life, would be defined as major neurocognitive disorder, possible Alzheimer's type. *Possible* or *probable* are the terms used to define the type of dementia disorder present, with *probable* being the most definitive the clinician can be with the diagnosis without performing a confirmatory brain biopsy.

The types of dementia are numerous, and it is not the intention of this chapter to discuss the diagnostic criteria required for defining all types of dementia, but it is worth mentioning the most prevalent forms of dementia and basic background of their defining characteristics.

Alzheimer's disease is by far the most prevalent of dementia disorders. The incidence and prevalence of Alzheimer's disease increases with age, with data suggesting that the prevalence of Alzheimer's doubles every 5 years after the age of 65 years. In 2011, 4.5 million people over the age of 65 years in the United States had Alzheimer's dementia. The number of patients in the United States with Alzheimer's disease is expected to rise to 13.8 million by the year 2050 (Hebert, Weuve, Scherr, & Evans, 2013). The pathogenesis for Alzheimer's is unclear. The disease is diagnosed by pathology showing extracellular amyloid plaques composed of amyloid beta peptides with 42 amino acids, as well as intracellular tau protein tangles. The diagnosis of Alzheimer's dementia clinically is dependent on the presence of the diagnostic criteria mentioned earlier of major neurocognitive disorder, with, specifically, cognitive impairments involving a minimum of two cognitive domains, specifically regarding visuospatial reasoning, executive function, memory, language, or personality changes. The initial and most prominent deficits noted in traditional Alzheimer's disease are related to the impairment of learning and recall of recently learned information, and problems with word finding, judgment, and problem solving.

Dementia with Lewy bodies is classically marked by visual hallucinations, which tend to be pleasant or nondistressing, often of small people. Parkinsonism, memory impairment, extreme sensitivity to neuroleptic agents, autonomic dysfunction, and REM sleep disorders are also classically linked with dementia with Lewy bodies. As with Alzheimer's disease, Lewy body dementia remains a clinical diagnosis owing to the inability to obtain pathologic samples premortem. Pathologic diagnosis of the disorder is notable for round, intracytoplasmic neuronal inclusions that are eosinophil predominant. These inclusions have since been named Lewy bodies, and are most commonly found within the substantia nigra (Forster & Lewy, 1912).

Parkinson's disease with dementia is often confused with dementia with Lewy bodies. They share similar features of parkinsonism, visual hallucinations, autonomic dysfunction, and REM sleep disorders, as well as memory deficits. The distinguishing characteristic of Parkinson's dementia is that the dementia component of Parkinson's disease arises late in the disease, often 10 or more years after development of the movement disorder symptoms. In contrast, the movement disorder symptoms of dementia with Lewy bodies develop at the same time as, or shortly thereafter, the time of onset of memory disturbance.

Frontotemporal dementia is a starkly different set of dementia disorders compared with the more amnestic dementias seen in Alzheimer's, Parkinson's, and dementia with Lewy bodies. Frontotemporal dementia is marked by prominent changes in social behavior and personality, with aphasia, often sexual disinhibition, and sometimes concomitant motor symptoms such as parkinsonism. Unlike the aforementioned dementia disorders, frontotemporal dementia is more commonly an early-onset dementia disorder, often presenting before the sixth decade of life.

Vascular dementia is the second most common form of dementia after Alzheimer's disease in most studies. It previously was limited to multi-infarct dementia wherein one saw a stepwise decline in cognitive domains with multiple strokes diagnosed by CT or MRI. The understanding of this disorder has grown rapidly over the turn of the 20th century, recognizing the high prevalence of chronic microvascular damage to the cerebral cortex, and the effect this has on cognition. The diagnosis of this disorder is clinical, with impairments in cognition resulting in impaired functionality with support of white matter lesions or stroke on imaging, as well as vascular risk factors and a symptom collection atypical for Alzheimer's dementia. More often, the presence of mixed dementia disorders, with a disorder such as Alzheimer's disease, compounded by the presence of vascular disease, is being recognized.

Other Forms of Cognitive Impairment

Many other forms of cognitive disorders exist, such as HIV dementia, prion disease, progressive supranuclear palsy, and cerebral amyloid angiopathy, to name a few; however, discussion of these disorders is beyond the scope of this chapter. The importance of dementia disorders, however, is clear with the high and rising prevalence of disease. The management of such cognitive disorders is difficult on a societal level, with limited pharmacotherapeutic interventions that provide clinical improvement, and high costs associated with care of the dementia population. The behavioral and functional disturbances common to these disorders are associated with increased risk of entry into assisted living or skilled nursing facilities. With the rising prevalence of disease, we must look toward modalities to focus on maintaining functionality for as long as possible, both for patient quality of life, as well as for curbing the exponentially rising health care costs. As such, a great deal of effort has been spent on researching how technological advances can aid in the functionality of patients with cognitive impairment. What follows is a discussion of the technologies that exist, as well as a look toward the future at ongoing areas of research to aid in the treatment of those with cognitive disorders.

OVERVIEW: USE OF TECHNOLOGY IN MANAGEMENT OF COGNITIVE IMPAIRMENT

Technology is growing rapidly and can be considered an important aid in providing care for elderly people with dementia. However, significant lack of clinical trials regarding intelligent assistive-technology devices, specifically involving their applications for elderly people with dementia, limits their use for this population (Bharucha et al., 2009). Therefore, we can only assume their usefulness based on their utility.

Currently, there are few studies conducted to show the effects of using technology in providing care for patients with dementia.

One study was published in the *Journal of NeuroEngineering and Rehabilitation* in May 2014 regarding computer-based cognitive stimulation applications to help the elderly population maintain and improve their cognitive skills. This study showed that their model was effective in improving attention and planning skills (Rute-Perez et al., 2014).

Another study compared iPad applications with traditional activities using a person-centered care approach. This study evaluated the impact of iPad application on well-being for persons with dementia. It showed that using an iPad group activity has a potential to be as effective and engaging as using other conventional activities in person-centered care approach in achieving well-being (Leng, Yeo, George, & Barr, 2014).

Increasingly, we are facing new challenges to provide care for our elderly population. One of the most significant challenges is caring for our seniors with dementia. Approximately 28 million people worldwide suffer from dementia. In the United States, 4.5 million persons have the diagnosis of Alzheimer's disease, the most prevalent type of dementia. The number of Americans with Alzheimer's disease and related dementias will triple to 13 million by 2050. Therefore, it is crucial to examine all modalities that can assist us in providing care for patients with dementia.

Although there have been extensive efforts to find effective medications to treat dementia, we still cannot rely on pharmacotherapy to cure this progressive and devastating disease. In some cases, medications can improve the function and behavior of the patient, but medications alone are not sufficient to manage this overwhelming disorder. Therefore, nonpharmacological therapies have always been an important asset to manage symptoms of dementia. These therapies are sometimes used in conjunction with medications, and sometimes used solely to control these symptoms.

The following are some nonpharmacological therapies for dementia:

- **Reminiscence,** which is recalling events in the patient's life.
- **Reality orientation** is reorientating the patient about time, place, and person.
- **Cognitive stimulation therapy** uses games and quizzes that can stimulate cognitive function. It can be used in mild to moderate dementia.
- **Validation therapy** is a technique that emphasizes the patient's inner reality and feelings, instead of focusing on external facts.
- **Music therapy** can decrease anxiety when used as individual music therapy, and can improve speech content and fluency when used as group music therapy.
- **Relaxation therapy** can decease behavioral disruptions and might help memory.
- **Snoezelen therapy** involves combining multisensory stimulation like using lights, tactile objects, music, and aromas. Regular use of this technique can improve behavior and mood in moderate to severe dementia.
- **Creative activities** can provide mental stimulation and make patients feel positive. (Bayer, 2010)

Providing nonpharmacological therapies needs extensive time and dedication. It can be costly to hire staff and can be exhausting for caregivers to provide these services. Here is where technology can be deployed to assist caregivers providing care to patients. In addition to such use, technology can be used directly to help with functional losses that patients face every day. These utilities are discussed further in this section.

Practical Use of Intelligent Assistive Devices

Applications for Nonpharmacological Therapies

We can explore the possible effectiveness of some computer applications and devices in nonpharmacological therapies for dementia. For example, there are some applications that provide a personalized life storybook and can be customized to design personal story pages for each patient. The application can also upload family photos, accompanied by text or voice narratives. These types of applications can provide reminiscence, which will help the patient recall his or her memories. The story pages can be filled with patient's interests, such as entertainers, films, politics, and other topics that are interesting for the patient. Some applications can play customized music by creating a customized music playlist, which can be played while the patient is reviewing other pages like story pages. These types of applications might be helpful in music and relaxation therapy. Other devices/applications can be used to reorient the patient to time and place at determined frequencies. Therefore, they can be used for reality orientation. There are some creative applications and games that could be used as creative stimulation.

Applications for Daily Struggles Secondary to Functional Losses

Aside from the use of intelligent assistive technology as a nonpharmacological modality for patients with dementia, there are technological innovations that can help these patients with day-to-day living challenges.

As memory impairment is the main cognitive concern in most types of dementia, especially Alzheimer's disease, most of these devices target this area.

Reminder messages are a good example. The messages are recorded on a device at home and then played back at appropriated times.

Phone pictures are other means that can assist patients who cannot remember the numbers.

Medication management is an important challenge for patients with dementia. There are special pillboxes designed for patients with dementia with an audible alarm that can be set to notify the patient or the caregiver.

Special clocks can also help patients with dementia. These clocks do not show the actual time but show the time of the day as morning, afternoon, evening, and night.

GPS location and tracking devices can assist patients with advanced stages of dementia with risk of wandering. They can be worn by or attached to patients. Some of them can alert emergency personnel immediately for assistance. However, in some cases, these devices should not be used as a substitute for more committed supervision (Sauer, 2014).

Although intelligent assistive technology cannot provide the human touch and cannot be recommended as a substitute to interpersonal interactions, it can definitely play a major role in supporting the caregivers, and be used as an aid to improve care for elderly people with dementia.

EVIDENCE FOR AND AGAINST MEMORY TRAINING FOR DEMENTIA

In light of the relatively minimal efficacy of existing pharmaceuticals for dementia, many researchers have begun looking beyond pills to investigate other means for preserving and enhancing cognition (AD 2000 Collaborative Goup, 2004). There has been a boom of memory-enhancing games created as applications, puzzle books, and more, with the intended purpose of regaining cognitive abilities lost through dementia, as well as holding onto those memories that remain. Studies of these interventions have been limited, leading to a misconception about the effect that they have. Initial studies of such interventions were performed on persons without dementia, and showed improved cognitive abilities in those individuals who routinely used the studied intervention. These early studies did not assess the effect of memory training on functional outcome, rather, they only assessed whether the individuals performed better on the tested intervention after a period of training with the intervention (Derwinger, Stigsdotter Neely, MacDonald, & Bäckman, 2004; O'Hara et al., 2007; Willis, 1987). Based on these interventions showing cognitive improvement, many geriatricians latched onto memory-enhancement games and puzzles, including them in the routine recommendations for patients with a new diagnosis of dementia. From puzzle books, such as Sudoku, to applications for phones, such as Lumosity, or even video games, such as Nintendo's Brain Age, there has been an explosion of memory-enhancement puzzles and games over the last decade. The question that has since been raised is, "Do they work?"

In order to answer the question of "Do they work," one must first determine what outcome is of interest. The outcome of any of these interventions is obviously not to cure dementia, but rather to mitigate the damage done by the disease on one's life. When thinking of the impact dementia has, it is best described as a loss of function. The *DSM*, in fact, defines dementia, or major neurocognitive disorder, as different from mild cognitive impairment, or mild neurocognitive disorder, based on dementia being a disorder not only of a memory decline, but also a loss of function. Hence, when assessing whether to recommend a memory game to a patient, one should ask the important question "Will this lead my patient to have an improvement in functional abilities?"

One study that set out to answer this question looked at the effects of cognitive training in a different way than had been done previously. Rather than just assessing patients' scores on the studied test before and after training, the Advanced Cognitive Training for Independent and Vital Elderly (ACTIVE) study group set out to assess patients in terms of their daily function before and after cognitive training. The ACTIVE study group is the largest independent trial to date for the assessment of cognitive training. In contrast to many prior studies on cognitive training, this study randomized its patient population in a single-blind trial. As had occurred in previous studies of cognitive training, this study excluded individuals who had cognitive impairment defined as a Mini-Mental State Exam score of less than or equal to 22. While still not answering the question we pose of whether cognitive training is of benefit to those with dementia, this study was unique in its assessment of functional impact, which brings us somewhat closer to the answer we seek. The study participants were randomized to undergo memory training, reasoning training, speed of processing training, or a control group. It was found that speed of processing training and memory training did not have a statistically significant effect on performance of IADLs, while there was a mild statistically significant benefit in IADL performance in the reasoning training group. This reported IADL improvement in the reasoning group, however, was based on a self-report of IADLs, and, ultimately, training of any type had no general effect on performance-based IADLs. The major finding of this study was that cognitive training resulted in an improvement in the ability to perform the task that was being trained in the exercises when compared with the control group. In other words, those who were assigned to memory training performed better on the memory training exercise, while those who were assigned to reasoning training performed better on the reasoning training exercise, and those assigned to the speed of processing training performed better on the speed of processing training exercise. While the cognitive training allowed the patients to perform better on the task they were trained on, they ultimately did not have a clear clinically significant change in their functional abilities as a result of this training (Willis et al., 2006).

Other studies have since attempted to provide the answer we seek, assessing whether cognitive training has any benefit in patients with dementia. Many of these studies, unfortunately, fell prey to confounders, or had other issues, such as small sample size or, again, investigating outcomes other than functional improvements (Moore, Sandman, McGrady, & Kesslak, 2001; Requena, Maestu, Campo, Fernandez, & Ortiz, 2006). It is clear from studies such as the ACTIVE study group's trial that cognitive training can help patients perform better on specific tests, but it is not clear if they also promote functional improvement.

A systematic review was published in 2011 assessing studies of cognitive training for patients with mild cognitive impairment to determine if cognitive training in this population could possibly delay or prevent development of dementia. Unfortunately, a systematic review is only as good as the studies that it summarizes, and the studies used in the systematic review were subject to the flaws of many studies performed for the assessment of cognitive training, most notable being small sample size. The largest sample size study included in the systematic review was a 2007 study of 59 patients. Some of the studies analyzed did not even include mental status scores to verify a cognitive disorder, and of the studies that did report Mini-Mental State Exam scores, the scores ranged from 17.2 to 28.9. A score of 28.9, of course, does not meet a diagnosis of mild cognitive impairment, hence muddying the interpretation of this systematic review of effects of cognitive training on mild cognitive impairment. The systematic review found wide variability in outcome measures, with the two studies that attempted to assess functional outcomes showing results similar to the ACTIVE group: improved performance on the training-specific outcome but no evidence of improvement in functional ability (Gates, Sachdev, Singh, & Valenzuela, 2011).

It is important to know the limitations of cognitive training. To date, few trials exist that have studied the effects of cognitive training alone for the treatment of dementia, and much of what we know about cognitive training is extrapolated from data assessing the training in patients without cognitive disorders. To date, the best evidence we have about cognitive training is that it will improve one's ability to perform the tasks of the training exercise, but has not shown consistent and clinically significant improvements in functional ability. Studies that exist are often limited by sample size (Gates et al., 2011), confounders (Berger et al., 2004; Requena et al., 2006), lack of randomization (Derwinger et al., 2004; O'Hara et al., 2007), or lack of inclusion of patients with cognitive disorders (Derwinger et al., 2004; O'Hara et al., 2007; Willis, 1987; Willis et al., 2006).

Unfortunately, despite this lack of clear evidence of benefit, many false claims exist in the community as to the benefits received from cognitive training. One such example is that of Lumosity, a brain-training program. This program was marketed as having the ability to delay or protect against memory decline including the prevention and delay of progression of dementia disorders. The Federal Trade Commission filed a complaint against the creators of Lumosity, resulting in a court case with Lumos Labs paying a $2 million settlement and being forbidden from making any claims or implications that the product could, in any way, delay or protect against cognitive disorders (*Federal Trade Commission v. Lumos Labs, Inc.*, 2015). Cases such as this highlight the dangers of cognitive training, as many people paid for this program under the false impression that it would correct cognitive deficits when no such evidence existed to suggest this.

A recent study published in *The Lancet* in 2015 assessed individuals aged 60 to 77 years with a moderate risk of development of dementia, assigning patients randomly to an intervention group of diet, exercise, cognitive training, and vascular risk monitoring versus a control group who just received general health advice. It was found that there was a mild improvement in cognition based on a neuropsychiatric battery of tests in the intervention group, arguing that a multimodal approach to dementia treatment may be of benefit (Ngandu et al., 2015). The limitation of this study, with regard to cognitive training, is that it grouped such an activity with other interventions, thus limiting the interpretability of the effect the addition of cognitive training had. It is argued by many researchers that cognitive training should be advocated for in addition to other lifestyle modifications, including physical exercise, as the risk of harm from cognitive training is low, even if the benefit from cognitive training is controversial and unproven (Karp et al., 2006; Wilson, Scherr, Schneider, Tang, & Bennett, 2007).

The potential harm to cognitive training in dementia is primarily one of cost. Should it be advocated by physicians to encourage patients to spend money on unproven interventions like cognitive training, knowing there is not sufficient evidence to argue for or against the intervention? It is recommended to have a careful discussion with patients about the evidence that exists for and against cognitive training, and making an individualized recommendation based on the patient's preferences and goals (Butcher, 2008). Clearly, there is evidence that cognitive training in isolation will not remedy dementia disorders. Perhaps, they may improve a patient's ability to perform specific tasks, but it remains unclear if it will improve a patient's ability to function in life. In summary, if a patient wishes to undergo cognitive training, the risks and benefits should be carefully discussed before a recommendation is made.

HOW TO ASSESS NEW TECHNOLOGIES

Increased human longevity brings with it increased rates of dementia and other cognitive disorders associated with aging. While a great deal of time and energy underlies the development of numerous technological advances designed to assist individuals with dementia and their caregivers, comparatively little thought has gone into the assessment of these tools. This section provides theoretical perspectives on the assessment of technologies for cognitive impairment.

Successful user-friendly technological innovations are developed through collaborations with behavioral scientists, engineers, and older adults. In fact, elder user preferences, patterns of use, and technology use goals must be delineated at the system-design stage if we are to design technologies to more effectively meet the needs of cognitively impaired older adults (Bouwhuis, Meesters, & Berentsen, 2008).

Lindenberger and his colleagues proposed three main principles for the evaluation of assistive technologies from a successful aging perspective (Lindenberger, Lövdén, Schellenbach, Li, & Krüger, 2008). They posited that net resource release, person specificity, and proximal versus distal frames of evaluation would allow for both useful and thorough assessment of assistive technologies. Although they did not specify cognitive impairment, this method of evaluation can easily be applied to this area.

Models exploring technology use among older adults' utilization of technology generally suggest that perceived usefulness, ease of use, and attitude toward technology, all factor into the acceptance and eventual use of that technology (Bouwhuis et al., 2008). Given that research suggests that older adults' decision-making process roughly equates to assessing how and where to expend potentially limited resources, technology's perceived usefulness is of particular relevance because older adults are less likely to allocate cognitive and financial resources into areas from which they expect fewer benefits (Baltes & Baltes, 1990). Similarly, ease of use weighs more heavily on those with cognitive or physical deficits, as resources and technological experience may be limited.

To utilize technology, the user must invest some degree of time and effort. From the perspective of an aging individual, the determination of how much time and effort and for what beneficial yield is vital because most people possess fewer internal and external resources as they grow older. Therefore, the use of a given technology is only adoptive if the costs of operation are lower than the expected benefits or gains. Described as a mathematical concept, no one wants to exert 10 units of energy to do something that saves or gains them only 5 units of energy. On the contrary, people would rather use their time and energy (personal resources) as efficiently as possible so that they may get a maximum benefit wherein 5 units of energy can yield 10 units of energy benefit. For example, learning to use a computer program can be a time-consuming and effortful process. The benefits gained from learning to use that computer program must eventually outweigh the time and effort put in for it to be considered a positive net resource release. In the area of cognitive impairment, the same thing holds true. Any technology that purports to assist a cognitively impaired individual must be evaluated in terms of net resource release. How much time/energy/effort does the use of this technology save versus the amounts used to learn that technology? In broader terms, we must determine if the use of this technology will be a wise investment for the individual with cognitive impairment (or their caregiver) given diminished resources.

Technologies addressing cognitive impairment must be also flexible and adaptable to a wide range of behaviors. Aging is highly variable both across and within individuals. Therefore, technologies developed for older adults are most effective when they can meet a wide range of highly specific and sometimes idiosyncratic needs. In terms of cognitive impairment, this means that technologies should be flexible, adaptable, and easy to use for maximum benefit. For higher order technologies, the ability to predict user goals on the basis of past behavior and/or habits is also important. Further, useful technologies must effectively adapt to the user, which can be extremely difficult in the face of cognitive decline. According to Lindenberger and his colleagues, it is preferable to learn the user's behavioral ecology before sensory, motor, or cognitive impairments occur so that newly introduced technologies can better maintain the user's lifestyle whenever possible.

Beyond assessing net resource release and highlighting person specificity, any assessment technologies for older adults with cognitive impairments must also properly weigh potential short-term and long-term benefits to the user to guard against excess disability. *Excess disability* refers to the loss of an ability that is not caused by the disease or impairment itself. In the case of cognitive decline, this commonly refers to the loss of abilities that go beyond the physiological changes that are caused by the dementia. In other words, the person suffering from cognitive decline will refuse to engage in previously mastered behaviors that should not be negatively impacted by the disease. In this situation, a balance must be struck such that the assistive technology does not create premature dependence or excess disability, but provides the user with just enough assistance to allow important goals to be reached. Over the long term, chronic disuse of certain skills or abilities will be to the user's detriment. Navigation systems can illustrate this point. In the short term, using a navigation system provides the user multiple benefits. A global positioning system (GPS) can free up cognitive resources, efficiently highlight the best routes to one's destination, and lessen stress associated with navigating unfamiliar territory. However, long-term dependence on GPS aids may ultimately weaken spatial abilities and damage navigational skills by reducing the size and efficiency of the brain structures responsible for such activities. The most effective technologies prevent excess disability and loss of autonomy by enhancing user motivation and providing some degree of challenge.

CONCLUSION

The aging population is growing at a rapid rate and seniors are actively seeking out innovative solutions for preserving physical and mental capabilities and preventing further decline. Within the past decade, a sudden influx of software, online programs, and applications has flooded the market with one goal—memory enhancement. Despite limited research supporting the efficacy of such products, developers continue to create and consumers continue to buy, with cognitive training software becoming an estimated $2 billion industry (Anderson, 2015; Lampit, Hallock, & Valenzuela, 2014). Together, researchers and developers are looking beyond rote brain training to enhance the user experience, with the goal of improving outcomes and transference of skills to authentic situations.

As developers aim to enhance current technology, understanding what has been proven to improve cognitive functioning in the elderly is critical. Much has been learned about the effects of physical activity on cognitive function, and a recent meta-analysis further supported these claims, as it was determined that physical activity does, in fact, have overall positive effects on cognitive function in dementia populations (Groot et al., 2016). This knowledge has led video game developers and researchers to create games that require users to perform both physically and cognitively challenging tasks. Maillot, Perrot, and Hartley (2012) assessed the efficacy of such products, also known as *exergaming*, predicting positive outcomes in cognitive functioning. The study revealed improvements in executive control and processing speed tasks on posttest measures, along with significant transference of skills on all measures. Although further research is needed to compare outcomes between physical activity training groups and exergaming groups, this study serves as a compelling launching pad for the further development of products aimed at enhancing cognitive skills by incorporating physical activity.

In addition to improving overall outcomes, future technology must address transference of skills into authentic settings. While past "brain game" participants have demonstrated improvements on targeted computerized cognitive training tasks, Owen et al. (2010) and Ackerman, Kanfer, and Calderwood (2010) learned that these improvements failed to cross over to similar activities not directly addressed in training. Advancements in video game technology have led to the creation of games that have the ability to place users in realistic, interactive scenarios. A 2014 observatory study analyzed the effectiveness of Xbox 360 Kinect to provide such an environment in which seniors could safely improve their driving skills. Researchers found the Kinect required users to engage beyond the cognitive skills necessary for driving, as the console closely replicated many of the visual and physical demands placed upon drivers on the road (Sue, Ray, Talaei-Khoe, Jonnagaddala, & Vichitvanichphong, 2014). These games not only allow users to practice cognitive skills with relevant tasks, but closely assess one's safety while performing such tasks in the real world. One can assume cognitive training within authentic settings will lead to improved outcomes beyond the games; however, rigorous comparative studies are still needed to support this assumption further.

Researchers are not only looking into video games as a means of improving cognitive performance in authentic situations, but also analyzing transference of skills beyond these virtual settings (Tsukayama, 2017). Virtual reality is capable of creating environments in which users focus on training the cognitive skill sets required for particular circumstances, relevant to the user's reality. For this to be of benefit, developers must have an understanding of the user's personal context, knowing the various situations encountered by the person in the real world, and the kinds of cognitive skills required to maintain functional independence (García-Betances, Jiménez-Mixco, Arredondo, & Cabrera-Umpiérrez, 2015). If successful, users have the potential to improve overall cognitive functioning while preserving the skills necessary to age safely in place at home.

As developers are redesigning and improving brain game content, researchers are analyzing how such products should be accessed and implemented. For instance, a meta-analysis found group-based computerized cognitive training was more effective than individual home-based training. Additionally, the presence of a trainer or supervisor was helpful for ensuring user compliance, providing encouragement and motivational support, pushing users to tackle more challenging tasks, and troubleshooting when technical issues arose (Lampit et al., 2014). A group setting may especially be most beneficial for users with mild cognitive impairment, as these participants were less adherent and required greater supervision for initiation and completion of tasks (Gigler, Blomeke, Shatil, Weintraub, & Reber, 2013).

While a facilitator-led group may garner better outcomes, this may be expensive and logistically impossible for many aging seniors. Researchers in Korea are attempting to solve this problem by creating robots utilized to provide instruction, motivation, and supervision. Kim et al. (2015) used brain imaging to measure changes in cortical thickness following traditional cognitive training and robot-assisted cognitive training. While cortical thinning over time was less than the control group (participants receiving no cognitive training), there was no significant difference between robot-assisted and traditional cognitive training. Results indicate robots may be capable of replacing group facilitators without impacting outcomes. Studies on the effectiveness of robotics are still few and far between, but the technology is becoming increasingly sophisticated and has the potential to lead to a cost-effective strategy for community-dwelling seniors and residential care communities to access cognitive training in mass.

As brain game content and implementation evolve, developers must also consider cost and accessibility with the design of future iterations. Users of such technology are currently responsible for covering the costs associated with the software and hardware discussed in this chapter. A lack of evidence-based research demonstrating the positive effects these devices may have on functional outcomes, or reducing health care expenditures, prevents Medicare and other insurance providers from justifying reimbursement for their cost. The out-of-pocket expense for many of these items is simply too much for a majority of aging Americans living on a fixed income. As health care providers, one must consider the cost and benefit before making such recommendations to patients.

Although seniors are increasing the incorporation of technology into their daily lives, many simply do not have access to personal computers and electronic devices, or a reliable Internet connection. As of 2015, 55% of U.S. adults aged 65 years and older reported owning a desktop or laptop, 32% reported owning a tablet, and just over half of seniors reported accessing the Internet "at least occasionally" (Anderson, 2015; Perrin, & Duggan, 2015). Technology use among the elderly population is expected to increase over time, but even those seniors with extensive experience will find it difficult to keep up financially and skills wise owing to the rapid rate at which technology improves. Exergaming, virtual reality, and robots are exciting prospects, but if users are unable to afford or operate such devices, their outcomes will be as limited as their predecessors.

Looking forward, researchers must increase the rigor of their methodology and closely evaluate all variables impacting performance and efficacy of technology-based cognitive training for aging populations. Training scenarios in which the user can practice in authentic, virtual environments may result in improved skill transference, while incorporating physical activity may just lead to better outcomes. What must not be overlooked as researchers and developers create novel and innovative products, however, are the users themselves.

REFERENCES

Ackerman, P., Kanfer, R., & Calderwood, C. (2010). Use it or lose it? Wii brain exercise practice and reading for domain knowledge. *Psychology and Aging, 25*, 753–766.

AD 2000 Collaborative Goup. (2004). Long-term donepezil treatment in 565 patients with Alzheimer's disease (AD2000): Randomised double-blind trial. *The Lancet, 363*(9427), 2105–2115.

American Psychiatric Association. (2013). *Diagnostic and statistical manual of mental disorders* (5th ed.). Arlington, VA: American Psychiatric Publishing.

Anderson, M. (2015, October 15). Demographics of device ownership. Technology Device Ownership: 2015. Retrieved from Pew Research Center: http://www.pewinternet.org/2015/10/29/the-demographics-of-device-ownership

Baltes, P. B., & Baltes, M. M. (1990). Psychological perspectives on successful aging: The model of selective optimization with compensation. In P. B. Baltes & M. M. Baltes (Eds.), *Successful aging: Perspectives from the behavioral sciences* (pp. 1–30). New York, NY: Cambridge University Press.

Bayer, A. (2010). Presentation and management of dementia. *Brocklehurst's textbook of geriatric medicine and gerontology* (7th ed., pp. 392–401). Philadelphia, PA: Saunders Elsevier.

Berger, G., Bernhardt, T., Schramm, U., Müller, R., Landsiedel-Anders, S., Peters, J., . . . Frolich, L. (2004). No effects of a combination of caregivers support group and memory training/music therapy in dementia patients from a memory clinic population. *International Journal of Geriatric Psychiatry, 19*(3), 223–231.

Bharucha, A., Anand, V., Forlizzi, J., Dew, M. A., Reynolds, C. F. 3rd., Stevens, S., & Wactlar, H. (2009). Intelligent assistive technology applications to dementia care: Current capabilities, limitation, and future challenges. *American Journal of Geriatric Psychiatry, 17*(2), 88–104.

Bouwhuis, D. G., Meesters, M. J., & Berentsen, J. (2008). Technology acceptance models in gerontechnology. *Gerontechnology, 7*(2), 78.

Butcher, J. (2008). Mind games do they work? *British Medical Journal, 336*(7638), 246–248.

Derwinger, A., Stigsdotter Neely, A., MacDonald, S., & Bäckman, L. (2004). Forgetting numbers in old age: Strategy and learning speed matter. *Gerontology, 51*, 277–284.

Federal Trade Commission v. Lumos Labs, Inc. Case No. 3:16-cv-00001-sk. 2015. (United States District Court for the Northern District of California, San Francisco Division).

Forster, E., & Lewy, F. H. (1912). *Handbuch der Neurologie: Paralysis agitans* (p. 920). Berlin, Germany: Springer-Verlag.

García-Betances, R., Jiménez-Mixco, V., Arredondo, M., & Cabrera-Umpiérrez, M. (2015, February). Using virtual reality for cognitive training of the elderly. *American Journal of Alzheimer's Disease and Other Dementias, 30*(1), 49–50. doi:10.1177/1533317514545866

Gates, N., Sachdev, P., Singh, M., & Valenzuela, M. (2011). Cognitive and memory training in adults at risk of dementia: A systematic review. *BioMed Central Geriatrics, 11*, 55.

Gigler, K., Blomeke, K., Shatil, E., Weintraub, S., & Reber, P. (2013, January 1). Preliminary evidence for the feasibility of at-home online cognitive training with older adults. *Gerontechnology, 12*(1), 26–35.

Groot, C., Hooghiemstra, A., Raijmakers, P., Berckel, B., Scheltens, P., Scherder, E., . . . Ossenkoppele, R. (2016, January). The effect of physical activity on cognitive function patients with dementia: A meta-analysis of randomized control trials. *Aging Research Reviews, 25*, 13–23. doi:10.1016/j.arr.2015.11.005

Hebert, L. E., Weuve, J., Scherr, P. A., & Evans, D. A. (2013). Alzheimer disease in the United States (2010–2050) estimated using the 2010 census. *Neurology, 80*(19), 1778–1783.

Karp, A., Paillard-Borg, S., Wang, H. X., Silverstein, M., Winblad, B., & Fratiglioni, L. (2006). Mental, physical and social components in leisure activities equally contribute to decrease dementia risk. *Dementia and Geriatric Cognitive Disorders, 21*(2), 65–73.

Kim, G., Jeon, S., Im K., Kwon, H., Lee, B. H., Kim, G. Y., . . . Na, D, L. (2015). Structural brain changes after traditional and robot-assisted multi-domain cognitive training in community-dwelling healthy elderly. *PLOS ONE, 10*(4), e0123251. doi:10.1371/journal.pone.0123251

Lampit, A., Hallock, H., & Valenzuela, M. (2014, November 18). Computerized cognitive training in cognitively healthy older adults: A systematic review and meta-analysis of effect modifiers. *PLOS Medicine, 11*(11), e1001756.

Leng, F. Y., Yeo, D., George, S., & Barr, C. (2014). Comparison of iPad applications with traditional activities using person -centered care approach: Impact on well-being of person's with dementia. *Dementia, 13*(2), 265–273.

Lindenberger, U., Lövdén, M., Schellenbach, M., Li, S. C., & Krüger, A. (2008). Psychological principles of successful aging technologies: A mini-review. *Gerontology, 54*(1), 59–68.

Maillot, P., Perrot, A., & Hartley, A. (2012). Effects of interactive physical-activity videogame training on physical and cognitive function in older adults. *Psychology and Aging, 27*(3), 589–600.

Moore, S., Sandman, C., McGrady, K., & Kesslak, J. (2001). Memory training improves cognitive ability in patients with dementia. *Neuropsychological Rehabilitation: An International Journal, 11*(3–4), 245–261.

Ngandu, T., Lehtisalo, J., Solomon, A., Levälahti, E., Ahtiluoto, S., Antikainen, R., . . . Kivipelto M. (2015). A 2 year multidomain intervention of diet, exercise, cognitive training, and vascular risk monitoring versus control to prevent cognitive decline in at-risk elderly people (FINGER): A randomised controlled trial. *The Lancet, 385*(9984), 2255–2263.

O'Hara, R., Brooks, J. O., Friedman, L., Schröder, C. M., Morgan, K. S., & Kraemer, H. C. (2007). Long-term effects of mnemonic training in community-dwelling older adults. *Journal of Psychiatric Research, 41*(7), 585–590.

Owen, A., Hampshire, A., Grahn, J. A., Stenton, R., Dajani, S., Burns, A. S., & Ballard, C. G. (2010, June 10). Putting brain training to the test. *Nature, 465*(7299), 775–778. doi:10.1038/nature09042

Perrin, A., & Duggan, M. (2015, June 26). Americans' internet access: 2000–2015. Retrieved from http://www.pewinternet.org/2015/06/26/americans-internet-access-2000-2015

Requena, C., Maestu, F., Campo, P., Fernandez, A., & Ortiz, T. (2006). Effects of cholinergic drugs and cognitive training on dementia: 2-year follow-up. *Dementia and Geriatric Cognitive Disorders, 22*(4), 339–345.

Rute-Perez, S., Santiago-Ramajo, S., Vistacion Hurtado, M., Jose Rodriguez-Fortiz, M., & Caracuel, A. (2014). Challenges in software applications for the cognitive evaluation and stimulation of the elderly. *Journal of NeuroEngineering and Rehabilitation, 11*, 88.

Sauer, A. (2014, September 24). 7 technological innovations for those with dementia. Retrieved from Alzheimers.net: http://www.alzheimers.net/9-22-14-technology-for-dementia

Sue, D., Ray, P., Talaei-Khoe, A., Jonnagaddala, J., & Vichitvanichphong, S. (2014). Assessing video games to improve driving skills: A literature review and observational study. *Journal of Medical Internet Research, 2*(2), e5. doi:10.2196/games.3274

Tsukayama, H. (2016, November 17). This physician is using virtual reality to treat patients with dementia. *The Washington Post*. Retrieved from https://www.washingtonpost.com/news/the-switch/wp/2016/11/17/this-physician-is-using-virtual-reality-to-treat-patients-with-dementia/?utm_term=.363b6936ca3b

Willis, S. L. (1987). Cognitive training and everyday competence. *Annual Review of Gerontology and Geriatrics, 7*, 159–188.

Willis, S. L., Tennstedt, S. L., Marsiske, M., Ball, K., Elias, J., Koepke, K. M., . . . ACTIVE Study Group. (2006). Long-term effects of cognitive training on everyday functional outcomes in older adults. *Journal of the American Medical Association, 296*(23), 2805–2814.

Wilson, R. S., Scherr, P. A., Schneider, J. A., Tang, Y., & Bennett, D. A. (2007). Relation of cognitive activity to risk of developing Alzheimer disease. *Neurology, 69*(20), 1911–1920.

8

Advances in Medication Adherence Technology in the Elderly Population

Kevin M. Krcmarik

Caring for the geriatric population can be a challenging endeavor, especially when considering the numerous issues that they may have to cope with on a daily basis. Chronic debilitating illnesses, sustainable nutrition, physical deconditioning and weakness with subsequent loss of independence, depression or other psychiatric illnesses, and cognitive integrity are some challenges, to name a few. Oftentimes, elderly individuals find themselves in a situation where they are faced with the responsibility of taking multiple medications to address their numerous health concerns. The issue of medication adherence can be a complicated one, especially in light of these factors.

ISSUES IN MEDICATION ADHERENCE AMONG THE ELDERLY POPULATION

So what is meant by "adherence"? The term has been previously defined by WHO as "the extent to which a person's behavior—taking medication, following a diet, and/or executing lifestyle changes, corresponds with agreed recommendations from a health care provider" (WHO, 2003). Numerous and diverse studies have consistently identified that problems with medication adherence contribute to major public health challenges, especially within the scope of chronic disease state management, which is most characteristic of older adults. Consequences of poor adherence may include (but are not limited to) increased rates of emergency department visits, lengthy and multiple readmissions to hospitals, and increased morbidity and mortality, which collectively burden our health care system and consume valuable resources (Butler, Davis, Johnson, & Gardner, 2011).

Indeed, medication adherence is a major global challenge as more than half of individuals with chronic diseases do not take any or all of their medications correctly (Haynes, McDonald, & Garg, 2002; WHO, 2003). In one quantitative review of 50 years of research, DiMatteo (2004) reports an average nonadherence rate of 24.8% across 17 diseases conditions. As an example of some of the extremes, higher mean adherence rates were found in HIV disease (88.3%), arthritis (81.2%), and gastrointestinal (GI) disorders (80.4%), while relatively lower adherence rates were found in diabetes (67.5%), pulmonary diseases (68.8%), and sleep disorders (65.5%). Obviously, there is no constant number that can embody a singular rate of adherence or nonadherence, as the rate estimates vary according to both demographic and disease-specific variables. Regardless, the problem of medication adherence is a significant one with important consequences. Besides the sheer magnitude of nonadherent users, the financial and health-related costs of nonadherence are also significant. As reported by Osterberg and Blaschke (synthesized from earlier reports), in a widely quoted 2005 report in the *New England Journal of Medicine*, 33% to 69% of all medication-related hospital admissions in the United States were due to poor medication adherence, constituting a direct financial cost of $100 billion per year. Computing in indirect costs, the total estimate rises to a staggering $290 billion annually. Keeping these costs in mind (which likely constitutes a significant underestimate in today's terms), it is already well established that optimizing medication adherence across a wide range of chronic disease states correlates with lower medical and hospital costs (Bitton, Choudhry, Matlin, Swanton, & Shrank, 2013; Kane & Shaya, 2008; Roebuck, Liberman, Gemmill-Toyama, & Brennan, 2011; Pinsky et al., 2009; Sokol, McGuigan, Verbrugge, & Epstein, 2005; Wan, Kozma, Slaton, Olson, & Feagan, 2014). In addition to the financial implications, health outcomes must also be considered in appreciating the value of modern advances toward improving medication adherence. Numerous examples of increased morbidity and hospitalization abound in the literature in terms of medication nonadherence. A few more recent examples include:

- An increased fracture risk in patients noncompliant with bisphosphonate therapy in osteoporosis (Eisenberg, Placzek, Gu, Krishna, & Tulsi, 2015; Mikyas, Agodoa, & Yurgin, 2014; Modi, Siris, Tang, & Sen, 2015; Siris et al., 2009)

- Increased resource utilization, reduced metabolic control, poorer physical and mental conditioning, and increased morbidity and mortality in diabetic individuals with poor adherence to oral hypoglycemic therapy (Asche, LaFleur, & Connor, 2011; Ho et al., 2006; Jha, Aubert, Yao, Teagarden, & Epstein, 2012; Wild, 2012)
- Higher risk of adverse outcomes, including all-cause hospitalization and cardiovascular disease (CVD) hospitalization in patients with poor adherence to antihypertensive medicines (Shin et al., 2013; Wu et al., 2010)

Thus, the huge financial ramifications and the increased morbidity and mortality described previously become drivers in the development of adherence technologies in the quest to change or reinforce behaviors that will ultimately lead to improvements in the lives of our elderly population. In their 2003 report calling for action to address nonadherence, WHO emphasized that advancing the current state of adherence interventions may produce a significantly greater impact on public health compared with any other singular improvement in specific medical treatment (WHO, 2003). Therefore, it becomes imperative to become aware of and to understand the technology available to both monitor and optimize medication adherence, especially in the elderly population.

So, what is at the root of medication nonadherence in the geriatric population? The answer is quite complex, embodying a large spectrum of causes identified in many published investigations. One recent systematic review of the barriers affecting medication adherence in older adults by Yap, Thirumoorthy, and Kwan (2015) narrowed down a group of 65 articles from over 17,000, identifying 80 factors that they subsequently grouped into five different categories: patient, physician, medication related, systems based, and all other factors—all of which contribute to poor medication adherence. For the sake of this topic we do not expound on such categorization, but note that a sampling of various "barriers" to adherence includes:

- Lack of financial resources (Wheeler, Roberts, & Neiheisel, 2014)
- Disability (sight and hearing; Vlasnik, Aliotta, & DeLor, 2005)
- Isolation/lack of caregivers (generally, patients with inadequate social support do poorly and have worse medication adherence; Catz, Kelley, Bogart, Benotsch, & McAuliffe, 2000; Scheurer, Choudhry, Swanton, Matlin, & Shrank, 2012; Zullig et al., 2015)
- Frequent changes and limited confidence in medications, anger or denial about the illness, and avoidance of adverse side effects (Hincapie, Taylor, Boesen, & Warholak, 2015; Ho et al., 2006; Vlasnik et al., 2005)

- Existential uncertainty involved in the self-management of medications caused by the fear of side effects and medical errors. Summer and Engstrom (2015) conducted a study via interviews exploring the experiences of elderly persons 75 years old with multimorbidity. They concluded that a good relationship between health professionals and elderly patients was a prerequisite to reduce stressors related to medication management and adherence
- Inadequate doctor–patient relationship (Martin, Mellotte, & O'Neill, 2005)
- Polypharmacy. As life expectancy has increased, so have the number of chronic diseases and comorbidities that the elderly population must cope with. As these accumulate, so do the number of accompanying medications inevitably prescribed to address these issues. One feasibility study of a systemic approach for discontinuation of multiple medications in 70 elderly adults reported an average use of 7.7 medications per adult (Garfinkel & Mangin, 2010). Ultimately, this issue of polypharmacy becomes significant because medication adherence decreases as the number of medications increases (Vlasnik et al., 2005)
- Cognitive impairment/forgetfulness (especially in elderly subjects) inclusive of memory and knowledge of medications (Campbell et al., 2016)

Drawing from this idea of barriers to medication adherence, care providers can be better prepared to identify and address nonadherence, whether it overtly becomes apparent or not. Perhaps a tremendous amount of financial resources may be otherwise spared if subsequent interventions can be further developed to address the problem of nonadherence. Despite these hopeful gains, one idea is earning increasing attention: No one type of technological intervention may optimally satisfy a patient's specific barriers to adherence. Utilizing multifaceted interventions to target multiple adherence determinants may prove to be the most reliable strategy in this effort (Kardas, Lewek, & Matyjaszczyk, 2013).

Many of the innovations and technologies that are discussed are not necessarily unique in their application to any one demographic or age group, as problems with medication adherence are common to all age groups. But, in considering the unique challenges that the elderly population must cope with—whether directly from morbidity of chronic disease states, socioeconomic factors, or from general sensory or cognitive disabilities—these modern and evolving endeavors to identify, characterize, and optimize adherence become immediately relevant.

ELECTRONIC MONITORING DEVICES AND REMINDER TECHNOLOGY

Traditionally, evaluating medication adherence has included pill counting, checking prescription refill rates, using self-report tools, and clinically following symptoms under the assumption that improvements or stability of such can be attributed to adequate adherence (Park, Howie-Esquivel, & Dracup, 2015). These more indirect methods have not proven as accurate when compared with directly observed therapy, where a health care worker watches a patient swallow each dose of medication. Collectively, however, all of these traditional methods require time, money, and resources to be successful, and are not always scalable or practical for chronic disease state management in the general population. Furthermore, they have been shown to be inaccurate in some cases (Laine et al., 2000; Osterberg & Blaschke, 2005). Nonetheless, they continue to play a role in our current state of medication therapy management (MTM), and their effectiveness is optimized and complemented by the use of relatively newer technologies of electronic monitoring.

The market for electronic devices geared toward monitoring and optimizing adherence has been rapidly developing in the past few years with the technological advancement of various electronic sensors and wireless devices. Traditional devices presently in use are continuously evolving to rapidly collect, organize, store, and/or analyze adherence events and patterns while providing feedback to patients and their providers (Park et al., 2015). Despite these advancements, special attention has been called to further delineate the functional capabilities of these technologies in both clinical and research settings (Ingerski, Hente, Modi, & Hommel, 2011). A list of several of these types of electronic monitoring devices or platforms more commonly described in the literature includes:

- Electronic medication dispensers (bottles and boxes) and blister packs
- Wirelessly observed therapy (WOT)
- Tactile, pulse-stimulation medication reminders[1]
- Digital medicine via ingestible sensors
    - Smartphone applications
    - Mobile short message service (SMS) reminders
- Video- and photo-assisted observation
- Electronic health records

[1]The MemoPatch® is an additional device designed to optimize medication adherence. Unlike the others, however, it serves predominantly as a reminder tool rather than a means to identify or aid in characterizing adherence.

For the sake of staying focused on the general concepts of evolving MTM adherence technology rather than providing a detailed explanation of all possible devices, let us take a closer look at some of the more representative of the technologies previously mentioned, as they illustrate the basic advances behind today's current and upcoming adherence technologies.

Pill Bottle and Pill Box Dispenser Technologies

Attempts at empowering patients toward medication adherence have traditionally been addressed with the application of pill box organizers and blister packs, which are still widely used today owing to their easy availability, low cost, and relatively straightforward concept. However, in their conventional state, pill organizers do not always address the problem of patient forgetfulness to take medication(s). Over time, these simple tools have evolved in the wake of persistently poor adherence rates and the need for more sophisticated interventions. Abbey, Alipour, Camp, and Hofer (2012), in their published work on constructing an ideal, organized dispensing mechanism, denote the ideal picture of what pill-dispensing technology should offer—an intuitive, portable design that is user friendly, yet flexible in its operational and programming capabilities. They attempted building an electronic model that would address the functional issues of adherence, portability, monitoring, notification, and cleaning—all of which, even at present, may variably pose challenges even in updated versions. If we keep the ideas of Abbey et al. in mind, we can now look more closely at the technological advances of newer versions of pill bottles and pill boxes.

When simple pill bottles and boxes become paired with programmable reminder capabilities, they acquire the capacity to address unintentional nonadherence (also known as forgetfulness; Browne, Behzadi, & Littlewort, 2015; Paterson, Kinnera, Bond, & McKinstrey, 2016). Depending on the particular device, upgraded capabilities of these newer generation pill-organizing devices may include (Ayoade & Oladipo, 2012; Comstock, 2013; Paterson et al., 2016; Vitality, 2010):

- Prompting patients to take a medication using audible and/or visual cues such as alarms or flashing lights (in order to avoid missed or untimely doses)
- Dispensing medications automatically at proper times so as to prevent intentional or unintentional abuse
- Giving instructions to the patient, such as providing an electronic voice telling the patient how many pills to take when he or she opens the case

- Contacting a health care provider via text message or email if medicines were not removed or were taken at the wrong time
- Connecting to smartphone applications involving schedules, a calendar, and having the ability to notify family members about missed doses
- Generating reports for remote caregivers, and calling them when a dose is missed, or if a medication requires refilling
- Allowing for reminders and alerts to be programmed by caregivers or health care professionals (to integrate other care providers and ensure correct dosing)
- Locking and unlocking automatically on a programmed basis consistent with windows when patients should be taking the medication(s), so as to prevent abuse
- Sensing the amount of medication that may be left inside a bottle device to help in preventing overdose
- Running on spare battery pack power should the power in the patient's house go out

It should be noted, however, that well-documented limitations of these devices include the inability to account for discrepancies between electronic cap opening and actual intake, portability issues, and mechanical failure (Bova et al., 2005; Hamilton, 2003; Wendel et al., 2001). In addition, these devices cannot account for intentional or unintentional nonadherence if they decide to decant pills into a different container (Bova et al., 2005; Wendel et al., 2011). Despite their extra features, it is not known whether electronic or automated versions provide any advantage over their traditional counterparts in terms of better adherence to a medication plan (Paterson et al., 2016). Nonetheless, there is evidence in the literature that such devices may be of value for some patients who have been assessed as having practical problems in managing their medicines (Galloway, Coyle, Guillen, Flower, & Mendelson, 2011; Paterson et al., 2016). One interesting prospective, randomized study of 80 post–renal transplant patients (followed for 1 year), whose adherence was evaluated using an electronic medication dispenser with wireless tracking of medicine taking behavior, concluded that the use of the device was associated with high compliance and indications of a lower rejection rate (Henriksson, Tyden, Hoijer, & Wadstrom, 2016).

Several technology companies have built upon the pill bottle construct by designing progressively more sophisticated containers whose caps (referred to as "medication event monitoring systems" or "MEMS" for short) contain a computer chip that logs a date and time-stamped event each time the cap to the bottle is opened. Based on the particular device, this information registered in the cap is downloaded via a separate reader to a computer (Ailinger, Black, & Lima-Garcia, 2008; Park et al., 2015), and/or it is transmitted wirelessly through a mobile network to designated care providers (Vitality, 2010), who can then observe the cumulative log and possibly identify potential patterns of nonadherence. As evaluated in earlier adherence studies (Hamilton et al., 2003; Schwed et al., 1999), this electronic cap/reader system technology has become a common method of adherence measurement owing to its widespread acceptance by patients. While some of these devices may be purchased over the counter, it appears that many more advanced versions are obtainable via provision from hospitals and providers on behalf of their patients.

In an attempt to alleviate problems with adherence in patients taking multiple medications, various electronic medication organizers (enhanced versions of pill boxes) available today are capable of providing "real-time data on adherence" (Park et al., 2015). The most innovative of these also combine real-time electronic monitoring with text message, email, fax, automated phone call, or even customized electronic medical record reminders if they forget to take their medications. Additional features of specific devices may include use of Bluetooth technology interfacing with the Internet to create user profiles by patients and providers, and preprogrammed, timed relay of adherence data via communication with a modem/landline to a secure website that can be accessed by patients and providers alike (Haberer et al., 2012; Vervloet, Linn, et al., 2012).

Are these more technologically savvy electronic multicompartment medication devices of particular benefit to the elderly population in terms of improving rates of adherence? Although the answer may intuitively seem "yes," it has not been firmly established as far as this author is aware because of lack of sufficiently robust data. Interestingly, in an intensive systematic review by Paterson et al. (2016) gauging whether these devices actually improved adherence, the study authors found that elderly users with "cognitive problems" and those "with conditions where timing and adherence to medication regimens are critical were the groups *most likely* to benefit from these more sophisticated reminder devices." They also reported that ease of use, device portability, and flexibility with setting reminder times were issues that still needed to be addressed (Paterson, 2016). It should also be emphasized that despite the advantages that these newer devices offer over older designs, they still can neither directly monitor actual medication ingestion, nor can they pair their adherence data with more sophisticated physiological variables, as we see subsequently. The recent development of WOT is doing just this, and allowing providers to gain a fuller and unique picture of the adherence patterns of their patients.

WOT and Reminder Patch Technologies

In contrast to these more conventional and traditional methods, newer technologies are emerging to empower patients to take their medications on a timely prescribed basis, as well as to directly identify patterns of adherence. WOT has been studied in both healthy volunteers as well as in patients with chronic disease states, such as diabetes, heart failure, hypertension, renal transplantation, schizophrenia, bipolar disorder, and tuberculosis (TB). WOT carries a more objective accounting of patient adherence to medications, while providing the additional benefit of expanded data and remote-monitoring capabilities. In contrast, reminder patch technology, involving self-adhesive and fully automated dermal patches, offers solid support in reminding patients to take their prescribed medications via a delivery of timed stimuli to take the medication, as well as to change the patch. The driving hope is that both of these technologies, because of their more integrated relationship with the individual user, will uniquely empower, yet demand less of patients and caregivers in the quest for optimal adherence. Let us first consider a novel patch/reminder system that approaches the business of reminder technology from a different perspective that was described earlier with pill bottle/box dispenser technologies.

Therasolve MemoPatch

In an effort to address the pervasive problem of forgetfulness, which significantly contributes to nonadherence, a new technology utilizing tactile pulse stimulation to remind patients of a scheduled medication dose appears to have promising commercial use. Therasolve, a Belgian medical technology company based at Hasselt University campus in Belgium, has developed the concept of a wearable adhesive patch (MemoPatch) that delivers nonpainful pulsatile stimuli to discretely remind its users of the need to take medications on a prescribed basis. It is a preprogrammed product conventionally worn on the upper arm and marketed as "stick and play" by its creators. The product has a dedicated pair of unique, carefully researched, low-intensity electrical signals (impulse currents) that both notify users of their next upcoming dose, and of the need to remove and replace a new patch on a weekly basis.

Although rather straightforward in concept and having a proprietary technology, the MemoPatch offers unique advantages over traditional reminder systems, such as pillboxes and MEMS devices. First, the signal impulse is invisible, discreet, and soundless—this latter advantage is especially useful in elderly patients with hearing and visual impairments, and who may otherwise have to rely on audio or verbal cues to remember to take their next dose. The tactile impulse overrules the need for visual or auditory reminders as long as the patient is able to make the obvious connection between the impulse and the timely need to take the next medication dose. Although this technology could have variable benefits in older subjects with significant cognitive challenges who may not remember this link, it otherwise could play an indispensable role in medication adherence, considering other technologies may not be either as relevant or feasible in an elderly population. In their report on the description and specification of the MemoPatch technology, W. De Geest, J. De Geest, S. De Geest, and Abraham (2007) emphasize the utility of the MemoPatch as aiming

> to reduce the "psychological distance" between device and reminder event; to improve the privacy of both reminder system and reminder event; to increase the simplicity of the compliance-enhancing intervention; to offer a seamless integration of medication-taking into daily life; to shorten the cognitive chain involved in compliance behavior; to promote patient acceptance of and confidence in reminder systems; and to stimulate a sense of self-responsibility on the part of the patient. (p. 508)

Although clinical trial data are pending until mid-2016, previously conducted feasibility studies demonstrate convincing safety profiles. As detailed in a study by Abraham, J. De Geest, W. De Geest, De Troy, & MacDonald (2015), no serious adverse effects were noted in a study population of 147 healthy adult human volunteers whom the authors subjected to multiple randomly sequenced signals varying in rise and fall time, width, and current intensity. Minor skin rash from the patch itself was noted in five of the subjects. The researchers concluded that "this study yielded five effective and safe candidate signals for potential use in the MemoPatch device, which have since been adapted technically and tested under additional conditions and constraints." They further noted that "the [impulse] signals were found to be virtually independent from, and therefore highly robust relative to sex, BMI, upper body adiposity, and skin impedance at the patch site, lending additional generalizability to the signals and hence their potential relevance to broad commercial application" (Abraham et al., 2015).

As reported in *Business Wire*, Therasolve obtained a U.S. patent for its technology in September 2015, and clinical testing among elderly patients began in November of the same year, with results pending as of mid-2016 (*Business Wire*, 2015a, 2015b). The advent of this new technology appears very promising, as evidenced by its claim to "Best Medtech Innovation" at the European Life Sciences Summit Biomedica of 2015 (Therasolve Press Release, 2015). The future hope for this technology is that it will be integrated into the delivery of a wide variety of medication types such as "pill(s), inhalers, eye drops, ointments, injections" and possibly even "be combined or integrated with transdermal drug patches" (Therasolve Press Release, 2015). As of the end of 2016, the Therasolve MemoPatch was not yet commercially available. It has not yet been finalized as to how and through which channels the MemoPatch will be made available to end customers, or whether a prescription will be required or not.

Digital Medicine: Proteus Discover®

Until now, the electronic monitoring technologies that we have discussed constitute indirect methods of gauging adherence. One of the more interesting approaches that may find its way into widespread clinical use is Proteus Discover. Developed by Proteus Digital Health, Inc., this technology is the first of its kind cleared by the U.S. Food and Drug Administration (FDA) that can directly measure medication adherence. It consists of a tiny (1 × 1-mm sized) ingestible sensor composed of silicon, coated with traces of copper and magnesium (minerals that are part of our regular diet and safe to be ingested). This sensor can be coupled with medication and ingested in a number of ways: within a placebo tablet that is taken at the same time as the medication; coencapsulated with the medication in a capsule by the pharmacist; or integrated within the medication during the medication's manufacturing process—the first of these integrated digital medications is currently under FDA review.

Once the sensor is ingested, the magnesium and copper inside the sensor become wet, triggering an electrochemical reaction that powers the circuit inside the sensor (similar to the principle behind a "potato battery"). Once activated, the sensor sends a unique message to the adhesive wearable sensor patch worn by the patient on the left lower torso, which records the date and time of the sensor ingestion. The ingestible sensor data (time stamped) is paired with additional physiological data from the wearable patch related to body angle, exercise (step count, duration of activity/rest), and heart rate. The ingestible sensor passes through the digestive system and is eliminated in the feces. Ultimately, the composite information from the ingestible sensor and wearable patch sensor is encrypted and then transmitted wirelessly using Bluetooth technology to a designated mobile device with communication to a secure data server/cloud (Au-Yeung & DiCarlo, 2012; Au-Yeung et al., 2011; DiCarlo, 2012; DiCarlo et al., 2012; Enriquez, 2015). The software application on the mobile device can display information about medication-taking patterns including the type of medication, dosage and time of ingestion, and the user's physiological data. The Proteus data and analytics can be securely accessed via a web portal by those authorized by the patient (e.g., health care providers, family, or other caregivers). One study has detailed the usefulness of employing additional interpretive software, which can organize and visually display the multiple streams of data to show patterns of adherence that can be grasped quickly, and serve as a basis for designing interventions to help enhance and modify adherence behaviors (Browne, Behzadi, & Littlewort, 2015).

Described in a study published in the journal *IEEE Transactions on Biomedical Engineering* (Hafezi et al., 2015), the new ingestible sensor/patch technology is "the first instance of a micro-fabricated integrated circuit developed and approved for daily ingestion by patients" (Enriquez, 2015). This recent IEEE report details this new ingestible pill technology as safe, reliable, and highly accurate, with a positive detection accuracy of sensor-detected ingestions of approximately 99.1% under direct observation (Hafezi et al., 2015). Recently, this technology has been studied in patients with schizophrenia and bipolar disorder (Kane et al., 2013; Profit et al., 2016), TB (Au-Yeung & DiCarlo, 2012; Browne, Haubrich, et al., 2015), uncontrolled hypertension with or without type 2 diabetes (DiCarlo et al., 2015; Frias et al., 2016), post–renal transplant patients (Eisenberger et al., 2013), patients being treated for hepatitis C (Bonacini et al., 2016), and pulmonary hypertension (Corris, Day, Gibiansky, Kim, & DiCarlo, 2016). Throughout various recent studies, the technology has been referred to by various names such as digital health feedback system (DHFS), digital medicine system (DMS), or, more generally, WOT.

Some interesting findings in these studies include the following:

- Compared with directly observed ingestion, the system's positive detection accuracy, or ability to detect the ingestible sensor, is 99.3% (95% CI, 0.977, 0.999; DiCarlo, 2012).
- In a study with patients diagnosed with schizophrenia and/or bipolar disorder (Kane et al., 2013), 70% (19) of the 96% (27) of patients who completed the study found the Proteus DHFS concept easy to understand, and 89% thought that it could be useful to them in managing their health condition. The mean +/− standard deviation adherence rate was 74% +/− 25% (95% CI, 64%–86%). There were no documented serious adverse device effects. Mild and self-limited skin irritation from the patch was reported in 18% (5) of the patients (Kane et al., 2013).
- In a recent nonrandomized, prospective clinical trial (Profit et al., 2016) designed to rapidly assess the technical performance and safety of the Proteus DMS in patients taking aripiprazole, a high accuracy rate of

overall ingestion detection was noted (96.6%). The average time for signal transmission from ingestion to wearable sensor detection ranged from 1.1 to 1.3 minutes. Within 30 minutes of ingestion, approximately 90% of ingestions were registered by the smartphone charged with receiving the data from the sensor patch. As with the Kane study, no serious adverse effects were noted.

- In a simulated WHO-based treatment model (Au-Yeung & DiCarlo, 2012) of TB patients comparing the cost of WOT versus directly observed therapy (DOT) for adherence confirmation, using WOT demonstrated a number of potential advantages. Cost savings of WOT were reflected in reductions in resources and time which would normally be dedicated to treatment supervision with DOT. Providers would be able "to treat respectively 2.7 times and 1.4 times more patients compared to 7-day and 3-day DOT." Furthermore, it was hypothesized that WOT may reduce the need for patients to travel to a designated location for DOT, thus allowing for greater patient privacy and productivity, as well as a reduction in their travel expenses.
- Browne, Haubrich, et al. (2015), more recently investigated the safety and positive detection accuracy (PDA) of WOT with the Proteus technology via coencapsulation of the ingestible sensor with a combination TB drug using a gelatin capsule. In a randomized bioequivalence (BE) study comparing overencapsulated drugs with native forms of the drug in 12 patients with active TB, the authors determined that overencapsulation with the ingestible sensor was both safe and bioequivalent to the standard drug. Additionally, not only was the PDA of WOT shown to be equivalent to DOT, but WOT actually outperformed DOT by confirming more drug doses ingested than DOT, overall.
- DiCarlo et al. (2015), in their registry study evaluating the impact of Proteus Discover in 150 patients with uncontrolled hypertension (taking at least two antihypertensive medications), demonstrated that the technology platform was able to "help identify the root cause of persistent hypertension (for 100% of subjects) and help 37% achieve blood pressure (BP) control within 2 weeks." In this brief interval, the mean systolic BP decreased from 158 ± 16 to 143 ± 16, and the mean diastolic BP decreased from 83 ± 12 to 77 ± 10. The authors concluded that "the Proteus platform demonstrates the potential to help providers identify specific factors contributing to uncontrolled hypertension and facilitates interventions to improve disease management."
- Proteus (Frias et al., 2016—American Heart Association [AHA] and American Diabetes Association [ADA]) investigated the usefulness of the

Proteus Discover technology in patients with poorly controlled type 2 diabetes (A1c > 7%) and hypertension (systolic BP ≥ 140 mmHg). In their cluster-randomized study of non–insulin-using subjects, they concluded that the Proteus digital health offering supports patient self-management and activation, aids therapy optimization, and facilitates improvement in blood pressure and glycemic control. After 4 weeks of use, patients using Proteus Discover had a 22-mmHg reduction in systolic BP compared with 13-mmHg drop in the usual care arm. In patients whose (Hb)A1c was at or above 8% ($n = 62$), the baseline HbA1c was 9.4% ± 0.2% with an HbA1c change of –0.5% ± 0.1% in the digital health group and 0.2% ± 0.3% in the control (usual care) group. Average reduction in low-density lipoprotein (LDL) was also greater for patients using Proteus (–30 mg/dL vs. –4 mg/dL after 4 weeks); these differences were more pronounced in patients whose baseline LDL was 70 mg/dL or higher (–37 mg/dL for Proteus vs. –4 mg/dL for usual care). In the renal transplant population, the ingestible sensor accurately detected the ingestion of two sensor-enabled capsules taken at the same time with a detection rate of 99.3% ($n = 2{,}376$; Eisenberger et al., 2013).

- Bonacini et al. (2016) evaluated the role of Proteus Discover to optimize adherence and virologic outcomes in chronic hepatitis C virus (HCV)-infected patients taking a combination pill of sofosbuvir and ledipasvir tagged to a sensor. In their interim analysis of five patients, they reported an overall adherence rate of 94% using the Proteus Discover. Twelve instances of identified missed doses using this technology allowed for targeted adherence counseling. Two of the patients who completed treatment achieved a 95% adherence rate and related in follow-up questioning that actually having this opportunity to see their data provided by Proteus Discover empowered them in both managing their own care and allowing greater comfort in sharing their experiences with their health care team.
- Corris et al. (2016) found that Proteus enabled targeted treatment decisions in patients with pulmonary arterial hypertension (PAH), and prescribed sildenafil three times daily coingested with a placebo sensor pill with each dose of sildenafil. The average adherence in the 21 patients was 94%, and average daily step count was 1,890. High adherence was related to higher steps/day; 2,145 steps/day for patients with 95% adherence or higher versus 1,658 steps/day for 95% adherence or lower. Patients had a reduction in 381 steps/day when the previous day's adherence was low (0%–25%) versus high (>75%). Therapy was escalated in seven patients with high adherence, yet diminishing clinical status.

Indeed, the novel implication of this technology is that there is now a highly accurate and direct means of monitoring adherence that can be coupled with other physiological data to produce a unique profile of a patient's health behavior at home to ascertain patterns of medication taking, health behaviors, and degree of response to therapy. Providers cannot just glean information about their patient's relative rate of adherence, but use the coupled data from a wearable sensor and connected devices to tailor treatment plans unique to the habits and lifestyles of their users. A future direction with digital medicine technology is to evaluate its capacity to facilitate earlier and more targeted interventions for patients at risk for disease progression or relapse. According to a press release, Proteus reports that their ingestible technology has the potential to "speed clinical trials and improve the real-world effectiveness of medicines in community settings" (Enriquez, 2015). Going forward, the DHFS technology, coupled with interpretive analytical software could "provide the opportunity to extend the health care patient interview allowing broader personalized intervention to support treatment success beyond the use of medication reminders alone" (Browne, Behzadi, & Littlewort, 2015).

Afternote to the Proteus Technology

The Proteus technology received FDA approval in 2012, as well as Commonwealth of Europe (CE) mark in 2010 for use in Europe, and has more than 300 issued patents. This was a significant step in MTM as it is the only system thus far ever cleared by the FDA as "an aid to measure medication adherence." In April 2016, however, drug manufacturer Otsuka Pharmaceutical was issued an FDA complete response letter for a sensor-embedded Abilify® (aripiprazole) pill for use in patients with schizophrenia and bipolar disorder, and as an adjunctive treatment for major depressive disorder. Despite multiple studies thus far, the FDA is requesting further data to show "performance of the product under the specific conditions in which it is likely to be used, as well as further human factors investigations to evaluate use-related risks and confirm that users can use the device safely and effectively" according to the manufacturer (Lawrence, 2016). The Proteus technology has already been cleared in the United States and Europe for use in conjunction with existing medicines—coingested alongside their medications, or coencapsulated with their medicine by a pharmacist. The company is currently offering Proteus Discover through partnerships with health system customers in the United States.

Mobile Health Technologies

As with the electronic monitoring devices previously discussed, emerging mobile technologies could also potentially offer substantial benefits to patients and providers. Owing to a recent decline in the spending growth in health care technology, a new relationship between mobile technology and health care services is driving a shift toward efforts aimed at decreasing health care costs (Silva, Rodrigues, de laTorre-Diez, Lopez-Coronado, & Saleem, 2015). In the wake of these efforts, the rise of Mobile Health (also known as mHealth) embodies a new array of novel tools aimed at the more efficient transfer of health data and care via electronic means. Mobile phone technologies, including smartphone applications and SMS reminders, video- and photo-assisted observation, and development of electronic health records (EHRs), are all important advancements geared for improving medication adherence in the elderly population. The field of mobile health technology is growing at a tremendous rate with an estimated 97,000 mobile health applications ("apps") available to consumers as of March 2013, with an annual doubling of downloads and users (Cortez, Cohen, & Kesselheim, 2014). Quoting directly from Jahns Ralf-Gordon (2013) from the Research2Guidance website in 2013: "The market for mHealth services has now entered the commercialization phase and will reach $26 billion globally by 2017." Within this large array of available products, applications dedicated to medication adherence are becoming increasingly more sophisticated.

Smartphone Medication Adherence Applications

Smartphone applications provide multiple ways in which to improve medication adherence and empower patients to participate more effectively in their own medication management. They provide tremendous utility in educating patients not only about their background disease(s), but also about their health management by compiling and simplifying their medication-specific information. They have streamlined informational delivery systems complete with reminder alerts and integration with other educational databases. They can be downloaded at minimal or no cost, and potentially cater to multiple caregivers at once. Many of these mobile tools can also be tailored specifically to the patient in question. As quoted from Dayer, Heldenbrand, Andersen, Gubbins, and Martin (2003) in reference to earlier studies (Conn et al., 2009; Williams, Manias, & Walker 2008): "Depending on the type of non-adherence and patient characteristics, using a combination of tailored interventions such as patient education, patient self-monitoring of specialized care, and stimuli to take medications [has] the greatest potential for improving adherence." Keeping this important concept in mind, one can appreciate the logical suitability of integrating smartphone application technology into the sphere of MTM. Applications have the potential to employ all three of these interventions, with the extra caveat that smartphone availability and usage is becoming ubiquitous. Let us now examine more closely some of the unique features of mobile application technology.

In a comprehensive review from 2013 of over 160 smartphone medication adherence applications, various pragmatic features of these tools were identified (Dayer et al., 2003). For example, certain applications may have the capability to

- Interface with a companion website that allows remote entry from a computer;
- Schedule complex medication instructions;
- Allow users to backup and retrieve a medication regimen from a cloud storage system;
- Connect to a separate medication database that allows users to enter, search, and select medications with autopopulation features;
- Transmit, print, or export medication regimens and/or medication-taking behaviors for use by the patient or health care provider;
- Provide customizable audio or visual cues to remind patients to take their medications[2];
- Call or schedule refills;
- Record taken and missed doses;
- Allow authorized providers to input and maintain the patient's medication regimen and relay this information to the patient's device.

Obviously, patients who are visually impaired, who are not accustomed to smartphone technologies, or who do not own a mobile device will have a difficult time reaping the potential benefits of this technology. However, the growing rate of smartphone ownership looks promising. According to a Pew research study (Smith, 2015), 64% of American adults now own a smartphone of some kind, up from 35% in the spring of 2011. Smartphone ownership is especially high among younger Americans, as well as those with relatively high income and education levels. Although ownership among elderly adults is less than this reported number, it is trending upward as well.

Despite the present challenge of making smartphone applications more accessible to the elderly population,

---

[2]Because of their inherently greater capacity for customizable audio and visual prompts that are capable of providing more robust reminders, the efficacy of applications may be equal to or greater than conventional text messaging reminder systems (Dayer et al., 2003).

> adherence applications represent a low-cost strategy that could be incorporated into a variety of pharmacy services, including medication reconciliation and discharge planning in institutional settings, [as well as] MTM or other services in . . . outpatient practice settings. Some community pharmacy chains already have incorporated adherence features into their brand applications; however, the extent to which these are being incorporated into pharmacists' practices in these settings is unknown. (Dayer et al., 2003)

Future directions for smartphone application technology will be focused on integrating health care provider accessibility and support, as well as broadening the convenience of autopopulation features (to deal with manual data entry) via better integration with other drug databases. Ultimately, personal use of mHealth smartphone applications will fulfill their technological potential if ways are found to integrate them directly into the use of other electronic monitoring technologies, as well as prescription and medical record databases (Dayer et al., 2003). Although the efficacy of smartphone technologies to reduce nonadherence rates or improve clinically relevant outcomes has not been well established, there are data that support the use of more conventional SMS text messaging to improve patient adherence over a short interval, especially in chronic states, which are highly relevant to our elderly population (Vervloet, Linn, et al., 2012).

SMS Reminders

According to a 2014 report from the International Telecommunications Union (2014), global mobile–broadband penetration was projected to reach 32% that year, doubling from the penetration rate reported in 2011. Developed countries would constitute a penetration rate of 84%—four times higher than that of developing countries. As mobile phone technology ownership and use continues to increase worldwide, its impact on health care must not be underestimated.

"Text messaging interventions using short message service [reminders are the] most widely applied" mobile phone technologies designed to address adherence (Park et al., 2015). Wald, Butt, and Bestwick (2015) report that "the use of text messaging is increasing as a means of communication between patients and their physicians to arrange appointments, increase immunization, and adjust treatment." It is also serving a unique role in optimizing patient adherence, although further research is necessary to characterize its effectiveness and identify specific target patient groups (including the elderly) for whom it is best tailored (Park et al., 2015). Various studies investigating the effectiveness of text messaging reminders on medication adherence have produced variable results. A meta-analysis published in the *American Journal of Medicine* in 2016 demonstrates a possible reason why: SMS reminder interventions (including mobile phone applications) that employ a "two-way" approach (described subsequently) greatly improve medication adherence over a "one-way" (notification reminder only) approach (Wald et al., 2015).

The process of two-way SMS is conceptually simple: Preprogrammed alerts are first sent to patients reminding them to take their medication(s). Patients are then expected to take the respective medication(s) in response to the alert, after which they then respond either by directly responding to the alert, or using a phone application that provides the response. The foremost encouraging aspect of this adherence technology is that mobile phone use today has skyrocketed and pervades all age groups in all areas of the globe. To date, multiple studies support the effectiveness of mobile reminder technologies in monitoring and promoting adherence in managing acute and chronic diseases (de Jongh, Gurol-Urganci, Vodopivec-Jamsek, Car, & Atun, 2012; Kamal et al., 2015; Strandbygaard, Thomsen, & Backer, 2010; Vervloet, vanDijk, et al., 2012; Wei, Hollin, & Kachnowski, 2011). However, the evidence is more robust in substantiating the positive effect on adherence only in the short term, as longer term follow-up adherence studies are presently lacking. Furthermore, as with other reminder technologies, this unique tool is not without its own drawbacks and challenges.

Text messaging reminder systems are built upon a foundation of trust. There can be 100% compliance with the actual responding to the alerts, but whether the medication is actually ingested is another question. Although the technology allowing for the daily reminder and the patient verification of adherence is novel, it in no way guarantees actual adherence. In contrast to the WOT described earlier, it remains, at best, an indirect means of monitoring adherence. It should also be remembered that although text messaging engages the patient in a convenient way, some elderly folks who are typically more technologically challenged may have difficulty using mobile phones for medication monitoring. Less familiarity with text messaging and mobile phone applications, waning interest if the technology rapidly evolves, compromised fine-motor skills, and general resistance to using mobile phones are all practical challenges to implementing this adherence technology in the elderly patient sector (Park et al., 2015). Factors that maintain engagement of participants remain unknown and serve as important areas of further research (Park et al., 2015).

Video- and Photo-Assisted Observation

What if it were possible to remotely visualize patients actually taking their medications, or in the least, obtain time-stamped photos of their medication(s) in hand prior to ingestion? SMS mobile technology has several advantages to offer, as previously detailed, but it is still considered an indirect method of measuring medication adherence, as ingestion itself cannot be verified. Through video- and photo-assisted observation, however, which expands upon simple mobile phone technology, we move closer to a scenario of more direct monitoring. These newer and more advanced methods of adherence monitoring can be further strengthened when they are paired with other methods such as pill counting, or electronic pill bottle caps that remotely send time stamps of pill bottle openings. Furthermore, remote adherence monitoring methods address the time and distance issues that patients may face, especially in remote settings, where in-person direct adherence monitoring may not be realistic.

In a comparative study by Galloway et al. (2011), multiple modes of adherence monitoring were followed prospectively over 8 weeks in 20 patients taking once a day modafinil for the treatment of methamphetamine dependence. Their medications were issued in MEMS cap–equipped bottles, additional pill counts were recorded on a weekly basis, and they were instructed to take a daily photo just prior to taking their pill out of their issued bottle. Pill bottle openings were sent as time-stamped events to a computer accessed by the study authors. The daily capsule photographs were transmitted via issued cell phones to a remote location as well. The three methods of adherence monitoring were then analyzed side by side with interesting results. Cellular telephone time-stamped images appeared to be the most accurate measure of adherence, as many of the MEMS caps transmitted adherence in a delayed fashion when tested by the study authors themselves after the study was finished. In addition, because photos were collected and sent in real time, this method allowed for more frequent assessment of adherence than either MEMS devices or pill counts. For now, photo-stamped cellular monitoring remains a very powerful and practical tool of monitoring adherence owing to the increasing use of cell phone technology throughout the world. Can cell phone technology, however, offer us anything more sophisticated? Moving beyond photocapture, what if recorded video technology could be implemented using cell phones to analogously, and more directly, monitor medication adherence?

A newer tool appropriately called mobile direct observation treatment (MDOT) is also showing promising results. MDOT has been piloted in a remote setting involving TB patients in Kenya who live considerable distances from a dispensing center that traditionally verifies adherence. In one proof-of-concept validation study by Hoffman et al. (2010), 13 patients were individually paired with "treatment supporters" (chosen by a district hospital in Nairobi, Kenya) who obtained daily short videos of their respective patients swallowing their TB medications. The patients then submitted the videos to a secure central database to be logged and time stamped for review by medical nurses. The study subjects also periodically received motivational videos of recovered patients' testimonials, advice from physicians, and TB prevention messages. Twelve of the study participants completed the program successfully, and 11 of these fully completed a series of questionnaires reflecting their opinions and eliciting feedback of the tested adherence intervention. Overall, the responses and ratings of the patient participants reflected an appreciation for the health messaging, a sense of no longer feeling isolated owing to the daily reminders, and a high level of satisfaction with the MDOT process once various technical difficulties were overcome. The authors of this study pointed out that "using mobile health technology may be a substitute for face-to-face visits with health care workers in remote areas where the incidence of tuberculosis and HIV/AIDS is high and medication adherence levels are suboptimal" (Hoffman et al., 2010). Encouraged with these results from the feasibility study, the authors pointed to the need for a larger clinical trial to assess whether MDOT would improve adherence (as well in other diseases besides TB) and be cost-effective against other adherence technologies.

Use and Integration of EHRs

Perhaps there is no better way at the moment of documenting, tracking, and avoiding potential issues with medication adherence than the prospect of building and integrating a national/worldwide system of shared electronic medical records. As of 2011, an estimated 55% of physician providers in the United States were working with EHR system platforms (Jamoom, Beatty, Bercovitz, Woodwell, & Reichsteiner, 2011). According to the Office of the National Coordinator for Health Information Technology (ONC), based on revised estimates, that number has increased substantially to well over 80% up and through 2014 (Heisey-Grove & Patel, 2015). There may be several contributors to this rapidly growing acceptance and use of EHR technology. As quoted by Dormuth, Miller, Hunag, Mamdani, and Juurlink (2012), "such systems [EHRs] provide a measure of safety with regard to medication errors, therapeutic duplication, and drug interaction." These electronic databases also assist with tracking how patients comply with and use their medications (Vollmer et al., 2012), and have the potential to be integrated with other monitoring systems (Park et al., 2015).

Over the last decade, the perceptions of the financial, personal, and social benefits of EHRs have varied considerably among both patients and providers. Some of the best data to date reflects the experience of EHR users in the Canadian and European health systems, as well as from the Veterans Affairs (VA) Health Care System here in the United States. One survey by Tharmalingam, Hagens, and Zelmer (2016), examining the perceptions of users of an integrated EHR system across Canada, demonstrated generally positive views in regard to the quality of care and user productivity offered by this technology. Some users, however, did cite concerns about the compatibility of the EHR into daily workflow, as well as the relative availability and helpfulness of technical support and training of users.

If we look at the impact that EHR technology has had in the United States, a number of survey findings from a national poll of physicians (currently using EHR technology) documented by Jamoom et al. (2011) cites a significant percentage of respondents who believe that their respective EHR produces clinical benefits for their practice, allows them to deliver better patient care, and makes records readily available at point of care. According to the ONC (2014), referring to numerous previous sources (Bell & Thornton, 2011; Couch, 2007; Kern et al., 2013), EHRs may be able to provide benefits, such as the following, far beyond just documenting patient adherence:

- Easier access to patient health records for more informed, accurate, patient-centered management, as well as improved communication among providers, hospital systems, pharmacies, and patients. This translates into more coordinated, efficient, higher quality care and lower health care costs by optimizing preventive medicine and reducing costs of redundant testing and treatment.
- Various benefits to providers including safer, more reliable prescribing, as well as improved productivity by streamlining documentation, coding, and billing.
- Optimized risk management and liability prevention through electronic documentation of informed consent, adherence with best evidence-based practices, and reduction in medical errors.

The value of EHRs in the United States cannot be overemphasized, especially when looking back over the last 30 years of experience of integrating health information technology systems with the VA. According to Byrne et al. (2010), the total estimated initial cost of developing, implementing, and maintaining the entire health information technology infrastructure (including the EHRs system, which constituted the largest portion of this cost at $3.09 billion) was $4.07 billion. Despite this enormous investment, however, the government had reaped an estimated net savings of $3.09 billion in health care costs by the 2007 fiscal year. According to the same authors, the streamlined computerized patient records system (CPRS) was the greatest contributor toward both the benefits and costs. Other contributing aspects of the EHR to high performance savings included electronic reminders to primary providers in providing prevention services (vaccines, cancer screenings, etc.), as well as care reminders for chronic conditions such as diabetes and heart failure.

At present, patient computer records localized to individual health care networks and pharmacies are the chief means by which a considerable cohort of health providers store and access their patients' information (Hing, Hall, & Ashman, 2010). Our present worldwide network of fragmented health information poses several problems to patient health care and optimizing adherence. Most patient databases today remain isolated from one another, leaving a substantial gap in communication between separate prescribers (Dormuth et al., 2012). This lack of system integration can result in significant safety issues, medication duplication errors, and problems with abuse and misuse that plague patients and providers alike. Fortunately, EHRs have been shown to solve such dilemmas. A good example can be found in a published timed-series analysis of prescription records from a centralized prescription network in British Columbia (Dormuth et al., 2012). This study demonstrated a marked reduction in inappropriately filled prescriptions for opioids and benzodiazepines (which was noted particularly among residents who were 65 years or older) as a consequence of the presence of an EHRs system. Can efforts to optimize medication adherence also benefit from the use of EHR technology?

With an EHR, barriers to adherence, as well as documentation of misuse and abuse can be detailed in a shared contiguous electronic format without having to restart a process of investigation, especially as patients may change providers frequently, engage in destructive behaviors, or mislead care providers about their medication use. Regardless of the availability or proposed effectiveness of such technology, however, successful operation of an EHR still depends on the reliability of accurate documentation by providers, and truthful accounting of medication use by their patients. Although the use of EHRs is limited at this time to large health organizations, there remains an important need for their expansion to a broader network of providers and patients (Park et al., 2015). With the predominance of organization-specific health records systems, considerable legal, ethical, and financial challenges stand in the way of this goal. Patient privacy issues, a myriad of various other legal concerns, and the lingering quandary of who would contribute to the enormous potential costs of creating and maintaining a national or multinational integrated system are just some to consider. Obviously, the technology of integrating EHRs both among individual networks and with other monitoring devices has a significant way to go toward achieving its true potential. This concerted effort at EHR integration will demand tremendous will and cooperation between national and private entities to overcome many obstacles.

CONCLUSION

We have provided a brief review of the topic of medication adherence and have described several promising technologies aimed at improving such within the larger scope of MTM. The tools at our disposal today greatly benefit our elderly population in particular, by better equipping them to manage their chronic health conditions and addressing their unique challenges. As improvements in adherence monitoring technology become more affordable and available, the business of health care will evolve into a more integrated enterprise between patients and their health care providers. Although the future direction and successful impact of many of these adherence technologies looks promising, they will only be possible if both medical and nonmedical professionals find ways to safely and effectively adopt them.

REFERENCES

Abbey, B., Alipour, A., Camp, C., & Hofer, C. (2012). *The smart pill box*. Resna Annual Conference—2012. Retrieved from https://www.resna.org/sites/default/files/legacy/conference/proceedings/2012/StudentDesign/SmartPillBox.html

Abraham, I., De Geest, J., De Geest, W., De Troy, E., & MacDonald, K. (2015). Detectability and acceptability of continuous pulse signals for the MemoPatch® device: An electronic skin patch intended to deliver tactile medication reminder signals. *Medical Devices: Evidence and Research, 8*, 119–129.

Ailinger, R. L., Black, P. L., & Lima-Garcia, N. (2008). Use of electronic monitoring in clinical nursing research. *Clinical Nursing Research, 17*(2), 89–97.

Asche, C., LaFleur, J., & Connor, C. (2011). A review of diabetes treatment adherence and the association with clinical and economic outcomes. *Clinical Therapeutics, 33*(1), 74–109.

Au-Yeung, K. Y., & DiCarlo, L. (2012). Cost comparison of wirelessly vs. directly observed therapy for adherence confirmation in anti-tuberculosis treatment. *International Journal of Tuberculosis Lung Disease, 16*(11), 1498–1504. doi:10.5588/ijtld.11.0868

Au-Yeung, K. Y., Moon, G. D., Robertson, T. L., DiCarlo, L. A., Epstein M. S., Weis, S. E., . . . Engel, G. (2011). Early clinical experience with networked system for promoting patient self-management. *The American Journal of Managed Care, 17*(7), e277–e287.

Ayoade, A., & Oladipo, I. (2012). Evaluation of the correlation between self-report and electronic monitoring of adherence to hypertension therapy. *Blood Pressure, 21*(3), 161–166.

Bell, B., & Thornton, K. (2011). From promise to reality: Achieving the value of an EHR. *Healthcare Financial Management, 65*(2), 50–56.

Bitton, A., Choudhry, N. K., Matlin, O. S., Swanton, K., & Shrank, W. H. (2013). The impact of medication adherence on coronary artery disease costs and outcomes: A systematic review. *The American Journal of Medicine, 126*(4), 357.

Bonacini, M., Yoona, A. K., Reichert, M., Travis, E., Virdi, N., Raja, P., & Savage, G. (2016). A new digital health feedback offering to keep patients adherent to oral hepatitis C therapy. *Gastroenterology, 150*(4), S1159. doi:10.1016/S0016-5085(16)33916-6

Bova, C. A., Fennie, K. P., Knafl, G. J., Dieckhaus, K. D., Watrous, E., & Williams, A. B. (2005). Use of electronic monitoring devices to measure antiretroviral adherence: Practical considerations. *AIDS and Behavior, 9*(1), 103–110.

Browne, S., Haubrich, R., Moser, K., Tucker, A., Vaida, F., Peloquin, C., & Benson, C. (2015). *Wirelessly observed therapy (WOT): A new paradigm in TB therapy monitoring*. Abstract and Poster Presentation at the CROI Conference, Seattle, Washington. Retrieved from http://www.croiconference.org/sessions/wirelessly-observed-therapy-wot-new-paradigm-tb-therapy-monitoring

Browne, S. H., Behzadi, Y., & Littlewort, G. (2015). Let visuals tell the story: Medication adherence in patients with type II diabetes captured by a novel ingestion sensor platform. *Journal of Medical Internet Research mHealth and uHealth, 3*(4), e108.

Business Wire. (2015a). Therasolve announces start of patient study with MemoPatch®. Retrieved from http://www.businesswire.com/news/home/20151103005901/en

Business Wire. (2015b). Therasolve announces US patent for MemoPatch®. Retrieved from http://www.businesswire.com/news/home/20150915005948/en/TheraSolve-Announces-Patent-Issuance-MemoPatch%C2%AE

Butler, R. J., Davis, T. K., Johnson, W. G., & Gardner, H. H. (2011). Effects of nonadherence with prescription drugs among older adults. *American Journal of Managed Care, 17*(2), 153–160.

Byrne, C. M., Mercincavage, L. M., Pan, E. C., Vincent, A. G., Johnston, D. S., & Middleton, B. (2010). The value from investments in health information technology at the US Department of Veterans Affairs. *Health Affairs (Millwood), 29*(4), 629–638.

Campbell, N. L., Zhan, J., Tu, W., Weber, Z., Ambeuhl, R., McKay, C., & McElwee, N. (2016). Self-reported medication adherence barriers among ambulatory older adults with mild cognitive impairment. *Pharmacotherapy, 36*(2), 196–202.

Catz, S. L., Kelly, J. A., Bogart, L. M., Benotsch, E. G., & McAuliffe, T. L. (2000). Patterns, correlates, and barriers to medication adherence among persons prescribed new treatments for HIV disease. *Health Psychology, 19*(2), 124–133.

Comstock, J. (2013, March 13). Slideshow: 8 pillboxes that connect to your phone. *MobiHealth News*. Retrieved from http://mobihealthnews.com/20795/slideshow-8-pillboxes-that-connect-to-your-phone

Conn, V. S., Hafdahl, A. R., Cooper, P. S., Ruppar, T. M., Mehr, D. R., & Russell, C. L. (2009). Interventions to improve medication adherence among older adults: Meta-analysis of adherence outcomes among randomized controlled trials. *The Gerontologist, 49*(4), 447–462.

Corris, P. A., Day, M., Gibiansky, M., Kim, Y. A., & DiCarlo, L. (2016). A pilot study of digital feedback to guide therapeutic decisions in pulmonary hypertension. *European Respiratory Journal, 48*(Suppl.), 2407.

Cortez, N. G., Cohen, G., & Kesselheim, A. S. (2014). FDA regulation of mobile health technologies. *New England Journal of Medicine, 371*(4), 372–379.

Couch, J. B. (2007). CCHIT certified electronic health records reduce malpractice risk. *Certified Commission for Healthcare Information Technology.* Retrieved from https://www.texmed.org/WorkArea/DownloadAsset.aspx?id=19497

Dayer, L., Heldenbrand, S., Andersen, P., Gubbins, P.O., & Martin B. C. (2003). Smartphone medication adherence apps: Potential benefits to patients and providers. *Journal of the American Pharmacists Association, 53*(2), 172–181.

De Geest, W., De Geest, J., De Geest, S., & Abraham, I. (2007). Description, specifications, and ASIC configurations of MEMOPATCH, a transdermal pulse generator medical device to promote patient compliance with medication regimens. *Conference Proceedings IEEE Engineering in Medicine and Biology Society, 2007*, 508–511.

de Jongh, T., Gurol-Urganci, I., Vodopivec-Jamsek, V., Car, J., & Atun, R. (2012). Mobile phone messaging for facilitating self-management of long-term illnesses (Review). *Cochrane Database of Systematic Reviews*, (12), CD007459.

DiCarlo, L., Moon, G., Intondi, A., Duck, R., Frank, J., Hafazi, H., . . . Zdeblick, M. (2012). A digital health solution for using and managing medications: Wirelessly observed therapy. *IEEE Pulse, 3*(5), 23–26.

DiCarlo, L., Naik, R., Macey, N., West, R. J., Godbehere, P., Thurston, R., . . . Kim, Y. A. (2015). A real-world registry study evaluating the impact of an ingestible sensor and wearable patch to track adherence and activity patterns in patients with uncontrolled hypertension. *Journal of Hypertension, 33*, 1.

DiCarlo, L. A. (2012). Role for direct electronic verification of pharmaceutical ingestion in pharmaceutical development. *Contemporary Clinical Trials, 33*(4), 593–600.

DiMatteo, M. R. (2004). Variations in patients' adherence to medical recommendations: A quantitative review of 50 Years of research. *Medical Care, 42*(3), 200–209.

Dormuth, C. R., Miller, T. A., Hunag, A., Mamdani, M. M., & Juurlink, D. N., (2012). Effect of a centralized prescription network on inappropriate prescriptions for opioid analgesics and benzodiazepines. *Canadian Medical Association Journal, 184*(16), E852–E856.

Eisenberg, D. F., Placzek, H., Gu, T., Krishna, A., & Tulsi, B. B. (2015). Cost and consequences of noncompliance to oral bisphosphonate treatment. *Journal of Managed Care and Specialty Pharmacy, 21*(1), 56–65.

Eisenberger, U., Wuthrich, R. P., Bock, A., Ambuhl, P., Steiger, J., Intondi, A., . . . De Geest, S. (2013). Medication adherence assessment: High accuracy of the new ingestible sensor system in kidney transplants. *Transplantation, 96*(3), 245–250.

Enriquez, J. (2015, July 6). FDA clears first ingestible device for medication adherence. *Med Device Online News Feature.* Retrieved from http://www.meddeviceonline.com/doc/fda-clears-first-ingestible-device-for-medication-adherence-0001

Frias, J., Virdi, N. S., Raja, P., Kim, Y., Savage, G., Unger, J., Raikhel, M., & Osterberg, L. (2016). Evaluation of a digital health offering to optimize blood pressure and lipid control in patients with uncontrolled hypertension and type 2 diabetes: A pilot, cluster randomized study. *Circulation, 134*(Suppl. 1), A17375.

Galloway, G. P., Coyle, J. R., Guillen, J. E., Flower, K., & Mendelson, J. E. (2011). A simple, novel method for assessing medication adherence: Capsule photographs taken with cellular telephones. *Journal of Addictive Medicine, 5*(3), 170–174.

Garfinkel, D., & Mangin, D. (2010). Feasibility study of a systematic approach for discontinuation of multiple medications in older adults: Addressing polypharmacy. *Archives of Internal Medicine, 170*(18), 1648–1654.

Haberer, J. E., Robbins, G. K., Ybarra, M., Ragland, K., Johnson, M. O., & Bangsberg, D. R. (2012). Real-time electronic adherence monitoring is feasible, comparable to unannounced pill counts, and acceptable. *Aids and Behavior, 16*(2), 375–382.

Hafezi, H., Robertson, T., Moon, G. D., Au-Yeung, K., Zdeblick, M., & Savage, G. (2015). An ingestible sensor for measuring medication adherence. *IEEE Transactions on Biomedical Engineering, 62*(1), 99–109.

Hamilton, G. A. (2003). Measuring adherence in a hypertension clinical trial. *European Journal of Cardiovascular Nursing, 2*(3), 219–228.

Haynes, R. B., McDonald, H. P., & Garg, A. X. (2002). Helping patients follow prescribed treatment. *Journal of the American Medical Association, 288*(22), 2880–2883.

Heisey-Grove, D., & Patel, V. (2015). *Any, certified, and basic: Quantifying physician HER adoption through 2014*. ONC Data Brief, No. 28. Retrieved from https://www.healthit.gov/sites/default/files/briefs/oncdatabrief28_certified_vs_basic.pdf

Henriksson, J., Tyden, G., Hoijer, J., & Wadstrom, J. (2016). A prospective randomized trial on the effect of using an electronic monitoring drug dispensing device to improve adherence and compliance. *Transplantation, 100*(1), 203–209.

Hincapie, A. L., Taylor, A. M., Boesen, K. P., & Warholak, T. (2015). Understanding reasons for nonadherence to medications in a Medicare Part D beneficiary sample. *Journal of Managed Care & Specialty Pharmacy, 21*(5), 391–399.

Hing, E., Hall, M. J., & Ashman, J. J. (2010). Use of electronic medical records by ambulatory care providers. *National Health Statistics Report*, (22), 1–21.

Ho, P. M., Rumsfeld, J. S., Masoudi, F. A., McClure, D. L., Plomondon, M. E., Steiner, J. F., & Magid, D. J. (2006). Effect of medication nonadherence on hospitalization and mortality among patients with diabetes mellitus. *Archives of Internal Medicine, 166*(17), 1836–1841.

Hoffman, J. A., Cunningham, J. R., Suleh, A. J., Sundsmo, A., Dekker, D., Vago, F., . . . Hunt-Glassman, J. (2010). Mobile direct observation treatment for tuberculosis patients: A technical feasibility pilot using mobile phones in Nairobi, Kenya. *American Journal of Preventative Medicine, 39*(1), 78–80.

Ingerski, L. M., Hente, E. A., Modi, A., & Hommel, K. A. (2011). Electronic measurement of medication adherence in pediatric chronic illness: A review of measures. *Journal of Pediatrics, 159*(4), 528–534.

International Telecommunications Union. (2014). *The world in 2014: ICT facts and figures*. Geneva, Switzerland: ITU Telecommunication Development Bureau. Retrieved from http://www.itu.int/en/ITU-D/Statistics/Documents/facts/ICTFactsFigures2014-e.pdf

Jamoom, E., Beatty, A., Bercovitz, D., Woodwell, K. P., & Reichsteiner, E. (2011). Physician adoption of electronic health record systems: United States. *NCHS Data Brief*, (98), 1–8.

Jha, A. K., Aubert, R. E., Yao, J., Teagarden, J. R., & Epstein, R. S. (2012). Greater adherence to diabetes drugs is linked to less hospital use and could save nearly 5 billion annually. *Health Affairs, 31*(8), 1836–1846.

Kamal, A. K., Shaikh, Q., Pasha, O., Azam, I., Islam, M., Memon, A. A., . . . Khoja, S. (2015). A randomized controlled behavioral intervention trial to improve medication adherence in adult stroke patients with prescription tailored Short Messaging Service (SMS-SMS4Stroke study). *BMC Neurology, 15*, 212.

Kane, J. M., Perlis, R. H., DiCarlo, L. A., Au-Yeung, K., Duong, J., & Petrides, G. (2013). First experience with a wireless system incorporating physiologic assessments and direct confirmation of digital tablet ingestions in ambulatory patients with schizophrenia or bipolar disorder. *Journal of Clinical Psychiatry, 74*(6), e533–e5340.

Kane, S., & Shaya, F. (2008). Medication adherence is associated with increased health care costs. *Digestive Diseases and Sciences, 53*(4), 1020–1024.

Kardas, P., Lewek, P., & Matyjaszczyk, M. (2013). Determinants of patient adherence: A review of systematic reviews. *Frontiers in Pharmacology, 4*, 91.

Kern, L. M., Barron, Y., Dhopeshwarkar, R. V., Edwards, A., Kaushal, R., & HITEC Investigators. (2013). Electronic health records and ambulatory quality of care. *Journal of General Internal Medicine, 28*(4), 496–503.

Laine, C., Newschaffer, C. J., Zhang, D., Cosler, L., Hauck, W. W., & Turner, B. J. (2000). Adherence to antiretroviral therapy by pregnant women infected with human immunodeficiency virus: A pharmacy claims-based analysis. *Obstetrics and Gynecology, 95*(2), 167–173.

Lawrence, S. (2016). Updated: FDA rejects Otsuka, Proteus pill with medication adherence monitoring. *FierceBiotech.* Retrieved from http://www.fiercebiotech.com/medical-devices/updated-fda-rejects-otsuka-proteus-pill-medication-adherence-monitoring

Martin, A., Mellotte, G., & O'Neill, D. (2005). Chronic kidney disease in the elderly: A silent epidemic. *Irish Medical Journal, 98*(2), 46–47.

Mikyas, Y., Agodoa, I., & Yurgin, N. (2014). A systematic review of osteoporosis medication adherence and osteoporosis-related fracture costs in men. *Applied Health Economics and Health Policy, 12*(3), 267–277.

Modi, A., Siris, E., Tang, J., & Sen, S. (2015). Cost and consequences of noncompliance with osteoporosis treatment among women initiating therapy. *Current Medical Research and Opinion, 31*(4), 757–765.

Office of the National Coordinator for Health Information Technology. (2014). Data brief: Improved diagnostics and patient outcomes. Retrieved from https://www.healthit.gov/providers-professionals/improved-diagnostics-patient-outcomes#footnote-4

Osterberg, L., & Blaschke, T. (2005). Adherence to medication. *New England Journal of Medicine, 353*(5), 487–497.

Park, L. G., Howie-Esquivel, J., & Dracup, K. (2015). Electronic measurement of medication adherence. *Western Journal of Nursing Research, 37*(1), 28–49.

Paterson, M., Kinnear, M., Bond, C., & McKinstrey, B. (2016). A systematic review of electronic multi-compartment medication devices with reminder systems for improving adherence to self-administered medications. *International Journal of Pharmacy Practice, 25*(3), 185–194.

Pinsky, B. W., Takemoto, S. K., Lentine, K. L., Burroughs, T. E., Schnitzler, M. A., & Salvalaggio, P. R. (2009). Transplant outcomes and economic costs associated with patient noncompliance to immunosuppression. *American Journal of Transplantation, 9*(11), 2597–2606.

Profit, D., Rohatagi, S., Zhao, C., Hatch, A., Docherty, J. P., & Peters-Strickland, T. S. (2016). Developing a digital medicine system in psychiatry: Ingestion detection rate and latency period. *Journal of Clinical Psychiatry, 77*, 9.

Ralf-Gordon, J. (2013). The market for mHealth app services will reach $26 billion by 2017. Retrieved from https://research2guidance.com/the-market-for-mhealth-app-services-will-reach-26-billion-by-2017

Roebuck, M. C., Liberman, J. N., Gemmill-Toyama, M., & Brennan, T. A. (2011). Medication adherence leads to lower healthcare use and costs despite increased drug spending. *Health Affairs (Millwood), 30*, 91–99.

Scheurer, D., Choudhry, N., Swanton, K. A., Matlin, O., & Shrank, W. (2012). Association between different types of social support and medication adherence. *American Journal of Managed Care, 18*(12), e461–e467.

Schwed, A., Fallab, C. L., Burnier, M., Waeber, B., Kappenberger, L., Burnand, B., & Darioli, R. (1999). Electronic monitoring of compliance to lipid-lowering therapy in clinical practice. *Journal of Clinical Pharmacology, 39*(4), 402–409.

Shin, S., Song, H., Oh, S. K., Choi, K. E., Kim, H., & Jang, S. (2013). Effect of antihypertensive medication adherence on hospitalization for cardiovascular disease and mortality in hypertensive patients. *Hypertension Research, 36*(11), 1000–1005.

Silva, B., Rodrigues, J., de la Torre Diez, I., Lopez-Coronado, M., & Saleem, K. (2015). Mobile-health: A review of current state in 2015. *Journal of Biomedical Informatics, 56*, 265–272.

Siris, E., Selby, P., Saag, K., Borgstrom, F., Herings, R. M. C., & Silverman, S. (2009). Impact of osteoporosis treatment adherence on fracture rates in North America and Europe. *The American Journal of Medicine, 122*(2, Suppl.), S3–S13.

Smith, A. (2015). U.S. smartphone use in 2015. Retrieved from http://www.pewinternet.org/2015/04/01/us-smartphone-use-in-2015

Sokol, M. C., McGuigan, K. A., Verbrugge, R. R., & Epstein, R. S. (2005). Impact of medication adherence on hospitalization risk and healthcare cost. *Medical Care, 43*(6), 521–530.

Strandbygaard, U., Thomsen, S. F., & Backer, V. (2010). A daily SMS reminder increases adherence to asthma treatment: A three-month follow-up study. *Respiratory Medicine, 104*(2), 166–171.

Summer, M. M., & Engstrom, G. (2015). Experience of self-management of medications among older people with multimorbidity. *Journal of Clinical Nursing, 24*(19–20), 2757–2764.

Tharmalingam, S., Hagens, S., & Zelmer, J. (2016). The value of connected health information: Perceptions of electronic health record users in Canada. *BMC Medical Informatics and Decision Making, 16*(1), 93.

Therasolve Press Release. (2015). Therasolve wins Biomedica 2015 Award for best Medtech innovation. Retrieved from http://media.wix.com/ugd/44ff5b_7e62d37958a543a4a87150f6ce6db4d4.pdf

Vervloet, M., Linn, A. J., van Weert, J. C., de Bakker, D. H., Bouvy, M. L., & van Dijk, L. (2012). The effectiveness of interventions using electronic reminders to improve adherence to chronic medications: A systematic review of the literature. *Journal of the American Medical Informatics Association, 19*(5), 696–704.

Vervloet, M., vanDijk, L., Santen-Reestman, J., vanVlijmen, B., vanWingerden, P., Bouvy, M. L., & deBakker, D. H. (2012). SMS reminders improve adherence to oral medication in type 2 diabetes patients who are real time electronically monitored. *International Journal of Medical Informatics, 81*(9), 594–604.

Vitality. (2010). GlowCaps. Retrieved from http://www.nanthealth.com/vitality

Vlasnik, J. J., Aliotta, S. L., DeLor, B. (2005). Medication adherence: Factors influencing compliance with prescribed medication plans. *Case Manager, 16*(2), 47–51.

Vollmer, W. M., Xu, M., Feldstein, A., Smith, D., Waterbury, A., & Rand, C. (2012). Comparison of pharmacy-based measures of medication adherence. *BMC Health Services Research, 12*, 155.

Wald, D. S., Butt, S., & Bestwick, J. P. (2015). One-way versus two-way text messaging on improving medication adherence: Meta-analysis of randomized trials. *American Journal of Medicine, 128*(10), 1139.

Wan, G. J., Kozma, C. M., Slaton, T. L., Olson, W. H., & Feagan, B. G. (2014). Inflammatory bowel disease: Healthcare costs for patients who are adherent or non-adherent with infliximab therapy. *Journal of Medical Economics, 17*(6), 384–393.

Wei, J., Hollin, I., & Kachnowski, S. (2011). A review of the use of mobile phone text messaging in clinical and healthy behaviour interventions. *Journal of Telemedicine and Telecare,* 17(1), 41–48.

Wendel, C. S., Mohler, M. J., Kroesen, K., Ampel, N. M., Gifford, A. L., & Coons, S. J. (2001). Barriers to use of electronic adherence monitoring in an HIV clinic. *Annals of Pharmacotherapy, 35*(9), 1010–1015.

Wheeler, K. J., Roberts, M. E., & Neiheisel, M. B. (2014). Medication adherence part two: Predictors of nonadherence and adherence. *Journal of the American Association of Nurse Practitioners, 26*(4), 225–232.

Wild, H. (2012). The economic rationale for adherence in the treatment of type 2 diabetes mellitus. *American Journal of Managed Care, 18*(3, Suppl.), S43–S48.

Williams, A., Manias, E., & Walker, R. (2008). Interventions to improve medication adherence in people with multiple chronic conditions: A systematic review. *Journal of Advanced Nursing, 63*(2), 132–143.

World Health Organization. (2003). *Adherence to long term therapies: Evidence for action.* Geneva, Switzerland: Author. Retrieved from http://www.who.int/chp/knowledge/publications/adherence_report/en

Wu, P. H., Yang, C. Y., Yao, Z. L., Lin, W. Z., Wu, L. W., & Chang, C. C. (2010). Relationship of blood pressure control and hospitalization risk to medication adherence among patients with hypertension in Taiwan. *American Journal of Hypertension, 23*(2), 155–160.

Yap, A. F., Thirumoorthy, T., & Kwan, Y. H. (2015). Systematic review of the barriers affecting medication adherence in older adults. *Geriatrics Gerontology International, 16,* 1093–1101.

Zullig, L. L., Stechuchak, K. M., Goldstein, K. M., Olsen, M. K., McCant, F. M., Danus, S., . . . Bosworth, H. B. (2015). Patient-reported medication adherence barriers among patients with cardiovascular risk factors. *Journal of Managed Care & Specialty Pharmacy, 21*(6), 479–485.

9

Technological Advancements in Pain Management in the Elderly Population

Muhammad A. Waqar, Kelly Conright, Dawn R. Currie, and Jessica C. Cate

Population trends show that the elderly population (defined as the age of 65 years or older) continues to grow at a staggering rate. It is estimated that elderly adults will make up about 21.7% of the U.S. population by the year 2040 (Administration on Aging, 2015). Despite advances in medicine, aging results in an irreversible decline in physiological function. Altered physiology and increases in degenerative disease prevalence have an influence on the health of older adults. In one estimate, 30% to 50% of adults 65 years and older have two or more health problems affecting their lives. For those 85 years and over, this statistic rises to 50% to 75% (Rastogi & Meek, 2013). Pain is not considered a normal part of aging, although the prevalence of pain increases with advancing age, ranging from 50% to 75% (Ferrell, 1995).

Pain is a complex phenomenon caused by noxious sensory stimuli or neuropathological mechanisms. Persistent pain, by definition, continues for a prolonged period of time and may or may not be associated with a well-defined disease process. The most common types of pain syndromes in the elderly population include musculoskeletal disorders, fibromyalgia, claudication, cancer, and neuropathies (Abdulla et al., 2013). Pain is more difficult to recognize and manage in the elderly population (Hanks-Bell, Halvey, & Paice, 2004; Rastogi & Meek, 2013). Barriers to effective management reported in the literature include challenges to proper pain assessment, underreporting of pain by patients, atypical manifestations of pain, and a need for increased appreciation of the pharmacokinetic and pharmacodynamic changes of aging (Abdulla et al., 2013).

Elderly individuals are more likely to underreport pain owing to misconceptions and personal beliefs regarding pain and medications utilized to treat pain. Often, older adults view pain as a normal part of aging, and do not want to be labeled as "weak" or a "complainer." Other barriers include fear of addiction, loss of independence, polypharmacy, adverse effects, and costs (Rastogi & Meek, 2013). Moreover, older adults with cognitive impairment are often unable to objectify pain. On the other hand, health care professionals also find it more difficult to assess and treat pain in elderly individuals owing to lack of adequate training, inability to interpret symptoms, personal biases, and lack of standardized guidelines/protocols for the management of persistent pain in older adults. Available guidelines and literature reviews have developed steps to follow in an attempt to standardize pain assessment in the geriatric patient (Abdullah et al., 2013; Kaye, Baluch, & Scott, 2010). Overall, the assessment and management of pain should be multidimensional and multidisciplinary.

Alterations in pharmacokinetics and pharmacodynamics in the elderly population affect tolerability of medications utilized for pain management. Elderly individuals are more vulnerable to adverse drug events (ADEs) and medication-related hospitalizations. Most notably, declines in hepatic and renal function prolong or intensify the action of analgesic medications. Owing to lack of clinical trials including elderly patients, recommendations for age-adjusted dosing are not available for most analgesics. However, untreated pain can result in functional impairment, falls, and mood changes, including insomnia, depression, and/or behavioral problems, which require treatment with other psychotropic medications. Thus, the goal has been to develop safer formulations of medications, novel drug delivery systems, and nonpharmacological alternatives for our elderly population to minimize drug toxicity and unwanted medications-related ADEs.

TECHNOLOGICAL APPLICATIONS TOWARD FORMULATION ADVANCES IN PHARMACEUTICALS FOR PAIN MANAGEMENT

As the understanding of pain pathophysiology and treatment increases, new routes of drug delivery are being discovered with the objective of attempting to block pain at peripheral sites, with maximum active drug and minimal systemic effects (Sastry, Nyshadham, & Fix, 2000). Most drugs are limited to only a few safe routes of administration, but new delivery systems are being developed each year. Some opioids, for example, can be administered through a variety of routes, including oral, subcutaneous, intravenous, transdermal, oral sublingual, intrathecal, and rectal. The least invasive method of drug administration should be used. Novel oral and topical preparations may prove to be helpful in minimizing ADEs in elderly patients.

Oral Drug Delivery

Oral drug administration remains the preferred route owing to convenience, cost, and invasiveness. There have been several novel technologies for oral drug delivery in the recent past. Oral disintegrating tablet (ODT) dosage forms, three-dimensional printing (3DP), and electrostatic coating are examples of a few existing technologies with the potential to accommodate various metabolic characteristics of drugs (Sastry et al., 2000). First of all, ODT dosage forms dissolve quickly in the mouth, and have proven most beneficial in elderly patients who have difficulty swallowing owing to neurological disorders. There are several medications available in ODT form for the treatment of pain, including fentanyl, tramadol, acetaminophen, meloxicam, and ibuprofen. Some disadvantages of ODTs are cost, lack of physical resistance, and limitations to active drug concentrations (Parkash et al., 2011). Second, 3DP technology was developed to address problems associated with drug-release mechanisms and release rates (Sastry et al., 2000). Ultimately, medications are printed by layering active medication and binders to form a matrix system. Use of 3DP technology to create pharmaceutical dosage forms may allow a precise control of the amount of active medication, as well as complex drug release profiles, which can be tailored on an individual-patient basis to minimize ADEs. Finally, electrostatic coating involves charging dry powder (active ingredient and substrate) to create a medicine with controlled size, morphology, uniform flow, and charging properties utilizing the principles of electrostatic deposition (Sastry et al., 2000).

Topical Drug Delivery

The skin is one of the most extensive and readily accessible organs of the human body. Drug delivery across the skin, otherwise known as *transdermal*, is a means for administration of medication that bypasses liver metabolism, and is able to maintain a relatively steady state of medication, similar to intravenous infusion (Gangarosa & James, 1995). The delivery of medication to the bloodstream through the skin does require a delivery mechanism, and many of those mechanisms utilize alternative forms of energy to facilitate medicine delivery through the skin (Dhote, Bhatnagar, P. K. Mishra, Mahajan, & D. K. Mishra, 2012).

Topical preparations are the result of such exploration. Topical analgesics, or anesthetics, are defined as liquids, gels, powders, creams, semisolids, emulsions, patches, foams, or aerosols containing an analgesic or anesthetic agent applied on or around the painful site (Bhowmik et al., 2012). Topical preparations are believed to avoid issues associated with oral or intravenous routes such as gastric disturbances, medication changes that result from liver metabolism, and variable concentrations in the blood. In addition, systemic absorption can be reduced without compromising the desired effect. In contrast, transdermal formulations act at the central level and use the skin as a vehicle for administration of the analgesic drug with gradual release of the medication into the bloodstream and resultant serum concentrations similar to levels obtained with intravenous/oral administration (Anitescu, Benzon, & Agroff, 2013). Topical analgesics are best used in peripheral pain conditions, like osteoarthritis and localized neuropathic pain.

The most commonly used topical medications are nonsteroidal anti-inflammatory drugs (NSAIDs), local anesthetics, and capsaicin. Other classes of medications available in topical preparations include tricyclic antidepressants, ketamine, baclofen, and gabapentin, which are used alone or in combination for refractory pain (Anitescu et al., 2013). Considering that the chronic use of oral NSAIDs is associated with gastrointestinal (GI), cardiac, and renal toxicity in older adults, it is important to minimize local GI toxicity, as well as the total dose of medicine typical with systemic absorption. Topical NSAIDs, most commonly diclofenac, has the most literature to support use for inflammation of joints and muscles (Altman, Bosch, Brune, Patrignani, & Young, 2015; Anitescu et al., 2013). Other topical medications such as ketamine, capsaicin, gabapentin, methadone, and local anesthetics have the most literature regarding use in neuropathic pain. Overall evidence to support compounded or mixed topical analgesics is limited, although case reports have demonstrated efficacy in elderly patients (Anitescu et al., 2013). Topical analgesics should be considered first-line in elderly patients owing to safer side-effect profiles.

Transdermal Drug Delivery System

The transdermal drug delivery system (TDDS) was developed to deliver medications via the skin to circulation; it is mainly useful for medications that are relatively small in molecular size and lipophilic in nature. TDDS is limited to delivery of peptides, proteins, and drugs that are charged ions and are hydrophilic (Dhote et al., 2012). Advances in transdermal drug delivery include iontophoresis and phonophoresis.

Iontophoresis

Derived from the Greek *ionto* meaning "ion" and *phoresis* meaning "to bear," iontophoresis is a process that allows increased penetration of medicine into the tissue by application of a low electric current (Dhote et al., 2012). Iontophoresis pushes ionized drugs across the skin's outmost layer, which is the main barrier when transporting medications across the skin. This is particularly important in the elderly population, owing to decreases in the permeability of the skin's outermost layer as a person ages. Iontophoresis uses like charges to repel the charged molecules across the skin. Once the medication crosses the skin barrier, natural diffusion and perfusion take over and distribute the medication. Pain management using iontophoresis includes reducing inflammation with dexamethasone and NSAIDs, as well as postoperatively with fentanyl.

Fentanyl iontophoretic transdermal system (ITS) is a patient-controlled analgesia (PCA) system that is approved for the management of acute, moderate-to-severe postoperative pain (Power, 2007). The fentanyl ITS was compared to morphine IV PCA and resulted in similar pain control to the standard regimen, with similar incidence of adverse events. The fentanyl ITS does have advantages over the standard morphine PCA including avoiding injections, thus decreasing risk of infection and injection injuries, as well as preprogrammed devices to avoid medication dosing errors with manual programming (Power, 2007). At this time, however, the evidence is limited to the postoperative setting; thus, future research is needed in the ambulatory care setting.

Phonophoresis

This is use of ultrasound to enhance the delivery of topically applied medications (Byl, 1995). This technique is used commonly in rehabilitation medicine, using anti-inflammatory or analgesic medications, to provide safe and painless alternatives to injections for treatment of inflammatory pain conditions (Saliba, Mistry, Perrin, Gieck, & Weltman, 2007).

Iontophoresis and phonophoresis both have evidence to support their use in pain management; however, the majority of evidence is in the adult population with the median age of 45 to 50 years, given this would need to take into consideration age-related changes when considering use of these technologies in treating pain in elderly patients.

Supersaturation

Skin penetration of medications using supersaturation can allow for increased penetration across the skin's outermost layer. The mechanism is based on increased drug driving force for transit out of the dosage form and into the skin (Cilurzo, Casiraghi, Selmin, & Minghetti, 2015). Supersaturated solutions found in the literature, using medications for pain, include diclofenac, fentanyl, ibuprofen, indomethacin, and salicylic acid. Supersaturation is obtained by mixing drugs with solvent and nonsolvent mixtures to obtain solutions, semisolid preparations, and for patch production using evaporation (Cilurzo et al., 2015). Unfortunately, owing to instability of the medications and solutions that leads to crystallization, causing decreased skin penetration, there is ongoing research for more stable options for drugs and solutions. Currently, there are no available products for pain management that utilize supersaturation for drug delivery; however, pharmaceutical researchers continue to work toward this.

TECHNOLOGICAL APPLICATIONS FOR PHARMACEUTICALS AND DEVICES FOR PAIN MANAGEMENT

Intrathecal Drug Delivery

Intrathecal drug delivery (ITDD) is an effective method of pain control for chronic nonmalignant pain (CNMP), pain associated with cancer, and spasticity. However, owing to the invasive procedure for placement of pumps, it is generally considered a last resort in pain management (Duarte et al., 2012). Owing to the metabolic changes seen in elderly individuals, use of oral and topical medications can result in increased risk of adverse drug reactions. ITDD allows for delivery of medication directly into the spinal route to achieve adequate pain control with smaller doses, which leads to reduction in side effects compared with systemic administration (British Pain Society, 2015). ITDD has been shown to be an effective treatment alternative in carefully selected patients with chronic pain that is unable to be controlled by medications and/or spinal cord stimulation. Unfortunately, there is no randomized controlled trial evidence for the use of continuous infusions in elderly patients, but there is supportive prospective open studies in all age groups (Abdulla et al., 2013).

Use of ITDD in both malignant and nonmalignant pain has been studied for many years as a means to decrease side effects of medications and improve control of pain. In 1979, Cousins and colleagues described the phenomenon of "selective spinal analgesia" in which opioids provided specific analgesic effect with few systemic side effects; use of epidural and intrathecal opioids followed shortly after (Cousins, Mather, Glynn, Wilson, & Graham, 1979). The opioid analgesic effect is due, mainly, to the uptake of the opioid directly into the spinal cord and cerebrospinal fluid. Opioids inhibit pain transmission by decreasing neurotransmitter release related to pain signals in the spinal cord. Other medications used in ITDD for malignant and nonmalignant pain include local anesthetics, clonidine, and ziconotide (British Pain Society, 2015). Intrathecal baclofen is used for severe pain and disability secondary to spasticity. Baclofen restores the balance between active and passive muscles, leading to relief from pain from muscle spasms and skeletal deformities (British Pain Society, 2015).

Indications for use of ITDD in CNMP are various types of intractable pain that has failed other management techniques, including spinal cord stimulation (British Pain Society, 2015). For pain associated with cancer, the majority of patients are able to be managed by oral medications; however, 10% to 20% of patients require more intensive interventions to manage pain, with about 3% of those requiring spinal analgesia (Zech, Grond, Lynch, Hertel, & Lehmann, 1995). Trials of ITDD are generally not recommended in malignant and nonmalignant pain; however, with use of baclofen for spasticity, a trial of either infusion or bolus is recommended to fully assess the effect on function (British Pain Society, 2015).

Spinal administration of medications for pain should be reserved for those with severe pain that has been refractory to all other appropriate treatments, with significant impact on quality of life. Selection of patients is important, especially when used for CNMP. The process should include a multidisciplinary team with a comprehensive understanding of the physical, psychological, and rehabilitation aspects of the patient's condition (British Pain Society, 2015). In patients with CNMP, the team should have a clear medical diagnosis, psychological assessment, and appropriate information regarding the long-term efficacy, as well as risks of therapy.

TECHNOLOGICAL DEVELOPMENTS IN NONPHARMACEUTICAL DEVICE USE IN PAIN MANAGEMENT

The literature is abundant with studies about electrotherapy applications for pain management. Unfortunately, the challenges with the multitude of studies are numerous: The broad array of study designs, electrotherapy applications (devices, modality), lengths of treatment, numbers of study participants, pain types, and conditions treated results in varying conclusions from different meta-analyses. However, the best evidence does support a multimodal and multidisciplinary approach for pain management, particularly for chronic pain. This includes the use of behavioral, pharmacological, and nonpharmacological approaches for the most successful management.

In this section, we discuss the technological advancements in nonpharmacological management of pain, both acute and chronic.

Background/History

It is interesting to note that the use of technology for the management of pain dates as far back as a couple of millennia ago, when the Romans, Egyptians, and Greeks first used electricity from an electric eel to treat medical conditions such as gout, arthritis, and headaches. More recently, in the 1800s, it is well documented that physicians were harnessing the power of electricity and applying it for a variety of ailments including the treatment of pain.

Nonpharmacological approaches include behavioral (cognitive behavioral therapy, biofeedback, and psychotherapy); physical or biomechanical (physical therapy, massage, chiropractic or osteopathic manipulations, exercise, thermal applications, such as heat and cold); interventional (e.g., surgery, acupuncture, injections such as botulin, nerve ablation, nerve blocks, epidural steroid injections); and finally neuromodulation approaches including the physical application of various electrical, ultrasound, and magnetic devices.

To better understand the concept of neuromodulation for pain control, we have broken it down into two distinct types of approaches and pathways: The first pathway focuses on cognitive behavioral approaches (through distraction techniques, cognitive behavioral therapy, biofeedback, etc.) and the second pathway focuses on a biophysical approach (via electrostimulation therapy of central nervous system, etc.). See Figure 9.1 for details of both these approaches of neuromodulation. Neuromodulation approaches are generally considered to be safe and have limited side effects.

Theory

Over the centuries, there have been a number of theories about the origins of pain, each with certain utilities and limitations. Perhaps the most recent, influential theory has been the gate control theory of pain (Melzack & Wall, 1965). Simply put, the gate control theory of pain hypothesizes that pain signals generated in peripheral nerves travel to the dorsal horn of the spinal cord, and are then sent to the brain to be interpreted as a conscious sensation. An area within the dorsal horn of the spinal cord acts as a "gate" that controls the transmission of pain signals to the brain, and different factors influence what signals the gate will permit to be further sent to the brain. Factors such as nonpainful input competes and overrides pain signals, and thus prevents pain signals from traveling to the brain.

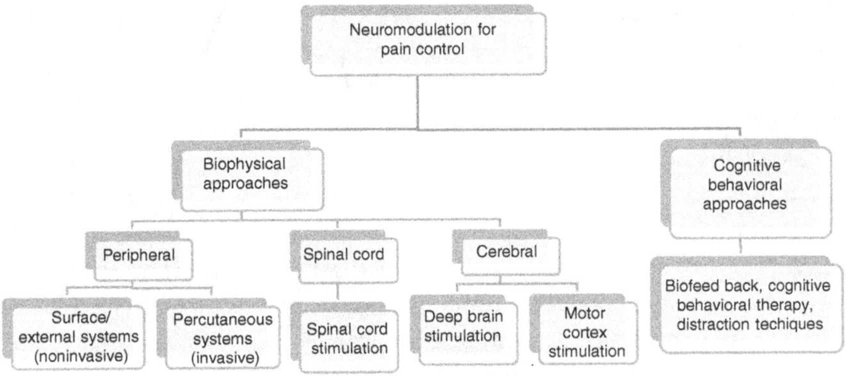

FIGURE 9.1 Pathways of neuromodulation for pain control.

The gate theory is the impetus for the production and use of transcutaneous electrical nerve stimulation (TENS) and other neuromodulatory devices for pain control. The efficacy of the TENS unit results from generated nonpainful electric impulses that interfere with the pain signals from the body that are simultaneously being transmitted. It should be noted that more invasive and cerebellar neuromodulation applications are screened and evaluated through a multidisciplinary team that includes a pain specialist, a neuropsychologist, and a neurosurgeon. These screenings are intended to identify potential barriers such as cognitive impairment and psychiatric disorders.

Types of Devices

The various neuromodulation devices currently available on the market with purported benefits of pain relief can certainly be mind boggling and overwhelming. We focus on a few general types of devices and approaches with applications to specific types of pain, for which the validity has been sufficiently supported in medical literature. We also discuss some treatments that are newly emerging, or are of limited scope such that they should be considered (but not firmly recommended), as they are still considered to be under investigation or experimental due to the low number of patients having been treated.

Peripheral Neuromodulation Applications

Peripheral neuromodulation devices can be divided into two subcategories: the noninvasive TENS devices and the minimally invasive peripheral electric nerve stimulation (PENS) devices.

TRANSCUTANEOUS ELECTRICAL NERVE STIMULATION One of the most widely used noninvasive peripheral neuromodulatory devices is a TENS unit. A TENS unit commonly has a battery pack, and two or more gel-pad electrodes that are applied to the skin. The TENS unit delivers electricity, and has settings to control the electric pulse width, frequency, and intensity. The settings can be adjusted to patient preference to achieve the optimal degree of pain relief.

TENS has proven to be effective for postoperative mild to moderate pain, by reducing the analgesic requirements and/or pain scores after procedures such inguinal hernia repair, tubal ligation, cardiac surgery, and thoracotomy. TENS has also shown to be effective for management of chronic pain, such as painful diabetic neuropathy, by reducing pain and improving quality of life. However, TENS has not been shown to be consistently effective enough to be recommended for uses such as neck pain, low back pain, phantom limb pain, or knee osteoarthritis. Some promising, yet not fully substantiated, other uses of TENS include applications for headaches such as migraines, cluster headaches, and trigeminal autonomic cephalalgias (Puledda et al., 2016).

Although generally considered safe and mostly free of side effects (aside from some skin irritation), there are several situations in which a TENS unit should not be used: over the eyes (as it can cause an increase of intraocular pressure), over the head, over the front of the neck (as it can cause hypotension), through the chest, on broken skin, and over cancers. TENS should also be avoided in people with pacemakers or implantable cardioverter defibrillators.

Owing to the challenges related to quality of study design and outcomes, many uses of TENS are considered investigational, and are not covered by major medical insurance agencies such as Medicare, Aetna, and Anthem. These types of insurance agencies only cover certain modalities for a defined condition under very specific circumstances.

PENS AND ELECTROACUPUNCTURE PENS devices operate by generating and sending electrical pulses through a needle that is inserted under the skin in an area of pain. The use of a PENS device may be considered where results from TENS have produced incomplete relief of pain. PENS devices may also be surgically implanted in certain patients where specialist consensus believes that the peripheral nerve stimulator would provide further significant relief from pain. Other applications in this category include electroacupuncture, with recent early evidence to support the use for pain relief in chemotherapy-induced neuropathy (Garcia et al., 2014) and carpal tunnel syndrome (Chung et al., 2016).

SPINAL CORD STIMULATION Spinal cord stimulation (SCS) is a neuromodulation treatment that has proven to be effective for failed back-surgery syndrome and complex regional pain syndrome. SCS can be permanently implanted with stimulating electrodes in the epidural space of the spinal canal, and an electrical pulse generator (battery) implanted in either the low abdominal area or gluteal region (Kumar et al., 2008).

CEREBELLAR NEUROMODULATION APPLICATIONS

Deep Brain Stimulation

Deep brain stimulation (DBS) is an approach of neuromodulation that is still in the early stages of use, with limited studies demonstrating efficacy for different pain syndromes. Preliminary evidence of efficacy for DBS has been demonstrated for intractable pain from conditions such as primary dystonia and cervical dystonia. It is recommended that DBS should only be performed in experienced centers.

Motor Cortex Stimulation

Motor cortex stimulation has been shown to be effective for neuropathic type pains such as central poststroke pain and facial pain (Cruccu et al., 2007). Good response rates have been demonstrated with motor cortex stimulation for both central pain (54% improvement) and facial pain (68% improvement); however, the side effect profile is increased with this neuromodulation modality. Risks include infections (~5%), hardware-related problems (~5%), and seizures in the early postoperative period (~12%), although chronic seizures are not noted (Fontaine, Hamani, & Lozano, 2009).

Vibration Therapy

The concept of focal muscle vibration, or whole-body vibration, is not a new one; in fact, it dates as far back as the late 19th century when John Harvey Kellogg first utilized vibrating bars, handles, and platforms to promote wellness in his patient population at his sanitarium. It is a form of noninvasive analgesia that has been gaining some traction and popularity in the geriatric population, particularly owing to evidence supporting its use in patients with fibromyalgia, multiple sclerosis, osteoporosis, sarcopenia, and Parkinson's disease (Perraton, Machotka, & Kumar, 2011).

Vibration therapy involves the application of vibrations through a platform of preset magnitude, oscillation, frequency, and amplitude while a patient is performing and maintaining various static exercise positions. There are a number of theories that postulate how vibration therapy actually works to produce neuromuscular adaptation, but they are beyond the scope of this book.

There is certainly evidence that supports the use of vibration therapy to decrease pain and fatigue in patients with fibromyalgia, as well as chronic lower back pain and osteoarthritis of the knee. Cooling vibration analgesia, when administered to individuals with cognitive impairment during certain invasive procedures, also has been shown to decrease the pain response (Schreiber et al., 2016).

However, it is important to also understand the risks associated with vibration therapy in the elderly population (Brooke-Wavell & Mansfield, 2009). Vibration therapy can lead to neurovascular damage and injury in the upper extremities (particularly the hands). It is interesting to note that vibration therapy is a known occupational hazard, and prolonged exposure has been linked to increased risk of lower back pain (the very symptoms that it has been postulated to treat). Vibration therapy is currently not a covered service under Medicare; similarly, vibration devices are also considered to be massage modalities, and are not eligible to be categorized as durable medical equipment (DME).

Pulsed Electromagnetic Field Therapy

Pulsed electromagnetic field therapy (PEMFT) was originally developed as a reparative technique to treat delayed or nonunion osseous fractures. However, this modality has since expanded its scope of treatment, and is currently being hailed as an innovative advancement in adjuvant noninvasive pain management (Markov, 2007). PEMFT relies on the delivery of nonionized, nonthermal electromagnetic energy to the painful areas of the body. The therapy is self-administered, usually within the comfort of the patient's own home through a portable device without the need for application of topical or invasive electrodes into the body. For these reasons, this form of analgesia holds much promise for the frail, debilitated, and homebound cohort of our older population.

There is strong evidence (both in vitro and in vivo studies) that supports the use of PEMFT for the treatment of a variety of localized pain syndromes (Harper, Schmidt, Kubat, & Isenberg, 2015). These include postsurgical pain, neuropathic pain, painful muscle spasms, and various rheumatological and orthopedic conditions. It is theorized that PEMFT is able to provide these analgesic effects by modulating factors involved in the inflammatory response and pain signaling pathway (Ross, Teli, & Harrison, 2016).

The PEMFT movement has been garnering massive interest in recent times, thanks in part to the extensive media, news, and television coverage it has been receiving. The recent U.S. Food and Drug Administration (FDA) approval of Optune (PEMFT device) for the treatment of brain cancers and pain related to brain tumors has been groundbreaking, and is pioneering a new era of PEMFT devices on the market. These devices are indeed classified as DME and are reimbursable through Medicare and other insurance providers.

Low-Level Laser Therapy

Low-level laser therapy (LLLT) or cold laser therapy is a modality of noninvasive analgesia that has been often employed by alternative medicine practitioners (particularly acupuncturists) for well over a couple of decades now. Unlike conventional (hot) laser therapy where the living tissue is burned and cut, proponents of LLLT claim that this form of nonthermal irradiation stimulates and encourages normal cell functioning by decreasing pain and inflammation at a cellular level.

The current literature is divided in terms of the effectiveness of LLLT and real-life clinical applications. This lack of consensus is, in part, due to the immense variation in the LLLT devices available on the market today, specifically related to the promised output for each individual device. Some controversial devices have been found to be no more than light-emitting diodes (LED lights) and in many cases the results were no better than placebo. However, certain meta-analyses and systemic reviews have conclusively demonstrated short-term analgesic effects, particularly in the management of various musculoskeletal and peripheral neuropathic conditions (Cg et al., 2015; Chow et al., 2009). Following these publications, the FDA has cleared them as "adjunctive devices for the temporary relief of pain" (FDA, 2015). Unfortunately, this form of analgesia probably holds little promise for geriatric patients, many of whom suffer from permanent and chronic forms of long-term pain syndromes.

Video Games and Other Distraction Techniques

Distraction techniques have widely been used as an adjunct to unpleasant procedures or discomfort in clinical practice for decades. The aim and hope of such adjunct therapies have been to avoid pharmacotherapy, particularly the prescribing of opiate and psychotropic medications. Both of these groups of medications have tremendous inherent risks and side effects. The goal with distraction techniques has been to draw the attention of the patient away from their pain by engaging them physically and psychologically in the therapeutic activity. Traditionally, the evidence-based distraction techniques have included guided imagery, music and aroma therapy, watching videotapes, relaxation, and deep breathing; all have been met with relative degrees of success.

Gone are the days when video games were considered to be childish. With the advent of role-playing games, it is now possible to create expansive virtual environments that allow users to explore rich and stimulating situations. The ability to navigate such imaginative territory and experience invigorating and energizing circumstances indirectly draws patients' attention away from their ongoing issues relating to chronic pain.

The effectiveness and sustainability of virtual reality as a form of adjunct pain therapy has been demonstrated successfully through real-time physiological monitoring (B. K. Wiederhold, Gao, Sulea, & M. D. Wiederhold, 2014). In addition to distraction from discomfort, video games have also been associated with other improved health outcomes, specifically physical therapy, psychological therapy, disease self-management, as well as skills training for clinicians (Primack et al., 2012).

Unfortunately, much of the literature in this regard has often focused on younger patients undergoing burn wound care, antineoplastic treatments, locally invasive procedures, and prolonged hospitalizations. However, it is reasonable to extrapolate that these same results can be replicated in older, but cognitively intact, patients. Unlike other fairly complicated pieces of technology (such as operating a personal computer), much of the newer generation of video game consoles are fairly straightforward and user friendly to operate. There is much evidence that supports this theory, particularly the studies involving consoles such as the Nintendo Wii, and its diverse uses by nursing homes, rehabilitation centers, and community-dwelling seniors across the nation (Donath, Rössler, & Faude, 2016; Godinho et al., 2016).

CONCLUSION

Pain management in the elderly remains a very complex and challenging issue to tackle. Much research is still required to assess the applicability and effectiveness of each of these described pain management modalities in our geriatric population. The advances in pharmacotherapy and drug delivery systems, while definitely promising, unfortunately do not bypass the uncertainty of drug pharmacokinetics and pharmacodynamics in the older population. Additionally, the recent epidemic of opiate-related deaths in the United States and efforts to minimize the use of controlled substances to address pain are worrisome. For these reasons, many practitioners are very hesitant to prescribe pharmacotherapy in the elderly population to address pain. As a consequence, this continues to result in improper and undertreatment of pain in the frailest of our population. Therefore, nonpharmacological advances in pain management might still be the safest and most effective way forward in addressing this very challenging issue for the majority of elders suffering from pain.

REFERENCES

Abdulla, A., Adams, N., Bone, M., Elliot, A. M., Gaffin, J., . . . Schofield, P. (2013). Guidance on the management of pain in older people. *British Geriatrics Society, 42,* i1–i57. doi:10.1093/ageing/afs200

Administration on Aging. (2015). A profile of older Americans: 2015. Retrieved from https://www.acl.gov/sites/default/files/Aging%20and%20Disability%20in%20America/2015-Profile.pdf

Altman, R., Bosch, B., Brune, K., Patrignani, P., & Young, C. (2015). Advances in NSAID development: Evolution of diclofenac products using pharmaceutical technology. *Drugs, 75,* 859–877. doi:10.1007/s40265-015-0392-z

Anitescu, M., Benzon, H. T., & Argoff, C. E. (2013). Advances in topical analgesics. *Current Opinion in Anaesthesiology, 26*(5), 555–561.

Bhowmik, D., Gopinath, H., Kumar, P. B., Duraivel, S., & Sampath Kumar, K. P. (2012). Recent advances in novel topical drug delivery system. *The Pharma Innovation, 1*(9), 12–31.

British Pain Society. (2015). Intrathecal drug delivery for the management of pain and spasticity in adults: Recommendations for best clinical practice. Retrieved from https://www.britishpainsociety.org

Brooke-Wavell, K., & Mansfield, N. J. (2009). Risks and benefits of whole body vibration training in older people. *Age and Ageing, 38,* 254–255.

Byl, N. N. (1995). The use of ultrasound as an enhancer for transcutaneous drug delivery: Phonophoresis. *Physical Therapy, 75*(6), 539–553.

Cg, S. K., Maiya, A. G., Hande, H. M., Vidyasagar, S., Rao, K., & Rajagopal, K. (2015). Efficacy of low level laser therapy on painful diabetic peripheral neuropathy. *Laser Therapy,* 24(3), 195–200. doi:10.5978/islsm.15-OR-12

Chow, R. T., Johnson, M. I., Lopes-Martins, R. A., & Bjordal, J. M. (2009). Efficacy of low-level laser therapy in the management of neck pain: A systematic review and meta-analysis of randomized placebo or active-treatment controlled trials. *The Lancet, 374*(9705), 1897–1908.

Chung, V. C., Ho, R. S., Liu, S., Chong, M. K., Leung, A. W., Yip, B. H., Hon, S. M., . . . Wong, S. Y. (2016). Electroacupuncture and splinting versus splinting alone to treat carpal tunnel syndrome: A randomized controlled trial. *Canadian Medical Association Journal, 188*(12), 867–875.

Cilurzo, F., Casiraghi, A., Selmin, F., & Minghetti, P. (2015). Supersaturation as a tool for skin penetration enhancement. *Clinical Pharmaceutical Design, 21,* 2733–2744.

Cousins, M. J., Mather, L. E., Glynn, C. J., Wilson, P. R., & Graham J. R. (1979). Selective spinal analgesia. *The Lancet, 1,* 1141–1142.

Cruccu, G., Aziz, T. Z., Garcia-Larrea, L., Hansson, P., Jensen, T. S., Lefaucheur, J. P., Simpson, B. A., & Taylor, R. S. (2007). EFNS guidelines on neurostimulation therapy for neuropathic pain. *European Journal of Neurology, 14*(9), 952–970.

DeSantana, J. M., Santana-Filho, V. J., Guerra, D. R., Sluka K. A., Gurgel, R. Q., & da Silva, W. M. Jr. (2008). Hypoalgesic effect of the transcutaneous electrical nerve stimulation following inguinal herniorrhaphy: A randomized, controlled trial. *The Journal of Pain, 9*(7), 623–629. doi:10.1016/j.jpain.2008.01.337

DeSantana, J. M., Sluka, K. A., & Lauretti, G. R. (2009). High and low frequency TENS reduce postoperative pain intensity after laparoscopic tubal ligation: A randomized controlled trial. *The Clinical Journal of Pain, 25*(1), 12–19. doi:10.1097/AJP.0b013e31817d1070

Dhote, V., Bhatnagar, P., Mishra, P. K., Mahajan, S. C., & Mishra, D. K. (2012). Iontophoresis: A potential emergence of a transdermal drug delivery system. *Scientia Pharmaceutica, 80*, 1–28. doi:10.3797/scipharm.1108-20

Donath, L., Rössler, R., & Faude, O. (2016). Effects of virtual reality training (exergaming) compared to alternative exercise training and passive control on standing balance and functional mobility in healthy community-dwelling seniors: A meta-analytical review. *Sports Medicine, 46*(9), 1293–1309. doi:10.1007/s40279-016-0485-1

Duarte, R. V., Raphael, J. H., Sparkes, E., Southall, J. L., LeMarchand, K., & Ashford, R. L. (2012). Long-term intrathecal drug administration for chronic nonmalignant pain. *Journal of Neurosurgical Anesthesiology, 24*, 63–70.

Ferrell, B. A. (1995). Pain evaluation and management in the nursing home. *Annals of Internal Medicine, 123*(9), 681–687.

Fontaine, D., Hamani, C., & Lozano, A. (2009). Efficacy and safety of motor cortex stimulation for chronic neuropathic pain: Critical review of the literature. *Journal of Neurosurgery, 110*(2), 251–256.

Gangarosa, L., & James, M. (1995). Modern Iontophoresis for local drug delivery. *International Journal of Pharmaceutics, 123*, 159–171. doi:10.1016/0378-5173(95)00047-M

Garcia, M. K., Cohen, L., Guo, Y., Zhou, Y., You, B., Chiang, J., . . . Wang, M. (2014). Electroacupuncture for thalidomide/bortezomib-induced peripheral neuropathy in multiple myeloma: A feasibility study. *Journal of Hematology and Oncology, 7*, 41. doi:10.1186/1756-8722-7-41

Godinho, C., Domingos, J., Cunha, G., Santos, A. T., Fernandes, R. M., Abreu, D., . . . Ferreira, J. J. (2016). A systematic review of the characteristics and validity of monitoring technologies to assess Parkinson's disease. *Journal of NeuroEngineering and Rehabilitation, 13*, 24. doi:10.1186/s12984-016-0136-7

Hanks-Bell, M., Halvey, K., & Paice, J., (2004). Pain assessment and management in aging. *Online Journal of Issues in Nursing, 9*(3). Retrieved from http://www.nursingworld.org/MainMenuCategories/ANAMarketplace/ANAPeriodicals/OJIN/TableofContents/Volume92004/No3Sept04/ArticlePreviousTopic/PainAssessmentandManagementinAging.aspx

Harper, W. L., Schmidt, W. K., Kubat, N. J., & Isenberg, R. A. (2015). An open-label pilot study of pulsed electromagnetic field therapy in the treatment of failed back surgery syndrome pain. *International Medical Case Reports Journal, 8*, 13–22. doi:10.2147/IMCRJ.S73068

Kaye, A. D., Baluch, A., Scott, J. T. (2010). Pain management in the elderly population: A review. *The Ochsner Journal, 10*, 179–187.

Kumar, K., Taylor, R. S., Jacques, L., Eldabe, S., Meglio, M., Molet, J., . . . North, R. B. (2008). The effects of spinal cord stimulation in neuropathic pain are sustained: A 24-month follow-up of the prospective randomized controlled multicenter trial of the effectiveness of spinal cord stimulation. *Neurosurgery, 63*(4), 762–770. doi:10.1227/01.NEU.0000325731.46702.D9

Markov, M. S. (2007). Expanding use of pulsed electromagnetic field therapies. *Electromagnetic Biology and Medicine, 26*(3), 257–274.

Melzack, R., & Wall, P. D. (1965). Pain mechanisms: A new theory. *Science, 150*(3699), 971–979.

Parkash, V., Maan, S., Deepika, Yadav, S., Hemlata, & Jogpal, V. (2011). Fast disintegrating tablets: Opportunity in drug delivery system. *Journal of Advanced Pharmaceutical Technology & Research,* 2(4), 223–235. doi:10.4103/2231-4040.90877

Perraton, L., Machotka, Z., & Kumar, S. (2011). Whole-body vibration to treat low back pain: Fact or fad? *Physiotherapy Canada, 63*(1), 88–93. doi:10.3138/ptc.2009.44

Power, I. (2007). Fentanyl HCl iontophoretic transdermal system (ITS): Clinical application of iontophoretic technology in the management of acute postoperative pain. *British Journal of Anaesthesia, 98*, 4–11.

Primack, B. A., Carroll, M. V., McNamara, M., Klem, M. L., King, B., Rich, M. O., . . . Nayak, S. (2012). Role of video games in improving health-related outcomes: A systematic review. *American Journal of Preventive Medicine, 42*(6), 630–638. doi:10.1016/j.amepre.2012.02.023

Puledda, F., & Goadsby, P. J. (2016). Current approaches to neuromodulation in primary headaches: Focus on vagal nerve and sphenopalatine ganglion stimulation. *Current Pain and Headache Reports, 20*, 47. doi:10.1007/s11916-016-0577-5

Rastogi, R., & Meek, B. D. (2013). Management of chronic pain in elderly, frail patients: Finding a suitable, personalized method of control. *Clinical Interventions in Aging, 8*, 37–46.

Ross, C. L., Teli, T., & Harrison, B. S. (2016). Electromagnetic field devices and their effects on nociception and peripheral inflammatory pain mechanisms. *Alternative Therapies in Health Medicine, 22*(3), 52–64.

Saliba, S., Mistry, D. J., Perrin, D. H., Gieck, J., & Weltman A. (2007). Phonophoresis and the absorption of dexamethasone in the presence of an occlusive dressing. *Yearbook of Sports Medicine, 42*(3), 349–354.

Sastry, V. S., Nyshadham J. R., & Fix J. A. (2000). Recent technological advances in oral drug delivery—A review. *Pharmaceutical Science & Technology Today, 3*(4), 138–145.

Schreiber, S., Cozzi, G., Rutigliano, R., Assandro, P., Tubaro, M., Cortellazzo, Wiel, L., . . . Barbi, E. (2016). Analgesia by cooling vibration during venipuncture in children with cognitive impairment. *Acta Paediatrica, 105*, 12–16.

U.S. Food and Drug Administration. (2015). Laser facts. Retrieved from http://www.fda.gov/radiation-emittingproducts/resourcesforyouradiationemittingproducts/ucm252757.htm

Wiederhold, B. K., Gao, K., Sulea, C., & Wiederhold, M. D. (2014). Virtual reality as a distraction technique in chronic pain patients. *Cyberpsychology, Behavior, and Social Networking, 17*(6), 346–352. doi:10.1089/cyber.2014.0207

Zech, D. F., Grond, S., Lynch, J., Hertel, D., & Lehmann, K. A. (1995). Validation of the World Health Organization guidelines for cancer pain relief: A 10 year prospective study. *Pain, 63*(1), 65–76.

10

Personalized Medicine and Wearable Devices

Andrew Michael and Thomas F. Osborne

As the Baby Boomer population ages and the pressure on the health care infrastructure becomes palpable, wearable devices have the potential to provide relief by not only empowering patients as active participants in their health, but also by extending the reach and efficiency of care providers. Wearable devices are positioned to disrupt the standard of care, and as a result, have become a hotly discussed topic among technology companies, universities, and government agencies.

In this chapter, we focus on the concepts of personalized medicine in relationship to wearable technology. We begin by reviewing the technical foundations of wearable devices, including sensor technology, big data, and the Internet of things (IoT). Next, we look at the benefits, challenges, and limitations of wearables in health care. Finally, we present specific case scenarios in which wearables have been, or could be, advantageous to an older population, applications in clinical research, the role of regulatory agencies, and the future direction of wearables in medicine.

OVERVIEW OF PERSONALIZED MEDICINE

The concept of personalized medicine is an attempt to break patients out of the one-size-fits-all approach to diagnosis and treatment. As such, personalized medicine is the tailoring of medical care to the individual characteristics, needs, and preferences of each patient (Food and Drug Administration [FDA], 2013). Personalized medicine is not new; in fact, it is arguably the oldest form of medicine. Although medicine can be greatly enhanced with technology, it is not essential to many forms of what may be considered personalized care such as multidisciplinary rounds in the hospital, home health visits, concierge services, and personalized health checkups.

Definitions of personalized medicine vary among scientific groups and government agencies. The Personalized Medicine Coalition defines it as "an evolving field in which physicians use diagnostic tests to determine which medical treatments will work best for each patient." The President's Council of Advisors on Science and Technology defines it as, "the tailoring of medical treatment to the individual characteristics of each patient." The American Medical Association (AMA) states that personalized medicine is "health care that is informed by each person's unique clinical, genetic, and environmental information." Finally, the National Cancer Institute says that it is "a form of medicine that uses information about a person's genes, proteins, and environment to prevent, diagnose, and treat disease" (FDA, 2013). The various definitions highlight a common philosophy: Personalized medicine attempts to harness the unique characteristics of each patient to provide more effective care. Wearable devices are a single, but growing, component of a much larger vision of personalized medicine.

WEARABLE DEVICES: THE ESSENTIALS

Broadly defined, wearable devices are electronic technologies worn on or attached to the body in the form of clothing and accessories. Wearable devices typically contain sensors capable of monitoring and tracking personal physiological data for health and fitness purposes. The information captured by a wearable device may be viewable in real time or near real time on the device itself, and may have the capability to transmit that information to other platforms such as a mobile phone, tablet, or computer. Connected wearables are also a component of the much larger IoT and big data universe. Wearable devices offer patients, providers, and research institutions new and exciting opportunities in clinical medicine and scientific research.

The wearables market is predicted to grow at an explosive rate over the next 10 years. A 2016 independent market research report outlined that the wearable technology market will reach over $30 billion in 2016, $40 billion in 2018, $100 billion in 2023, and eventually over $150 billion by 2026 (James Hayward, 2016). Analysts at Morgan Stanley expect that wearables will "become the fastest ramping consumer technology, outstripping even smartphones and tablets," and believe that they "will far surpass market expectations," which could eventually lead to a $1.6 trillion industry (Derrick, 2014; Morgan Stanley, 2015).

The Internet of Things

The IoT is a network of connected technologies capable of collecting and exchanging data. This growing group of connected "things" may be part of everyday objects that are digitally enabled including appliances, vehicles, and even buildings. Networking experts believe that IoT will reach close to 50 billion connected devices by 2020 (Evans, 2011). Wearable devices are an important component of the IoT universe, and will inevitably establish a deeper level of interconnectedness between individuals and organizations. IoT holds the potential for enhanced remote health monitoring, personalized care support, and emergency services. With the simultaneous integration of data obtained from multiple sources, there are exciting possibilities to unravel previously unknown correlations between health risk factors and comorbidities. However, there remain important considerations such as the safety of connected devices and security of personal data that are connected and shared with ever greater efficiency.

Securing the IoT infrastructure is crucial to the success of connected devices. Vulnerable IoT devices can potentially be exploited in various ways. For example, they can be used to build a hostile botnet, capable of carrying out a distributed denial-of-service (DDoS) attack by sending unmanageable amounts of data to a single network target in an attempt to cripple vital infrastructure. Simply put, a connected light bulb, car, smartwatch, pacemaker, or any other IoT device could be the ammunition in a cyber attack against critical infrastructure (e.g., electrical grids, water plants, air traffic controllers). Fortunately, this threat is becoming an actively researched topic by government agencies, technology companies, and security organizations (The President's National Security Telecommunications Advisory Committee, 2014).

Big Data

For decades, computers and networks have produced incredible scientific, business, economic, and social advancements—sometimes changing our entire way of life. These technological enhancements have created an unprecedented amount of data that is growing at an accelerated rate. At the time of this writing, each day, our digital world generates 2.5 quintillion bytes of data; in fact, 90% of the world's data was produced in the last 2 years (IBM, n.d.). The resulting datasets can become so vast and complex that traditional processing tools may struggle to evaluate the immense scope of information. However, data originating from a variety of sources, including computers, devices, sensors, and networks, generating datasets consisting of billions of records, can now be analyzed with advanced tools to reveal profound associations, trends, and patterns (Big data, n.d.). Although there are many definitions of Big data, the term often refers to this extraordinary bulk of information, and sometimes the definition also includes the advanced analytics tools used to gain insights from this volume of information. Wearable devices themselves will generate a seemingly unfathomable amount of data that will need to transformed into reliable and actionable insights for consumers, patients, and health care professionals.

Wearable Device Requirements

As the name would suggest, at a minimum, a wearable device must be wearable. However, other essential wearable device requirements such as being controllable, beneficial, and mobile will be specifically covered in the following sections.

Must Be Wearable

A wearable device is typically worn in the form of clothing or accessories. Digitally enhanced stand-alone devices such as fitness trackers, jewelry, and even clothing are leading examples. Solutions are not necessarily limited to a single wearable device; they may be comprised of multiple connected devices interoperating with each other. For example, a watch might interact with an earring to identify the proximity of the hand to the head; or a group of rings might interact with each other to translate sign language.

Fashion, comfort, durability, and safety are all crucial considerations while designing a wearable device. The intersection of fashion and technology is inevitable; in fact, various well-known designer labels and technology giants are actively involved in the integration of technology into their apparel. Fashion aside, failing to design comfortable and durable wearable devices may suffer similar consequences of poorly designed and manufactured clothing.

Safety is arguably the most important element in the design of any device, particularly one that is in continuous contact with the human body. Poor safety can be a health hazard and a costly financial recall risk, which may also damage a company's brand equity. In August 2016, McDonald's recalled almost 33 million wearable fitness trackers in the United States and Canada after more than 70 reports of skin irritation, burns, and blisters were reported (U.S. Consumer Product Safety Commission, 2016). These issues impact everyone in the field because reports of harmful wearable devices could potentially spread an irreparable message of distrust among consumers, thwarting the further advancement of wearables in the medical field. Other critical safety considerations include the reliability of the data itself, from which clinical decisions may be made. The vital oversight and safety evaluation processes provided by federal agencies such as the FDA are discussed later in this chapter.

Must Be Controllable

Ideally, a wearable device should be actively or passively controllable by the patient or provider. Some examples of ways to control a wearable device include power use, device mode, calibration, and communication settings. Positive and negative feedback algorithms can also be incorporated to automatically control the function of the instrument. For example, a device sensor may be able to detect a high glucose level in a patient, thereby automatically activating an implanted insulin pump. However, this case underscores the critical importance of accurate and reliable sensor information for medical decision making because inappropriate insulin treatment based on inaccurate blood glucose data can lead to acute life-threatening hypoglycemia or hyperglycemia.

Must Be Beneficial

Wearable devices should provide value, which may translate into improved personal health, decreased cost of care, or preferably both. Personal health value may take many forms including empowering patients to have greater participation in their own care, convenience, providing additional clinical data points, and potentially integrating data with primary health information systems.

A variety of portable wearable solutions are now available to do things that were previously only available in dedicated facilities. For example, wearable products are available, or are under development, such as hats that record EEG patterns, wristwatches that communicate cardiac arrhythmias, and socks that can detect risks of ulcers or gait abnormalities. Specific use cases are discussed later in this chapter.

Must Be Mobile

A wearable device should allow the user to move about freely without significant hindrance. However, meeting this requirement can be an engineering challenge. Fortunately, flexible electronics, smaller sensors, and extended battery life are providing innovators with the raw materials necessary to overcome mobility issues. Digital communication technologies further enhance movement by allowing the device to wirelessly interact with nearby smartphones, routers, location beacons, or other IoT devices. As an example, new Bluetooth low energy (BLE) technology automatically adjusts the wireless transmitter to stay in a low-power state until the device triggers the need for a short high-energy transmission. This configuration avoids the necessity of the standard always-on Bluetooth connection, which can drain batteries or require that larger batteries are incorporated into the device. Additional advancements continue to push the boundaries of what is possible. For example, the latest version of Bluetooth (version 5) offers two times the speed, four times the range, and eight times the bandwidth of the BLE profile, an endeavor designed to further facilitate mobility and the IoT experience (Bluetooth SIG, 2016). Lastly, wireless carriers are developing new network communication standards such as LTE-M and NB-IoT to handle low power, as well as infrequent communications with IoT and wearable devices (LinkLabs, 2015).

Sensors and Telemetry: Understanding Our Environments

A sensor is hardware technology that responds to a physical stimulus and transmits a resulting impulse (Sensor, n.d.). Sensors are an essential component of wearable devices, and many devices have several different types of miniature sensors built into the housing. However, there are detached options as well. For example, when a device is in proximity to a remotely placed sensor (4 cm or less), coupling with a near field communications (NFC) tag can provide data collection opportunities with little or even no energy required by the sensor (Near Field Communication, 2011). There are a variety of sensors that have the ability to detect and quantify various stimuli including, but not limited to, heat, light, sound, pressure, motion, and distinct chemical signatures. The following is an overview of some of the more common sensors available today.

Accelerometers, Motion, and Activity Tracking

Accelerometers are used in a variety of industries such as engineering, biology, medicine, transportation, navigation, and, most notably, consumer electronics. In consumer electronic applications, accelerometers provide motion, orientation, and digital image stabilization capabilities. Activity trackers are among the most popular wearable devices on the market today, using accelerometers and gyroscopes as their primary data collection tools (InvenSense, 2016). Because these sensors are so affordable, mobile device manufacturers often build accelerometers into their hardware designs even if it is not part of their current strategy, in the event that enhanced functionality would potentially benefit from the sensor at a later date. Possible medical applications for accelerometers are numerous and include fall detection, gait abnormality diagnosis, concussion detection, and obsessive-compulsive treatment (i.e., trichotillomania), to name a few.

Proximity and Ultrasonic Sensors

Ultrasonic sensors can be utilized to calculate distance between two or more points. The device will typically transmit a short burst of ultrasonic sound toward the target that is then reflected back to a sensor. Using the speed of sound, the sensor will calculate distance based on the time that the sound is echoed back from the target (Massa, 1999). In doing so, the technology leverages the same physics principles that help bats to fly at night, or for dolphins and whales to swim in dark water. There are numerous types of ultrasonic sensors available today, most of which have subtle differences in frequency, configuration, and feature sets. Depending on the environment under measurement, some ultrasonic sensors are more suitable than others and, therefore, much like any component, selecting the correct sensor for the task requires a thorough understanding of the goals and requirements of the particular device.

Several medical applications have been explored using ultrasonic sensors embedded in wearable devices. Examples include arm motion tracking, muscle contraction monitoring, and foot monitoring in diabetic patients (Trindade, Ono, Lemaire, & AlMohimeed, 2014). Ultrasonic sensors are ideally suited for applications that aid in spatial awareness for disabled individuals. For example, a visually impaired patient may be able to "feel" their surrounding environment with haptic feedback—that is, generating an electronic touch sensation to the patient as a result of the input from the sensor data (IEEE Robotics & Automation Society, n.d.).

Electrochemical Sensors: Blood, Sweat, and Tears

Real-time monitoring of human body fluids (blood, sweat, and tears) enables a wide variety of opportunities for noninvasive medical diagnostic applications. For example, a smart bandage might be able to detect subtle changes in pH and other markers, providing insight about wound healing, specific types of infections, and immune response. Measuring metabolites, electrolytes, and skin temperature using textiles may be used to calculate a sweat profile, providing useful information about hydration status and drug use/compliance. A smart contact lens could, for example, extract information from biomolecules in tears, providing a way to monitor blood glucose levels and other biomarkers without blood draws (Farandos, 2015; Miller, 2015).

While "Lab-on-a-Chip" electrochemical sensors are already used widely in biotechnology and analytical chemistry, their use in health devices remains limited for a variety of indications. Integrating electrochemical sensors into noninvasive monitoring devices presents a challenge because chemosensors and biosensors usually require direct molecular interaction with the substrate before a reaction is observable and recordable. When this substrate is blood, sweat, or urine, sensors can become limited by possible contamination or evaporation, which may render inaccurate measurements (Gao et al., 2016).

Electromagnetic Sensors: Capturing User Interactions

Electromagnetic (EM) fields are emitted by electrically charged objects, and each appliance we use throughout the day has a distinct EM footprint. EM sensors in the form of probes or antennae are capable of measuring EM fields and their unique signatures.

The University of Washington has recently collaborated with Microsoft Research on a low-power wrist-worn wearable system called *MagnifiSense*. Using the unique electromagnetic interference (EMI) footprint, the system can identify which electronics and appliances the user interacts with throughout the day. Tracking device usage can provide valuable information about the status of the user. Their research provides a use case example of an elder adult in a home or assisted living facility using *MagnifiSense*. For example, the system would be able to detect who and when someone turns a stove on or off, identify whether the individual leaves the stove unattended, and provide a reminder to the user or supervisor if the stove is left for an extended period (Wang, Lee, Mariakakis, & Goel, 2015).

Similar research conducted by Disney, in collaboration with Carnegie Mellon University, led to the development of *EM-Sense*, another wrist-worn wearable EMI sensing system capable of detecting what a user is touching. In a prototype demonstration, the wearable system was able to detect when the user picked up a toothbrush, and automatically started a 1-minute timer to promote improved dental hygiene practices (Laput, Yang, Xiao, Sample, & Harrison, 2015). These technologies may become particularly useful to the aging population by providing personalized safety and assistance with activities of daily living.

Flow Measurement

Within medicine, understanding blood flow characteristics provides unique insight into cardiovascular health and disease progression. Recently, an international team led by researchers at the University of Illinois at Urbana-Champaign and the U.S. National Institutes of Health developed a continuous blood flow monitor using flexible electronics. The wearable device detects subtle changes in heat patterns caused by blood flow just beneath the skin; additional details about blood flow is then calculated using a computer algorithm. Such a device has the potential to revolutionize the management of various vascular conditions that involve the skin, including diabetes, arteriosclerosis, and wound healing (Hsu, 2015).

Torque and Force Measurement

Torque sensors are used to measure the force on a rotating system, such as a car engine, bicycle, or human joint movement. Studying the subtleties of joint movement and strength may provide new insight into patients with various diseases including arthritis, nerve damage, muscular dystrophy, and traumatic injury. Using torque sensors, Italian researchers developed *ThimbleSense*, a system useful for studying grasp manipulation (Battaglia et al., 2016). Importantly, torque sensors may prove to be especially useful in physical rehabilitation efforts as they collect information about the forces related to specific body movements.

Ambient Sensors: Temperature, Humidity, and Light

Wearable devices equipped with temperature, humidity, and light sensors allow integrated systems to more efficiently adjust the ambient characteristics in an environment; this is sometimes referred to as ambient intelligence. For example, changing skin temperatures detected by a sensor may automatically trigger the adjustment of a heater or air conditioner; air moisture levels detected in the mask of a continuous positive airway pressure (CPAP) machine may appropriately modify humidity levels; sweat measurements may prompt fitness recommendations; and light sensors may provide alerts regarding the harmful effects of overexposure or underexposure. Ambient sensors generally do not require significant computational power, making them ideal for integration into wearable devices and surrounding IoT infrastructure (Sensirion, 2016).

Visual Systems and Augmented Reality

Wearable visual enhancement systems have been a hot topic in the media over the past several years. Google Glass, a head-mounted display, attempts to bring ubiquitous computing to the consumer—that is, real-time, always-on, always-present computing. The device discreetly projects an image into the visual field, enabling the user to augment everyday tasks. Practical medical applications using head-mounted optical systems could include hazard detection, reading assistance, and facial recognition.

More specifically, facial recognition software could identify an individual, search databases for information about that person, and present that information to the user, which may be particularly useful to those with memory impairments. However, these integrated visual technologies encounter political and societal obstacles owing to their potential to violate the privacy of individuals. Because privacy is a crucial concern among technology companies and regulatory bodies, Google has explicitly banned Google Glass applications that provide real-time facial recognition and voice print analysis (Google Developers, 2015).

Augmented reality (AR) represents a live view of the real world with computer-generated elements superimposed on the visual field in a way that they appear to be part of the environment. Augmented elements can be sensor driven or purely artificial. Wearable devices, and/or the functional components of wearable devices integrated into AR devices, will likely play a significant role in AR applications, as this technology effectively serves as the eyes, ears, and instruments of the system. Within medical education, AR may assist medical professionals and patients to learn complex concepts in a more intuitive visual way. Further discussion about the applications and potentials of these types of educational applications can be found in Chapter 13.

BENEFITS AND ADVANTAGES

Numerous benefits are observed by incorporating wearable devices in modern medical practice. Among the most notable advantages include real-time data collection, clinical decision support, convenience, decreased health care costs, safety, efficiency, standardization, and improved access to care.

Data Collection and Clinical Decision Support

Gaining insight into a medical condition typically requires that essential diagnostic tasks be completed by specifically trained medical professionals. With the introduction of wearables, providers may have access to additional real-time streaming patient telemetry collected from sensors from almost anywhere in the world with Internet access. In scenarios where real-time telemetry cannot be streamed (i.e., no Internet access), data can be stored on the device and forwarded at a later time, using "store-and-forward" operating procedures (Public Health Institute Center for Connected Health Policy, n.d.). As a result of these advancements, providers may have an unprecedented view into the health of their patients through the data that they generate. If systems are robust, caregivers will also have access to integrated clinical decision support systems and on-demand data analytics services, which add a layer of certainty in their judgments, and ultimately offering more optimized and timely care to their patients.

Potential to Decrease Health Care Costs

Data shared by the Centers for Medicare & Medicaid Services (CMS) show that national health expenditure (NHE) in 2014 reached an unprecedented $3 trillion, which accounted for 17.5% of the gross domestic product (GDP), and is projected to increase to 20.1% of the GDP by 2025. Of particular interest, per person, personal health care spending for the 65 years and older population was $18,988 in 2012, which is over five times higher than spending per child ($3,552), and approximately three times the spending per working-age person ($6,632) (CMS, 2016). It is evident that the current financial trajectory is unsustainable.

Wearable devices have the potential to be an important part of the economic health care solution. Specifically, the ability to reduce the numbers of caregivers necessary to collect health data, with wearable technology, offers direct cost savings. Furthermore, empowering patients with the personalized tools for improved wellness and prevention promises to reduce costs further. Importantly, analyzing the wealth of information available is likely to lead to more precise and accurate personalized care that ultimately reduces cost through improved chronic disease management, medication compliance, accelerated recovery, decreased readmission rates, and hopefully avoiding disease risks altogether. As a result of these appealing prospects, insurers and employers are already starting to use wearables in their wellness programs (UnitedHealthcare, 2016). More research is required in this area to determine how to best utilize wearables to optimize value. However, the future for such applications appears very promising.

Potential to Improve Access to Care

For those who have limited access to reliable transportation, have difficulty covering child care obligations, or have disabilities themselves, making the trip to a medical appointment may be a significant challenge. Fortunately, integrated telehealth solutions have begun to bridge this gap in a scalable way. Home telehealth also provides an infrastructure that opens access to medical expertise that would not otherwise be available to remote geographic locations. For those recovering from illness or managing chronic disease, home telehealth provides an opportunity to stay in the comfort of their homes longer with a decreased risk of nosocomial infections. Wearable health technology is optimally positioned to make remote and home telehealth a more successful and cost-effective solution for all stakeholders. Additional dedicated discussion about home telehealth is available in Chapter 4.

CHALLENGES AND LIMITATIONS

Wearable devices have tremendous potential; however, as with many emerging technologies, there are significant limitations to consider. A major overarching obstacle for the field is the relative lack of collaboration between the siloed expertise and perspectives of engineering, medical professionals, and payers. As a result, inventors and entrepreneurs are vulnerable to creating solutions that are not appropriately designed to the nuanced requirements of those who will be using them. The negative results could be product failure or worse, patient harm. More specific technical challenges for older adult populations include improved usability, accuracy/reliability, battery life, interoperability, and technical support of the wearable device. Determining how technology will be funded is a critical element. These overarching concepts are discussed further in Chapters 2 and 4.

Usability

Usability is critical to developing a successful wearable device. Today's consumer expects electronics to work straight out of the box, with minimal setup and configuration. Presenting new technology to older adults may require specific strategies and systems designed for the optimal user experience of this important and unique population. More specifically, older adults are more likely to have specific disabilities such as impaired vision requiring larger text, or reduced hearing requiring louder volume configuration options. Decreased dexterity can also be a significant issue with small buttons, device size, and complex interfaces. If a device is not user friendly, it risks utterly failing to achieve the goal of improving patient care. Dedicated discussion of technology usability is covered in Chapter 2.

Data Accuracy

For medical applications, wearable device accuracy is paramount, and should be highest on the list of priorities. Clinical decisions may be adversely influenced by inaccurate data, the consequences of which are potentially life-threatening. Evidence of this challenge is already apparent with activity trackers, each of which records footsteps slightly differently than the next. A recent study evaluated the accuracy of wearable devices and smartphone applications with the direct observation of 500 and 1,500 step counts. The study measured 14 participants, 10 applications, 10 devices, and 56 walking trials, and demonstrated variation among the different devices, with one device reporting 20% fewer steps than what was actually observed (Case, Burwick, & Volpp, 2015).

Similarly, a separate study monitored the heart rate of 50 stable intensive care unit patients equipped with both a personal fitness tracker (PFT) and continuous echocardiography (cECG), the accepted gold standard measurement. The results demonstrated that the PFT yielded a slightly lower heart rate than the reading captured from cECG. Those who did not have a sinus rhythm had worse results. The study concluded that further evaluation is necessary before PFTs can augment early warning systems in hospitals (Kroll, Boyd, & Maslove, 2016). While a few inaccurately recorded heartbeats may not appear to be life-threatening, the impact of inaccurate data on large-scale research projects may lead observers to false outcomes—inevitably corroding the foundations of evidence-based medicine. Also, minor variation in other biological metrics may have a significant impact in the care of a patient. Government agencies, such as the FDA, will play a fundamental role in establishing the necessary frameworks for approving wearable devices for safe and effective clinical use. Government oversight is discussed in greater detail later in this chapter.

Battery Life

Battery life is among the biggest technical weaknesses in today's wearable devices. Given the typically preferred thin, small, and lightweight design of most wearable devices, embedding a sufficiently sized battery is challenging. While simple activity trackers do not require a tremendous amount of power, more sophisticated medical devices may. Furthermore, devices with additional features such as back-lit displays, faster processors, and communication components need additional power and, therefore, larger batteries or more frequent recharging. To solve these problems, engineers are exploring solutions such as energy harvesting, a concept in which energy is generated from body movements or even body heat. Power management, such as BLE technology discussed earlier, is another solution in which the power use of devices can be intelligently augmented on the basis of use. Advances in the size, flexibility, and longevity of batteries themselves are also under active development (Chandler, 2016).

Technical Support

Users who encounter technical issues with their device or service will require access to technical support. This essential requirement must not be overlooked while deploying a device-based solution in any context, but this is especially critical in health care. For home-based care scenarios, patients must have clear instructions for contacting tech support, whether it be a dedicated team within a hospital system supporting the technology, or the device manufacturer itself. A central 24/7/365 contact number may be beneficial to triage the technical needs of patients and caregivers more appropriately. Optimally, technical support will be able to access the device remotely to reduce frustration and increase successful support encounters in a timely fashion.

USE CASE SCENARIOS: WEARABLE DEVICES AND THE OLDER ADULT

One in six consumers in the United States currently uses wearable technology. It is expected that 19 million fitness wearables were sold in 2016, a number which is projected to grow at an accelerated pace to 110 million devices in 2018 (Piwek, Ellis, Andrews, & Joinson, 2016). The following sections of this chapter review some common use case scenarios in which wearables are expected to aid patient health care in the older adult.

Continuous Vital Sign Monitoring

One of the greatest advantages of wearable devices is their inherent ability to capture a continuous stream of data. Monitoring vital signs using wearable echocardiograms, sphygmomanometers, and thermometers is becoming an affordable and accessible option for consumers. Vital signs no longer need to be manually captured in snapshot fragments by the provider or the patient, allowing the patient's home to become a virtual extension of a hospital or doctor's office.

Once the devices capture vitals, several actions can be performed depending on the medical necessity. Utilizing the latest technologies, vital sign data can be transmitted in real time over an encrypted channel to a cloud-based data service such as Amazon Web Services, Microsoft Azure, Google Cloud Platform, and IBM Watson. The service would then securely deliver the processed data directly to authorized providers, family members, friends, and of course, the patient. Data in various forms may potentially be transmitted to a secure onsite data warehouse or electronic health record. Alternatively, or perhaps in conjunction, the data might be transmitted to and be viewable on a web-based environment, requiring Internet access and authentication before the information is obtained. For those patients or devices without Internet access, data can be stored on a local device and forwarded to a final data management service at a later time (Public Health Institute Center for Connected Health Policy, n.d.). As discussed earlier in this chapter, devices will continue to gain connectivity to a larger network, making device communication a more standard feature.

Unfortunately, intensive continuous vital sign monitoring may carry legal liabilities. A provider or institution is typically responsible for the remote medical data in their possession (Chesanow, 2014). Having access to multiple continuous patient data streams would result in thousands, if not millions, of individual readings. If a doctor misses a critical value in an ocean of data, one could argue that the physician failed his or her responsibility to monitor the patient appropriately. This is a liability issue that vendors, government, and providers must address before health care providers become comfortable using such technologies. More research is needed in the area of continuous monitoring, so that we may be better prepared to handle unexpected events at inconvenient times, and effectively account for false alarms while also ensuring that critical events are addressed in a timely way. Appropriately designed data analytics software and artificial intelligence (AI) may help us understand when and where to set important thresholds.

Chronic Disease Management

As of 2012, chronic conditions affect 117 million people in the United States. Eighty-six percent of health care spending in 2010 was for people with one or more chronic medical conditions. In 2012 alone, the estimated cost of diagnosed diabetes was $245 billion (Centers for Disease Control and Prevention [CDC], 2016d). Using wearables to prevent, diagnose, and manage chronic diseases has great potential to reduce costs and help individuals obtain the personalized care that they need.

Glucose Management

Managing diabetes is different for every patient; one size does not fit all. Keeping up with constant fluctuations in glucose levels and resulting therapies has been a source of difficulty for both patients and providers. Device manufacturers have developed continuous glucose monitoring (CGM) products and services to ease the frustrations of diabetes management. Unfortunately, these devices still require a thin wire sensor to penetrate the skin to record an accurate reading, which can result in bleeding, skin rashes, and infection (Englert et al., 2014). Alternative options such as implanted CGM sensors often carry a limited life span owing to immune system response, resulting in inaccuracies (Nichols, Koh, Storm, Shin, & Schoenfisch, 2013).

Noninvasive approaches to glucose monitoring are often touted as the "holy grail" of diabetes management, and several teams are working toward this goal. International researchers led by the Institute for Basic Science in Seoul, South Korea, have developed a wearable patch that is capable of monitoring glucose levels and delivering metformin using a graphene-based electrochemical device with thermoresponsive microneedles (Lee et al., 2016). In 2014, Google and Novartis set out to develop a dual function wearable device—a smart contact lens featuring glucose-monitoring capabilities, while simultaneously providing accommodative vision correction to people with presbyopia (Miller, 2015). While large technology companies continue to research and develop noninvasive CGM solutions, assistive wearable devices may help to avoid chronic diseases, such as diabetes, through the promotion and support of healthy lifestyle activities.

Obesity and Weight Loss Management

More than one third of adults in the United States are obese. In 2008, the estimated annual medical cost of obesity was $147 billion (CDC, 2016a). Among the most popular wearable devices are activity trackers, capable of monitoring physical activity using accelerometers, global positioning system (GPS), and other sensors. Using activity data, individuals can gain insight into their habits, and make healthy lifestyle modifications in an attempt to control and hopefully reverse unhealthy weight problems. This personalized insight is particularly relevant as we move from the paradigm of treating illness toward promoting wellness.

Interestingly, while the idea of using a wearable device to encourage weight loss may seem logical, a recent study has suggested otherwise. Researchers at the University of Pittsburgh compared standard behavioral weight loss intervention and technology-enhanced weight loss intervention in 471 adult participants. They found that the intervention group using the wearable device differed significantly from the group using standard behavioral intervention, with the former group resulting in less weight loss over 24 months than the latter. They concluded that devices measuring physical activity may not offer advantages over standard behavioral weight loss strategies (Jakicic et al., 2016). There are several plausible explanations for these negative results. Perhaps the device was hard to use, did not provide information in a meaningful way, or did not provide the type of encouragement that a person could need. These outcomes emphasize that technology in isolation is not a solution to health care challenges and the necessity to objectively reassess assumptions. Implementing solutions with a fuller understanding of the patient's needs, health care requirements, and technological limitations is imperative to successful solutions.

Pain Relief and Drug Abuse Detection

Pain is a significant public health issue that costs society at least $560 billion to $635 billion annually in the form of medical expenses and lost productivity (The American Academy of Pain Medicine, n.d.). The opiate abuse epidemic is a critical side effect of our limited treatment options, and, unfortunately, drug abuse is rampant throughout the world, negatively affecting health, economies, and societies. It is estimated that one in 20 adults worldwide, or roughly 247 million individuals between the ages of 15 and 64 years, used at least one illicit drug in 2014. Twenty-nine million of those people suffer from drug use disorders, ultimately resulting in 207,400 drug-related deaths in 2014. Roughly one third to one half of those deaths were due to overdosing, with most cases attributable to opioids (United Nations Office on Drugs and Crime, 2016).

As a result, researchers and manufacturers continue to invest in innovative methods for providing pain relief. Specifically designed wearable devices may play a role in treating pain with fewer medications, or potentially even without any pharmacological intervention at all.

The device manufacturer NeuroMetrix conducted a peer-reviewed study of Quell, their wearable, fixed-site, high-frequency transcutaneous electrical nerve stimulation (FS-TENS) device that is attached to a user's calf and stimulates the body's opiate production. The study enrolled and observed 130 participants with chronic low back pain, lower extremity pain, or both. The participants were self-administered an FS-TENS device over a period of 60 days. At the 60-day follow-up, 80.7% of participants reported that their pain had improved. The study concluded that the treatment is a safe and effective option for treating chronic low back and lower extremity pain (Gozani, 2016).

Wearable devices may also play a role in drug abuse detection. A small pilot study with four emergency department patients receiving parenteral opioids and one individual with a 20-year history of daily cocaine use was conducted with the utilization of a wrist-worn wearable device capable of detecting drug use. The device continuously measured electrodermal activity (EDA), the property of the human body that causes continuous variation in the electrical characteristics of the skin, skin temperature, and acceleration. The results showed that both intravenous cocaine and opioid administration were temporally associated with notable biometric changes, primarily with an increase in measurable EDA (Carreiro et al., 2014). Other devices are under development to detect specific drug metabolites excreted in sweat (De Giovanni & Fucci, 2013). More research in this area is needed, as this type of technology may serve well the older population, where analgesic abuse may occur, or where drug administration is not regularly supervised.

Fall Detection

Falls cause severe injuries, especially when they occur when a patient is alone. Bone fractures, intracranial bleeding, and loss of consciousness can all lead to fatal or permanently debilitating outcomes. The ability to detect a fall and report it to an emergency medical service is invaluable to older adults. However, traditional fall detection systems are bulky and uncomfortable to wear (Baek, Kim, Bashir, & Pyun, 2013). Wearable devices are under development to provide superior fall detection and even prevention for the user, making them an ideal choice for the older adult.

A team of Korean researchers, funded by the Seoul National University Research Grant, demonstrated a wearable fall detection system using a wristband triboelectric generator in conjunction with a lithium-ion battery and integrated sensors, controllers, and wireless components. The intricate device can harvest electrical energy from daily human activity, which is then used to charge a battery, finally powering an accelerometer and Bluetooth communications. During an unexpected fall, the accelerometer is designed to automatically transmit an alarm to appropriate emergency services (Jung et al., 2015).

Wound Care Monitoring and Therapy

Skin ulcers and chronic wounds can lead to disfigurement, limb-threatening osteomyelitis, or life-threatening sepsis. In the United States, chronic wounds affect 5.7 million patients, and cost over $20 billion annually (Torre, 2015). These numbers are expected to grow tremendously owing to our aging population with multiple comorbidities, such as diabetes, peripheral vascular disease, neuropathy, and mobility limitations. Managing a chronic wound is often tedious and typically costly for patients, providers, and payers.

To address these issues, the European Union funded *SWAN-iCare*, a project aimed at developing an autonomous device for the monitoring and personal management of chronic wounds. The system works using wearable negative pressure technology, which is equipped with sensors, communication components, and microactuators. Optical and electrochemical sensors are intended to monitor for the presence of infection or inflammation (Texier et al., 2013). An effective wound care wearable can serve as an invaluable addition to treatment plans for people with diabetes and older adults, potentially helping hundreds of millions around the world. Furthermore, sensor-enhanced socks and shoes are under development to detect potential risks for ulcers to identify problems before they even begin (Perrier et al., 2014).

Heart Failure

Heart failure affects about 5.7 million adults in the United States. In 2009, one in nine deaths included heart failure as a contributing cause, and roughly half of all people with heart failure die within 5 years of diagnosis. Heart failure costs the United States an estimated $30.7 billion each year in health care services, medications, and missed days of work (CDC, 2016c).

To curb these statistics, researchers are revisiting older methods of measuring heart activity using modern technologies. Ballistocardiography (BCG) is a technique used to create a graphic representation of the movements of the body imparted by the ballistic forces associated with cardiac contraction and ejection of blood through the large vessels (National Library of Medicine, 2011). Seismocardiography (SCG), a similar technique, is a noninvasive recording of cardiac vibratory activity as a measure of cardiac contractile function. A wearable BCG or SCG monitor would make use of an accelerometer sensor, taped or attached to the user using textiles. According to a large multicenter trial, when BCG was combined with electrocardiogram, the predictive accuracy of detecting physiologically significant coronary artery disease was increased significantly over the results of the ECG alone (Inan et al., 2015). In the older adult, incorporating BCG and SCG into wearable technologies may allow providers to monitor the progression of heart failure, and deliver potentially lifesaving notifications to emergency services.

CLINICAL RESEARCH AND REGULATORY AGENCIES

Clinical trials are conducted to observe the safety and efficacy of investigational products or devices. In the United States, conducting a clinical trial for the purpose of seeking a new drug application requires significant resources across regulatory agencies, institutional review boards, and, sometimes, between different companies and countries. Apart from ensuring patient safety, study teams must verify that timely and accurate data are provided to the FDA in accordance with strict protocols. Patient recruitment, data collection, and verification are all laborious, cost-intensive tasks that will benefit from the introduction of wearable devices. With these benefits, using wearable devices to increase the speed and volume at which data are collected is expected to become commonplace in the industry.

Once clinical-grade wearable devices are approved by the FDA, they themselves can also be used to make other clinical research more efficient and cost-effective. Wearables are already starting to appear in clinical trials with Apple's ResearchKit, an open-source software development kit (SDK) capable of turning the iPhone into a powerful medical research device. iPhone applications designed with ResearchKit allow developers to create informed consents, participant procedures, and surveys. Working in conjunction with ResearchKit, HealthKit is another Apple SDK that securely centralizes data storage of personal health information. Using ResearchKit, Stanford University amazingly recruited 11,000 subjects for a heart disease study in only 24 hours. Achieving the same task using traditional methods would have required dozens of medical centers and over a year of work (Robinson, 2015).

With the introduction of wearable devices into clinical research, a standardized method for evaluating and approving new clinical-grade devices must be strictly adhered to. Fortunately, existing regulatory frameworks are established that can contribute to the advancement of these devices. Good Clinical Practice (GCP) is a unified international standard for ethically conducting clinical trials in the United States, Japan, and the European Union. Similarly, Good Manufacturing Practice (GMP) provides a framework in which new products are manufactured. GCP, GMP, and other regulations will play a fundamental role in the development of personalized medicine using wearable and IoT devices.

CONCLUSION

Wearables are still in the relatively early stages of development. Just as computers and smartphones have evolved, so will wearables. Advancements in sensors, connectivity, and battery technologies are expected to unearth new applications for wearables and potentials for medicine. Sensors will become more sophisticated, cheaper, smaller, and more capable of detecting existing physical properties with higher accuracy, or have the ability of sensing entirely new physical properties such as illness markers on the breath. Implantable sensors may aid those recovering from internal injuries or systemic illnesses, provided that they are safe and do not negatively interact with the body's immune system. Other sensors may feature biodegradability for monitoring sensitive environments without need for surgical removal. Self-powered sensors may not require batteries, potentially harvesting body heat and movement. Self-healing sensors will possibly repair themselves in the event that they are damaged. Useful for clinical trials, sensors may detect the effect of medicines and other interventions at a scale not previously possible, therefore revealing new insights about optimal personal treatment options.

Wearable devices show great promise for aiding the development of personalized medicine, particularly home-based use case scenarios for the older adult. There are numerous requirements for creating successful wearable solutions including aesthetic design, mobility, connectivity, and data analysis. Obstacles and limitations are a reality, but technology companies, universities, and governments are working to surmount issues such as accuracy, security, and engineering. Wearables are poised to impact society by democratizing access to personalized medicine while reducing hospital readmissions—potentially slowing the growth of our multitrillion-dollar health care expenditures.

REFERENCES

The American Academy of Pain Medicine. (n.d.). AAPM facts and figures on pain. Retrieved from http://www.painmed.org/patientcenter/facts_on_pain.aspx

Baek, W.-S., Kim, D.-M., Bashir, F., & Pyun, J.-Y. (2013). *Real life applicable fall detection system based on wireless body area network*. Proceedings of the 2013 IEEE 10th Consumer Communications and Networking Conference (CCNC) (pp. 62–67). Las Vegas, NV: IEEE.

Battaglia, E., Bianchi, M., Altobelli, A., Grioli, G., Catalano, M. G., Serio, A., . . . Bicchi, A. (2016). ThimbleSense: A fingertip-wearable tactile sensor for grasp analysis. *IEEE Transactions on Haptics, 9*(1), 121–133. Retrieved from http://ieeexplore.ieee.org/abstract/document/7294702

Big data. (n.d.). In *Dictionary.com*. Retrieved from http://www.dictionary.com/browse/big-data

Bluetooth SIG. (2016, December 7). *Bluetooth 5 now available*. Retrieved from https://www.bluetooth.com/news/pressreleases/2016/12/07/bluetooth-5-now-available

Carreiro, S., Smelson, D., Ranney, M., Horvath, K. J., Picard, R. W., Boudreaux, E. D., . . . Boyer, E. W. (2014). Real-time mobile detection of drug use with wearable biosensors: A pilot study. *Journal of Medical Toxicology, 11*(1), 73–79. Retrieved from https://www.ncbi.nlm.nih.gov/pmc/articles/PMC4371024

Case, M. A., Burwick, H. A., & Volpp, K. G. (2015). Accuracy of smartphone applications and wearable devices for tracking physical activity data. *Journal of the American Medical Association*, 625–626. doi:10.1001/jama.2014.17841

Centers for Disease Control and Prevention. (2016a). Adult obesity facts. Retrieved from https://www.cdc.gov/obesity/data/adult.html

Centers for Disease Control and Prevention. (2016b). Chronic disease overview. Retrieved from http://www.cdc.gov/chronicdisease/overview

Centers for Disease Control and Prevention. (2016c). Heart failure fact sheet. Retrieved from http://www.cdc.gov/dhdsp/data_statistics/fact_sheets/fs_heart_failure.htm

Centers for Medicare & Medicaid Services. (2016d). NHE fact sheet. Retrieved from https://www.cms.gov/research-statistics-data-and-systems/statistics-trends-and-reports/nationalhealthexpenddata/nhe-fact-sheet.html

Chandler, D. L. (2016, July 25). New lithium-oxygen battery greatly improves energy efficiency, longevity. Retrieved from MIT News: http://news.mit.edu/2016/new-lithium-oxygen-battery-greatly-improves-energy-efficiency-longevity-0725

Chesanow, N. (2014, October 22). Do virtual patient visits increase your risk of being sued? Retrieved from https://www.americanwell.com/wp-content/uploads/2014/12/www.medscape.pdf

De Giovanni, N., & Fucci, N. (2013). The current status of sweat testing for drugs of abuse: A review. *Current Medicinal Chemistry, 20,* 545–561. Retrieved from https://www.ncbi.nlm.nih.gov/pubmed/23244520

Derrick, J. (2014, November 20). Morgan Stanley: Wearable technology a potential $1.6 trillion business. Retrieved from http://finance.yahoo.com/news/morgan-stanley-wearable-technology-potential-131618384.html

Englert, K., Ruedy, K., Coffey, J., Caswell, K., Steffen, A., & Levandoski, L. (2014). Skin and adhesive issues with continuous glucose monitors. *Journal of Diabetes Science and Technology, 8,* 745–751. Retrieved from https://www.ncbi.nlm.nih.gov/pmc/articles/PMC4764227

Evans, D. (2011, April). The internet of things: How the next evolution of the internet is changing everything. Retrieved from http://www.cisco.com/c/dam/en_us/about/ac79/docs/innov/IoT_IBSG_0411FINAL.pdf

Farandos, N. M. (2015). Contact lens sensors in ocular diagnostics. *Advanced Healthcare Materials, 4,* 792–810.

Food and Drug Administration. (2013). Paving the way for personalized medicine. Retrieved from http://www.fda.gov/downloads/scienceresearch/specialtopics/personalizedmedicine/ucm372421.pdf

Gao, W., Nyein, H. Y., Shahpar, Z., Fahad, H. M., Chen, K., Emaminejad, S., . . . Javey, A. (2016, May 9). Wearable microsensor array for multiplexed heavy metal monitoring. *ACS Sensors,* 866–874. doi:10.1021/acssensors.6b00287

Google Developers. (2015, May 22). Google glass policies. Retrieved from https://developers.google.com/glass/policies

Gozani, S. N. (2016). Fixed-site high-frequency transcutaneous electrical nerve stimulation for treatment of chronic low back and lower extremity pain. *Journal of Pain Research, 2016*(9), 469–479.

Hsu, J. (2015, October 30). Flexible sensors measure blood flow under the skin. Retrieved from http://spectrum.ieee.org/tech-talk/biomedical/devices/flexible-sensors-measure-blood-flow-under-the-skin

IBM. (n.d.). What is big data? Retrieved from https://www-01.ibm.com/software/in/data/bigdata

IEEE Robotics & Automation Society. (n.d.). Haptics. Retrieved from http://www.ieee-ras.org/haptics

Inan, O., Migeotte, P., Park, K., Etemadi, M., Tavakolian, K., Casanella, R., . . . Di Rienzo, M. (2015). Ballistocardiography and seismocardiography: A review of recent advances. *IEEE Journal of Biomedical and Health Informatics, 19,* 1414–1427. Retrieved from https://www.ncbi.nlm.nih.gov/pubmed/25312966

InvenSense. (2016). Wearables. Retrieved from https://www.invensense.com/solutions/wearables

Jakicic, J. M., Davis, K. K., Rogers, R. J., King, W. C., Marcus, M. D., Helsel, D., . . . Belle, S. H. (2016). Effect of wearable technology combined with a lifestyle intervention on long-term weight loss: The IDEA randomized clinical trial. *Journal of the American Medical Association, 316*(11), 1161–1171.

James Hayward, G. C. (2016, July). Wearable technology 2016–2026. Retrieved from http://www.idtechex.com/research/reports/wearable-technology-2016-2026-000483.asp

Jung, S., Hong, S., Kim, J., Lee, S., Hyeon, T., Lee, M., & Kim, D.-H. (2015, November 24). Wearable fall detector using integrated sensors and energy devices. *Scientific Reports, 5*, 1.

Kroll, R. R., Boyd, J. G., & Maslove, D. M. (2016, September). Accuracy of a wrist-worn wearable device for monitoring heart rates in hospital inpatients: A prospective observational study. *Journal of Medical Internet Research, 18*(9), e253.

Laput, G., Yang, C., Xiao, R., Sample, A., & Harrison, C. (2015). *EM-Sense: Touch recognition of uninstrumented, electrical and electromechanical objects*. UIST '15, November 8–11, Charlotte, NC. Retrieved from https://www.disneyresearch.com/wp-content/uploads/EMSense-Recognizing-Handled-Uninstrumented-Electro-Mechanical-Objects-Using-Software-Defined-Radio-Paper.pdf

Lee, H., Choi, T. K., Lee, Y. B., Cho, H. R., Ghaffari, R., Wang, L., . . . Kim, D.-H. (2016, June). A graphene-based electrochemical device with thermoresponsive microneedles for diabetes monitoring and therapy. *Nature Nanotechnology, 11*, 566–572.

LinkLabs. (2015, December 10). LTE-M & 2 other 3GPP IoT technologies to get familiar with. Retrieved from https://www.link-labs.com/lte-iot-technologies

Massa, D. P. (1999, February 1). Choosing an ultrasonic sensor for proximity or distance measurement Part 1: Acoustic considerations. *Sensors Online*. Retrieved from http://www.sensorsmag.com/sensors/acoustic-ultrasound/choosing-ultrasonic-sensor-proximity-or-distance-measurement-825

Miller, J. (2015, September 5). Novartis to start human tests with Google lens in 2016. Retrieved from http://www.reuters.com/article/us-novartis-ceo-idUSKCN0R50E920150905

Morgan Stanley. (2015, January 23). When we wear the future. Retrieved from http://www.morganstanley.com/articles/coming-wave-of-wearable-device-technology

National Library of Medicine. (2011). Ballistocardiography. Retrieved from https://www.nlm.nih.gov/cgi/mesh/2011/MB_cgi?mode=&term=Ballistocardiography

Near Field Communication. (2011, November). Near field communication technology standards. Retrieved from http://nearfieldcommunication.org/technology.html

Nichols, S. P., Koh, A., Storm, W. L., Shin, J. H., & Schoenfisch, M. H. (2013, February 7). Biocompatible materials for continuous glucose monitoring devices. *Chemical Reviews*, 2528–2549. Retrieved from https://www.ncbi.nlm.nih.gov/pmc/articles/PMC3624030

Perrier, A., Vuillerme, N., Luboz, V., Bucki, M., Cannard, F., Diot, B., . . . Payan, Y. (2014). Smart diabetic socks: Embedded device for diabetic foot prevention. *IRBM, 35*(2), 72–76. doi:10.1016/j.irbm.2014.02.004

Piwek, L., Ellis, D. A., Andrews, S., & Joinson, A. (2016). The rise of consumer health wearables: Promises and barriers. *PLoS Medicine, 13*(2), e1001953.

The President's National Security Telecommunications Advisory Committee. (2014). *NSTAC report to the president on the internet of things*. Retrieved from https://www.dhs.gov/sites/default/files/publications/IoT%20Final%20Draft%20Report%2011-2014.pdf

Public Health Institute Center for Connected Health Policy. (n.d.). Store and forward. Retrieved from http://www.cchpca.org/store-and-forward

Robinson, R. (2015, June). Wearables in clinical trials. *PharmaVoice*. Retrieved from https://www.mdsol.com/sites/default/files/mHealth_Wearables-Clinical-Trials_20150601_PharmaVOICE_Article.pdf

Sensirion. (2016). Humidity and temperature sensors widen potential for wearable devices. Retrieved from https://www.sensirion.com/about-us/newsroom/newsletter/articles/humidity-and-temperature-sensors-widen-potential-for-wearable-devices

Sensor. (n.d.). In *Merriam Webster*. Retrieved from http://www.merriam-webster.com/dictionary/sensor

Texier, I., Marcoux, P., Pham, P., Muller, M., Benhamou, P.-Y., Correvon, M., . . . Lymperopoulos, L. (2013). *SWAN-iCare: A smart wearable and autonomous negative pressure device for wound monitoring and therapy.* Proceedings of the Samos Conference (pp. 137–144). IEEE. Retrieved from http://samos-conference.com/Resources_Samos_Websites/Proceedings_Repository_SAMOS/2013/Files/2013-IC-18.pdf

Torre, J. I. (2015, October 1). Chronic wounds. Retrieved from http://emedicine.medscape.com/article/1298452-overview

Trindade, B. M., Ono, Y., Lemaire, E. D., & AlMohimeed, I. (2014). *Development of a wearable ultrasonic sensor and method for continuous monitoring of mechanical properties of plantar soft tissue for diabetic patients. IEEE Xplore*. Chicago, IL: IEEE. doi:10.1109/ULTSYM.2014.0526

U.S. Consumer Product Safety Commission. (2016, August 23). McDonald's Recalls "Step-iT" activity wristbands due to risk of skin irritation or burns. Retrieved from https://www.cpsc.gov/Recalls/2016/McDonalds-Recalls-Step-iT-Activity-Wristbands

United Nations Office on Drugs and Crime. (2016). *World drug report 2016*. Retrieved from https://www.unodc.org/doc/wdr2016/WDR_2016_ExSum_english.pdf

UnitedHealthcare. (2016, January). Optum remote participant monitoring. Retrieved from https://www.uhc.com/ces/innovations/optum-remote-participant-monitoring

Wang, E. J., Lee, T.-J., Mariakakis, A., & Goel, M. (2015). MagnifiSense: Inferring device interaction using wrist-worn passive magneto-inductive sensors. *UbiComp '15/ASWC*, September 7–11. Osaka, Japan. Retrieved from http://homes.cs.washington.edu/~mayank/Papers/MagnifiSense.pdf

11

Social Robots and Other Relational Agents to Improve Patient Care

Victor H. S. Wang and Thomas F. Osborne

This chapter introduces the concept of a "relational agent," a technological entity that can build social relationships. Such an agent can be represented in many forms, ranging from a voice originating from a "black box," to a virtual animated nurse on a computer monitor, or even a robotic puppy. As we see in this chapter, the potential uses of relational agents are as varied as their potential embodiments. Relational agents hold the promise to help solve some of the fundamental challenges facing health care (such as limited human resources), to operationalize important follow-up care protocols, to provide the psychosocial support necessary to improve self-management, and to reduce overall costs in certain complex patient populations.

This chapter is organized into three main sections. First, we provide the context and general overview of the field. We then describe the different types of relational agents, and, finally, we present specific examples and scientific evidence for each category of relational agent.

THE MOTIVATION FOR RELATIONAL AGENTS

A variety of established and emerging health technologies have the potential to deliver improved care at a lower cost. Many of these innovations address the procedural and technical requirements of delivering health care more efficiently to large numbers of people. However, a key factor in the success and adoption of any intervention is psychological and social support. This sometimes overlooked factor is important for all populations, but is particularly relevant for older patients who may be more isolated owing to physical, social, and geographic factors.

More specifically, recent research has emphasized the role of social isolation and loneliness on health care outcomes, demonstrating that they are major contributors to functional decline, increased morbidity, and increased mortality, particularly among older adults (Cacioppo, Hawkley, Norman, & Berntson, 2011; Holt-Lunstad, Smith, Baker, Harris, & Stephenson, 2015; Perissinotto, Cenzer, & Covinsky, 2012). Evidence shows that the risk for mortality from a lack of social relationships is actually greater than that from obesity (Hold-Lunstad, Smith, Baker, Harris, & Stephenson, 2015). It is not surprising that loneliness, the subjective feeling of social isolation, has been linked to depression; however, loneliness is also correlated to physiological impairments such as poorer immune response and suppressed gene expression (Hawkley & Cacioppo, 2010).

In the United States, in 2016, 29% of noninstitutionalized older adults lived alone. This tendency to live alone increases with age, with almost half (46%) of women aged 75 years and over living alone (Administration on Aging, 2016). Furthermore, many high-risk older adults—those who tend to drive health care costs—have no meaningful family support whatsoever. It has been estimated that, of the respondents in the national Health and Retirement Study, 22.6% are at risk for being an "elder orphan" (Carney, Fujiwara, Emmert, Liberman, & Paris, 2016).

Traditional care and support for these at-risk older adults, with multiple health risk factors, rely largely on expensive labor resources that are in short supply. To complicate the challenge, from 2010 to 2030, the proportion of the U.S. population in their prime caregiving years is expected to increase by only 1%, while the number of people aged 80 years and older who need long-term health support and services is projected to increase by a staggering 79% (Redfoot, Feinberg, & Houser, 2013). Therefore, with our existing model of care delivery, there will not be enough caregivers to meet the need, even if we could afford it.

A 2016 meta-analysis explored the potential of information and communications technology (ICT) in the home, such as social networks or video calling platforms, to mitigate social isolation. However, the analysis found that the effect of ICT on social support seemed to be short lived, and noted that some studies found an insignificant, or even negative, impact on the subjective feeling of loneliness (Chen & Schulz, 2016). Moreover, older adults with multiple health risk factors often present with an additional challenge: an unfamiliarity, and sometimes even an aversion, to technology. Major obstacles to the success of ICT projects in older populations include lack of motivation and disinterest in learning ICT, as well as cognitive, eyesight, and other physical impediments (Chen & Schulz, 2016). Because not only functional impairment, but also disinterest and lack of motivation contribute to poorer outcomes and higher health care costs (Greene & Hibbard, 2012; Hibbard & Greene, 2013), it is critical to the sustainability of our health care system that technology adapt to the preferences of an individual or population, rather than requiring patients to adapt to unfamiliar software interfaces, which may not be designed for their specific perspectives, and their physical or cognitive limitations.

Enter the relational agent—a technological apparatus that is capable of building and maintaining social relationships with patients in a more intuitive way. Relational agents that have been developed and commercialized take various physical forms, or embodiments, and function differently behind the scenes (Campbell, Grimshaw, & Green, 2009). What they have in common, at least in theory, is the ability to form socially supportive relationships with patients, using an interaction modality that is typically more user friendly than traditional ICT interfaces. In some cases, relational agents can transcend what the user conceives of as technology, and instead be considered more as a friend or assistant. More specifically, evidence supports their efficacy for a variety of indications including mitigating delirium and falls risk in the hospital, providing hospital discharge instructions, basic postdischarge follow-up, coaching self-care tasks, diabetes management, medication adherence, exercise, and diet (Bickmore et al., 2010; Bickmore, Schulman, & Sidner, 2011; King, Bickmore, Campero, Pruitt, & Yin, 2013; Puskar, Schlenk, Callan, Bickmore, & Sereika, 2011; Thompson, Cullen, Redondo, & Anderson, 2016; Wang, 2016; Watson, Bickmore, Cange, Kulshreshtha, & Kvedar, 2012; Wexler & Drury, 2017; Wexler et al., in press).

In the following sections, we explore the various kinds of relational agents, their current state of the art, evidence of efficacy, and practical applications.

PHYSICAL FORM: DISEMBODIED VERSUS EMBODIED RELATIONAL AGENTS

The physical or nonphysical form of the relational agent determines whether we refer to it as "embodied" or "disembodied." An embodied agent is one that interacts with its environment through what a user would consider to be an expressive "body," which can take various forms such as a graphically animated depiction of a person or character on a computer screen, physical humanoid robot, or an animal-like robot. For our discussion, representations of a relational agent that do not have a visually expressive form will be considered disembodied.

Disembodied Relational Agents

In the most traditional sense, a phone can be considered the technological interface through which a case management team may maintain a relationship with a patient to support positive health care outcomes. Because the phone has no expressive capabilities other than the actual verbal dialogue and intonations of voice, the phone combined with its supporting team of support staff can be thought of as a disembodied relational agent.

Newer technologies, such as wearable telephonically connected pendants, or even camera-enabled "telesitter" systems in hospitals, can also serve as the interface of disembodied relational agents.

Disembodied relational agents can be relatively limited in their relationship-building capabilities because of the lack of a visual/physical component to the relationship, resulting in limitations in the ability to express nonverbal expressive emotional cues, and the potential lack of feeling of continuity or presence. This limitation may be particularly key for systems that use a synthesized voice generated in software by a "text-to-speech" system (Georgila, Black, Sagae, & Traum, 2012). A live, human voice can of course provide a greater fidelity of emotional response, and as anyone who has talked with friends or loved ones over the phone will have experienced, can provide a significant level of psychosocial support despite the lack of any physically expressive embodiment. It has, however, been shown that while telephone conversations can improve social isolation and loneliness, face-to-face social interactions are superior to telephone interactions in reducing the incidence of depression (Teo et al., 2015).

Embodied Relational Agents

Perhaps the most widely popularized form of the embodied relational agent is the social robot. A typical social robot is often only able to manipulate parts of its own physical body (e.g., by smiling, nodding, raising its eyebrow, or waving its hand), to express emotional states and communicate more effectively than through voice alone (Figure 11.1). The field of social robotics builds on prior research about how the bulk of human-to-human communication is actually nonverbal (Mehrabian & Epstein, 1972), combined with the much studied phenomenon of anthropomorphism, in which humans imbue nonhuman agents with humanlike characteristics, motivations, intentions, or emotions (Epley, Waytz, Akalis, & Cacioppo, 2008; Epley, Waytz, & Cacioppo, 2007).

An alternative solution to achieving the expressiveness of a physical robot is the virtual embodied agent, which has its "body" graphically represented

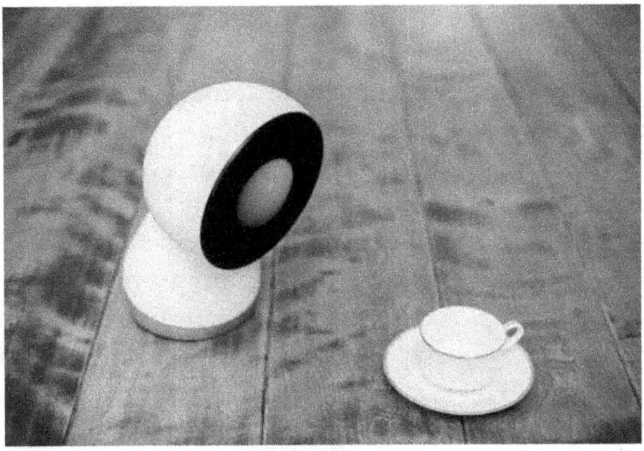

FIGURE 11.1 Jibo, a social robot with a very simple-looking physical embodiment, points its "eye" toward a cup and saucer placed next to it on a wooden table. The spherical portion of the robot physically articulates, and the flat portion is a display screen that enables the digitally displayed eye to "blink" and animate in other ways to indicate emotion and meaning as it talks.

Source: Jibo, Inc. (n.d.).

on a display screen. This alternative may be a much more cost-effective solution because it utilizes existing technology such as a computer monitor or smart mobile device.

Nonetheless, early research in social robotics suggests an advantage of physical, robotic relational agents over virtual embodiments for the purposes of building trust and influencing decisions (Kidd & Breazeal, 2004; Shinozawa, Naya, Yamato, & Kogure, 2005). Interestingly, studies experimenting with various possible physical representations of relational agents have shown that even agents with highly minimal and abstract physical appearances can elicit social and emotional responses from patients (Paauwe, Keyson, Hoorn, & Konijn, 2015), and that when rating the likeability of a potential agent, people may prefer humanoids or toy robots over real humans (Bartneck, Kanda, Ishiguro, & Hagita, 2007).

SOURCE OF INTELLIGENCE: ARTIFICIAL VERSUS HUMAN

Artificial Intelligence

Artificial intelligence (AI) has been defined as "the capability of a machine to imitate intelligent human behavior" (Artificial intelligence, n.d.). In practice, this usually refers to a piece of software running on a computer, and the ability of that software to perform some limited subset of what a human brain can do, such as visual perception, speech recognition, or decision making. Modern AI can, in some cases, exceed human performance at specific tasks, such as specific types of image recognition, or even playing games such as chess or *Jeopardy!*. However, AI is insufficient for other, less-constrained tasks, such as creative writing or free-form conversation.

AI-powered relational agents seek to capture elements of human social intelligence and relational behaviors in software. For example, using knowledge of how human relationships are built and maintained, a relational agent may be programmed to refer to information from previous conversations, or to gradually share more "personal" information about itself as it emulates a deepening relationship (Campbell et al., 2009).

Functionally, a relational agent driven by AI uses some mechanism to receive input from the user. This may take the form of voice recognition software, a computer touch screen with multiple-choice options (Figure 11.2), or simply a touch-tone telephone interface.

The AI then uses its programmed algorithms and retained knowledge to generate an appropriate response back to the user. Often, this response is generated through a form of AI known as an "expert system," which emulates the decision-making abilities of an expert human. At its most basic, this

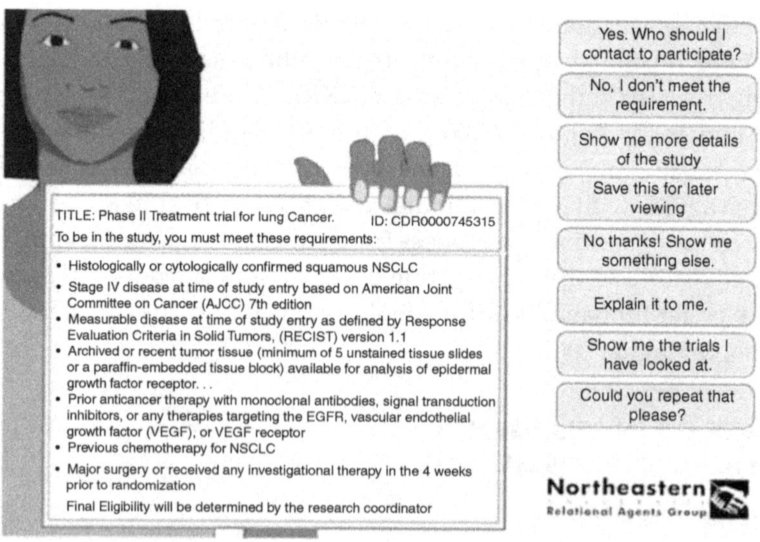

FIGURE 11.2 An example of an AI-driven relational agent showing multiple-choice options for its user to select from.

Source: Bickmore, Utami, Matsuyama, and Paasche-Orlow (2016).

decision making can be represented as a series of "if . . . then . . . else . . ." logic branches. For example, in human-readable logic, "if the user indicates adherence to the medication regimen, then say 'Good job,' else begin a follow-up conversation about medications and alert a care provider."

In other cases, more sophisticated machine intelligence is implemented. However, even with the most technologically advanced AI systems, the limitations of human–machine interaction become quickly apparent in the setting of unstructured social conversations (i.e., outside of a conversation about a specific, limited topic). As a reflection of our current capabilities, there is a famous challenge within the field of computer science known as the "Turing Test," which was originally proposed in 1950 as "The Imitation Game" by Alan Turing, a pioneering computer scientist. This game is won when a computer can exhibit intelligent behavior that is indistinguishable from that of a human during an unstructured conversation (Turing, 1950). To date, no AI system has passed that test, and even optimistic futurists estimate 2029 as the date when the most advanced AI might approach the conversational abilities of a human (Marvin, 2016). Despite this limitation, AI-driven relational agents can be cost-effective and beneficial for automating conversations with motivated patients about specific health care topics or self-care tasks (Bickmore et al., 2010).

Human Intelligence

In its most basic form, "disembodied human-driven relational agents" can simply be a colorful way of saying "follow-up phone calls." However, new technological embodiments lend exciting new capabilities to such human teams attempting to operationalize important follow-up care reminders and to encourage behaviors that save health care costs.

In the literature, using a human to directly control a relational agent that has an expressive physical or virtual form is sometimes referred to as the *Wizard of Oz model* (Vardoulakis, Ring, Barry, Sidner, & Bickmore, 2012), based on the fictional character who uses technology to project his visage as a fantastical embodiment of himself. A more popular term that may be used to describe such an "embodied" relational agent is an *avatar*, a pop culture term used to refer to any figure in a computer game or online forum that represents a real person (derived from a similar Sanskrit word describing the personal embodiment of a deity). In this case, the relational agent can respond in conversation with the same level of intelligence that a human could, because, indeed, a human is responding in real time through the avatar interface.

This approach, of course, offers the benefits of human conversational sophistication, flexibility, and compassion that are often required for complex patient populations. While these benefits come at the cost of the human workforce required to staff the avatar, the technology layer can be further leveraged to reduce the cost of this workforce and to grant it with new capabilities key to driving health care outcomes. For example, the workforce can be remote and hired in more economical locations. Regardless of the location of the workforce, the technology may allow caregivers to interact with, or at least to observe and check-in on, multiple patients at a time. In addition to extending the reach of any one team member, the effective skill level and training of each worker can be augmented through expert systems built into the software, for example, to guide evidence-based, protocol-driven health coaching and triage of care. Software can thus improve care with the help of a greater knowledge base, improved consistency, and, therefore, enhanced safety and quality.

EXAMPLES AND EVIDENCE

In the following sections, we examine several specific examples for each category of relational agent, including clinical evidence supporting their efficacy, strengths, and weaknesses.

Disembodied AI-Driven Relational Agents

Most people in industrialized countries have probably interacted with a disembodied AI-driven relational agent. In its most basic form, such a relational agent could be the interactive voice response (IVR) system that answers and redirects a customer support call to check on items such as a phone bill, flight status, credit card fraud alert, or even satisfaction with a previous customer support interaction. Such systems are customized to each organization, with the interactive voice exhibiting the tone, personality, and brand of the organization it represents. While a well-executed IVR system can help to deliver information at a lower cost, these systems are often relatively simplistic, with limited ability to answer unexpected questions, or to build the social relationship by referring to past conversations. In fact, if the system has no capability to reference past interactions, or to otherwise build a relationship over time, it may be considered a more simplistic "social agent" or "conversational agent," rather than a true "relational agent" (Bickmore & Cassell, 2001). In addition, because these systems require a certain patience and motivation to speak clearly or to press telephone buttons to indicate multiple-choice responses, they may cause frustration, and are generally considered inferior to live support by a human.

Very similar systems currently power some hospital postdischarge platforms, helping to call patients and screen them for risk of readmission, and to encourage them to adhere to self-management best practices, follow-up appointments with primary care, and other risk and cost-saving protocols. Examples of well-established commercial providers of such systems include Phytel, Vocantas, and Emmi. White papers supporting the efficacy of such interventions abound, but peer-reviewed publications on the subject do not all agree, with some demonstrating neutral results. One of the more successful studies showed that with a population of 875 Medicare patients, an IVR post–hospital discharge protocol implemented using a system called the Geisinger Monitoring Program (GMP) was associated with a 44% reduction in 30-day readmissions (Graham et al., 2012). More recently, a large meta-study updated in 2015 concluded that, at least for patients with heart failure, "structured telephone support" reduced the risk of all-cause mortality and heart failure–related hospitalization, while also improving health-related quality of life, heart failure knowledge, and self-care behaviors (Inglis, Clark, Dierckx, Prieto-Merino, & Cleland, 2015).

AI-driven personal assistants are also becoming increasingly advanced for consumer use. Leading commercial examples include Google's generic-sounding Assistant, as well as Apple's Siri, Amazon's Alexa, and Microsoft's Cortana, which strive to show off their own personality not just through their names, but often through humorous responses to certain commands or questions (if you have an Apple iPhone, try asking Siri, "Will you marry me?"). As recently as late 2015, Google's senior vice president of search was quoted in *Time* magazine (Luckerson, n.d.) explaining why the Google Assistant purposely was not designed to have a personality represented by elements such as gimmicky, preprogrammed jokes, stating "I'm not saying personality shouldn't come, but the science to get that right doesn't fully exist." As technology advances, these types of commercial products may one day be configured to provide social support and medical assistance for patients.

Disembodied Human-Driven Relational Agents

The earlier noted limitations of AI may be solved by incorporating humans, who are, of course, capable of true conversational understanding, and of building compassionate relationships with patients.

Many established care transitions programs such as Project RED (ReEngineered Discharge), Care Transitions Intervention, and Project BOOST incorporate postdischarge phone calls by a real person, generally a nurse or social worker (Berkowitz et al., 2013; Coleman, Parry, Chalmers, & Min, 2006; Williams et al., 2014). In fact, it is instructive to think of even a traditional, analog home phone as the interface of a human-driven relational agent. Although it is disembodied because the phone has no expressive body through which to interact with the patient, the phone is indeed serving as the conduit to a relationship between the patient and the care provider organization. Unfortunately, despite the widespread use of this kind of telephone-based follow-up, the evidence around its effectiveness as a stand-alone intervention is contentious. On a positive note, a study involving over 30,000 members of a Medicare Advantage health plan has shown that receipt of a discharge call is associated with reduced rates of readmission (Harrison, Hara, Pope, Young, & Rula, 2011). However, other studies were less encouraging. For example, a more recent research study conducted prospectively with over 5,000 patients by the University of California, San Francisco, and Cedars-Sinai Medical Center showed no significant benefit. In that study, after accounting for the observation that patients who answered the calls also naturally had a lower expected propensity for readmission, postdischarge phone calls from trained nurses led to no significant benefit to readmission rates (Harrison, Auerbach, Quinn, Kynoch, & Mourad, 2014). Another study, specifically comparing home visits with telephone calls for transitional support, found that to be effective, calls should be integrated with in-home visits (Wong, Chow, Chan, & Tam, 2014).

Perhaps one of the most well-known examples of a permutation to the follow-up telephone call paradigm is the personal emergency response system (PERS), popularized by the Philips Lifeline brand of wearable pendants, which has reportedly served over 7 million subscribers (The Lifeline Story, n.d.). Many competing products and services now exist in this space, but their basic premise is that the phone interaction has been transformed into a much more accessible, wearable form. In this context, the device is always available, and a conscious patient is therefore able to interact with a support team in a medical emergency with a single press of a button. While the labor utilization of these services is not well documented in the literature, the author has noted in conversations with senior management and other knowledgeable representatives of these service providers that the bulk of the calls fulfilled by the call centers are not for true emergencies, but rather to provide some level of social support, peace of mind, and ongoing relationship with the patient. As far as clinical outcomes, however, the literature is inconclusive, with one of the more widely cited publications on the topic, published in *Academic Emergency Medicine* (Lee et al., 2007), showing no evidence that a PERS reduced anxiety, fear of falling, or return to the emergency department (ED) among older adults discharged from the ED.

Yet another variation to the concept of a disembodied human-driven relational agent is the telesitter or "virtual patient observation" system, which has been quickly adopted by hundreds of hospitals across the country. These systems' primary purpose is to multiply the observational capabilities of a single hospital inpatient sitter, by placing that sitter behind a set of computer monitors to watch over multiple patients (Figure 11.3). Instead of sitting at the bedside of a single patient, the telesitter can now watch over, in practice, up to 12 patients. These systems are theoretically capable of patching the telesitter through to each patient by voice, not just to remind them to stay in

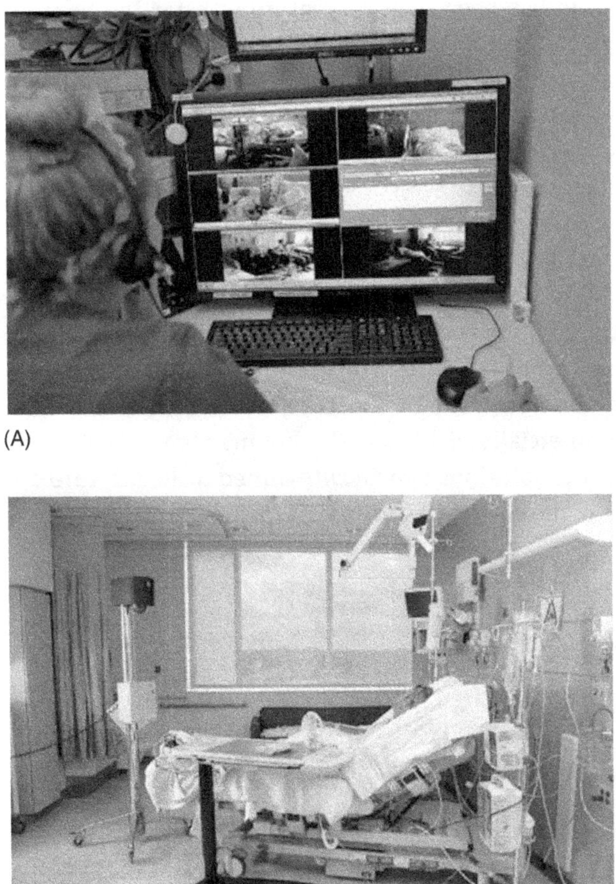

(A)

(B)

FIGURE 11.3 Example of AvaSys "Telesitter" system by AvaSure, showing the monitoring station (A) and the telesitter tower with the black box that incorporates a speaker, microphone, and high-definition camera dome (B).

Source: AvaSure (n.d.).

bed or stop pulling the IV lines, but potentially also to provide psychosocial support. Unfortunately, the high visual and cognitive load of observing so many patients simultaneously generally precludes any meaningful conversation and relationship building. Adoption of this technology has been relatively rapid owing to the presumed high value of substituting inpatient sitter costs. Early evidence suggests that when combined with a nursing-driven sitter protocol and administrative oversight, such a telesitter system can deliver significant return on investment (Burtson & Vento, 2015).

Embodied AI-Driven Relational Agents

The past decade has been one of great growth for the field of social robotics. Indeed, at the time of this writing, the International Conference on Social Robotics is going into its ninth year, and the industry is seeing the launch of multiple new social robot product lines backed by major global companies, including Pepper, the mobile humanoid robot by SoftBank, a multinational telecom company based in Tokyo (Vincent, 2014); and Sota, the miniature robot for elders by Nippon Telegraph and Telephone Corporation (Figure 11.4; Sota Home Robot to Care for Japan's Elderly, 2015), another major telecom company and competitor to SoftBank. In the world of start-ups, one of the more robustly funded ventures is Jibo, a spinout from the MIT Media Lab's Personal Robots Group, which has raised more than $60 million in equity investment, with the ambitious mission of putting a social robot in every home (Tilley, 2015). The rise of the commercially viable social robot may have finally arrived.

Looking at the solutions specifically aimed at health care and aging care, Sota's launch in the elder care industry is forthcoming, and has been marketed

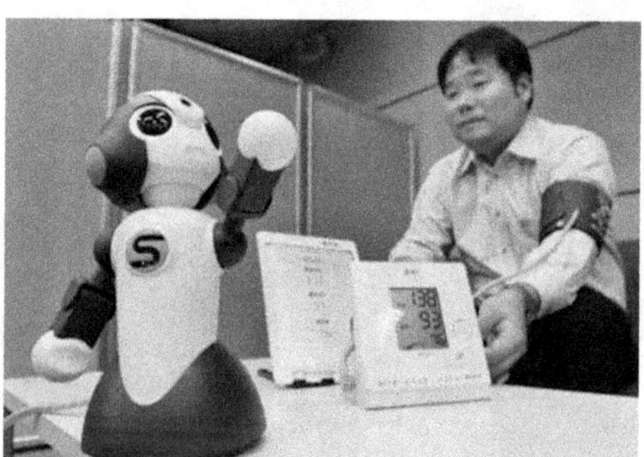

FIGURE 11.4 Sota, the elder care robot by Nippon Telegraph and Telephone Corporation.

Source: Yoshikazu Tsuno (n.d.).

by NTT in conjunction with televisions, blood pressure monitors, and other Internet of Things devices. Another product in the early stages of commercial launch is Mabu by Catalia Health (2016), slated to serve as a health coach at home. While both examples are founded on significant literature backing the feasibility of such social, emotional, expressive robotic solutions for patient engagement and care plan adherence, clinical validation to show robust outcomes with these products remains to be seen.

The adoption of social robotics in the market may also hinge on price. The cost of each of the previously mentioned robots is generally about $1,000, plus a smaller ongoing service fee. A potential alternative to help avoid the price tag of robot hardware is to emulate the physical expressiveness of the robot in software. An example of such a virtually embodied solution is the line of virtual nurses created by Sense.ly, a start-up that has an active partnership with the National Health Service (NHS) of the United Kingdom.

As an emerging field, there is promising evidence of the potential for these virtual relational agents. For example, a small-scale study conducted by Tim Bickmore at Northeastern University showed that 74% of hospital patients preferred receiving their discharge instructions from a virtual nurse over their regular doctors or nurses (Bickmore et al., 2010).

Nonconversational Relational Agents (Embodied AI-Driven)

As discussed, a major benefit of relational agents is the ability to guide patients to better care through the context of interactive conversations. However, there is a class of relational agents that can provide therapeutic and health care benefit without any conversational dialogue.

For example, PARO, the robotic puppy seal, is a nonconversational relational agent that has over 60 publications supporting its feasibility and efficacy as a therapeutic tool, primarily for dementia care, by simulating the benefits of animal-assisted therapy and by forming relationships with older adults (PARO Therapeutic Robot, n.d.). As a true relational agent, it is programmed to adapt its movement behavior and other nonverbal communication on the basis of how it has previously been touched by its user, and can learn and respond to new spoken names that its user gives it. PARO is licensed as a Class II medical device (Okita, 2013; Shibata, 2012), and costs about $5,000.

The application of nonconversational relational agents to aging care is commercially compelling. Hasbro, a multinational toy and board game company, recently launched a line of "Joy for All" robotic cat and dog "companion pets," also aimed at this elder care market, but marketed with a much more affordable price point in the neighborhood of $100, and without the medical claims (Joy for All Pets, n.d.). While there are anecdotal reports of positive relationships being built between older adults and Joy for All pets, the device does not have the same learning behavior or ability to reference the past that is key to a typical relational agent. Despite this relative simplicity and lack of clinical evidence, the device appears to be well received in the market.

Embodied Human-Driven Relational Agents

The *Wizard of Oz* technique of controlling a social robot using a human in the background is often used in research to test out the feasibility and user response to the robot. For example, Alice is a robot developed by Johan Hoorn of VU University in Amsterdam, designed to converse socially with older adults (Hoorn, Konijn, Germans, Burger, & Munneke, 2015). It has received much attention, and is featured in the documentary film "Alice Cares," which highlights several relationships that it builds with older adults. While the human control allows the relational agent to leapfrog current possibilities in AI and natural language processing, beyond small pilots and feasibility studies, the high cost of the human staffing model is challenging to scale, not only commercially, but even just to reach sufficient statistical power to generate robust clinical outcomes over the course of a research study.

A commercial example of such a (virtual) embodied and human-driven relational agent is care.coach, for which the first author of this chapter currently serves as CEO. The company solves the staffing challenge by leveraging a global workforce and online platform, enabling it to be very selective in sourcing high-quality and compassionate, yet cost-effective staff to work as a 24 × 7 team from around the world. The team members have their skills augmented through an expert system embedded into their online work interface, which guides them through evidence-based protocols to coach for multiple chronic conditions and mitigate other health care risks through a virtual avatar (Figure 11.5). To date, care.coach has multiple small-scale research publications suggestive of its larger scale potential in the community to improve self-management and care plan adherence (Chi et al., in press; Chi, Demiris, Thompson, Lazar, & Lin, 2016; Demiris, Thompson, Lazar, & Lin, 2016; Machesney et al., 2014; Wang, 2016), as well as a 95-patient clinical study that has shown, among hospitalized elderly inpatients, 70% to 85% fall rate reduction, and statistically significant mitigation of both delirium and loneliness by mounting the avatar onto patients' bed rails or bedside tray tables. At the bedside, the avatars support the nursing team by providing additional oversight, while conversationally engaging patients in evidence-based delirium and falls risk mitigation protocols (Wexler et al., in press; Wexler & Drury, 2017).

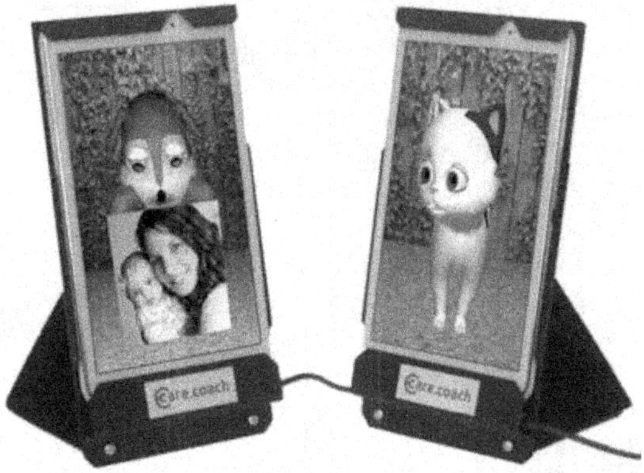

FIGURE 11.5 Examples of different care.coach avatars, designed to be engaging, joyful, and nonjudgmental. A hospital bedside version is also available for inpatient use.

Source: Courtesy of Victor Wang.

CONCLUSION

Exciting advances in technology can extend the capabilities of traditional care teams to not only provide the functional aspects of self-management support and monitoring, but also the very important and human need for psychosocial support and companionship. Using the framework described in this chapter, we can see that seemingly futuristic relational agents such as social robots or virtual health care avatars may be viewed in a similar light to traditional telephone calls supported by a care management team, but with advanced capabilities. While clinical evidence is building around some of these developing solutions, the literature to date is very promising. In the near future, pioneering practitioners and forward-thinking organizations have an opportunity to utilize relational agents to mitigate risks faced by our vulnerable older patient populations, while also alleviating the burden on our limited health care workforce.

REFERENCES

Administration on Aging. (2016). *A profile of older americans: 2016*. U.S. Department of Health and Human Services. Retrieved from https://www.acl.gov/sites/default/files/Aging%20and%20Disability%20in%20America/2016-Profile.pdf

Artificial intelligence. (n.d.). In *Merriam-Webster.com*. Retrieved from https://www.merriam-webster.com/dictionary/artificial intelligence

AvaSure. (n.d.). For the media. Retrieved from http://avasure.com/for-the-media

Bartneck, C., Kanda, T., Ishiguro, H., & Hagita, N. (2007, August). *Is the uncanny valley an uncanny cliff?* In RO-MAN 2007—The 16th IEEE International Symposium on Robot and Human Interactive Communication (pp. 368–373). doi:10.1109/ROMAN.2007.4415111

Berkowitz, R. E., Fang, Z., Helfand, B. K., Jones, R. N., Schreiber, R., & Paasche-Orlow, M. K. (2013). Project ReEngineered Discharge (RED) lowers hospital readmissions of patients discharged from a skilled nursing facility. *Journal of the American Medical Directors Association, 14*(10), 736–740.

Bickmore, T., & Cassell, J. (2001, March). *Relational agents: A model and implementation of building user trust.* In Proceedings of the SIGCHI Conference on Human Factors in Computing Systems (pp. 396–403). ACM, Vancouver, Canada.

Bickmore, T. W., Mitchell, S. E., Jack, B. W., Paasche-Orlow, M. K., Pfeifer, L. M., & O'Donnell, J. (2010). Response to a relational agent by hospital patients with depressive symptoms. *Interacting with Computers, 22*(4), 289–298.

Bickmore, T. W., Schulman, D., & Sidner, C. L. (2011). A reusable framework for health counseling dialogue systems based on a behavioral medicine ontology. *Journal of Biomedical Informatics, 44*(2), 183–197.

Bickmore, T. W., Utami, D., Matsuyama, R., & Paasche-Orlow, M. K. (2016). Improving access to online health information with conversational agents: A randomized controlled experiment. *Journal of Medical Internet Research, 18*(1), e1.

Burtson, P. L., & Vento, L. (2015). Sitter reduction through mobile video monitoring: A nurse-driven sitter protocol and administrative oversight. *Journal of Nursing Administration, 45*(7/8), 363–369.

Cacioppo, J. T., Hawkley, L. C., Norman, G. J., & Berntson, G. G. (2011). Social isolation. *Annals of the New York Academy of Sciences, 1231*(1), 17–22.

Campbell, R. H., Grimshaw, M. N., & Green, G. M. (2009). Relational agents: A critical review. *The Open Virtual Reality Journal, 1*(1), 1–7.

Carney, M. T., Fujiwara, J., Emmert, B. E., Liberman, T. A., & Paris, B. (2016). Elder orphans hiding in plain sight: A growing vulnerable population. *Current Gerontology and Geriatrics Research, 2016*, 1–11.

Catalia Health. (n.d.). Retrieved from http://www.cataliahealth.com

Chen, Y. R. R., & Schulz, P. J. (2016). The effect of information communication technology interventions on reducing social isolation in the elderly: A systematic review. *Journal of Medical Internet Research, 18*(1), e18.

Chi, N., Demiris, G., Thompson, H., Lazar, A., & Lin, S. (2016). The usability of a digital companion pet for older adults with mild cognitive impairment. *The Gerontologist, 56*(Suppl. 3), 566.

Chi, N., Sparks, O., Lin, S., Lazar, A., Thompson, H. J., & Demiris, G. (in press). Pilot testing a digital pet avatar for older adults. *Geriatric Nursing.*

Coleman, E. A., Parry, C., Chalmers, S., & Min, S. J. (2006). The care transitions intervention: Results of a randomized controlled trial. *Archives of Internal Medicine, 166*(17), 1822–1828.

Demiris, G., Thompson, H. J., Lazar, A., & Lin, S. Y. (2016). *Evaluation of a digital companion for older adults with mild cognitive impairment.* Presented at the American Medical Informatics Association 40th Annual Symposium, Chicago, IL.

Epley, N., Waytz, A., Akalis, S., & Cacioppo, J. T. (2008). When we need a human: Motivational determinants of anthropomorphism. *Social Cognition, 26*(2), 143–155.

Epley, N., Waytz, A., & Cacioppo, J. T. (2007). On seeing human: A three-factor theory of anthropomorphism. *Psychological Review, 114*(4), 864.

Georgila, K., Black, A., Sagae, K., & Traum, D. R. (2012). *Practical evaluation of human and synthesized speech for virtual human dialogue systems* (pp. 3519–3526). Retrieved from https://www.researchgate.net/profile/David_Traum/publication/267559748_Practical_Evaluation_of_Human_and_Synthesized_Speech_for_Virtual_Human_Dialogue_Systems/links/549087ed0cf214269f26b04e.pdf

Graham, J., Tomcavage, J., Salek, D., Sciandra, J., Davis, D. E., & Stewart, W. F. (2012). Postdischarge monitoring using interactive voice response system reduces 30-day readmission rates in a case-managed Medicare population. *Medical Care, 50*(1), 50–57.

Greene, J., & Hibbard, J. H. (2012). Why does patient activation matter? An examination of the relationships between patient activation and health-related outcomes. *Journal of General Internal Medicine, 27*(5), 520–526.

Harrison, J. D., Auerbach, A. D., Quinn, K., Kynoch, E., & Mourad, M. (2014). Assessing the impact of nurse post-discharge telephone calls on 30-day hospital readmission rates. *Journal of General Internal Medicine, 29*(11), 1519–1525.

Harrison, P. L., Hara, P. A., Pope, J. E., Young, M. C., & Rula, E. Y. (2011). The impact of postdischarge telephonic follow-up on hospital readmissions. *Population Health Management, 14*(1), 27–32.

Hawkley, L. C., & Cacioppo, J. T. (2010). Loneliness matters: A theoretical and empirical review of consequences and mechanisms. *Annals of Behavioral Medicine, 40*(2), 218–227.

Hibbard, J. H., & Greene, J. (2013). What the evidence shows about patient activation: Better health outcomes and care experiences; fewer data on costs. *Health Affairs, 32*(2), 207–214.

Holt-Lunstad, J., Smith, T. B., Baker, M., Harris, T., & Stephenson, D. (2015). Loneliness and social isolation as risk factors for mortality—A meta-analytic review. *Perspectives on Psychological Science, 10*(2), 227–237.

Hoorn, J. F., Konijn, E. A., Germans, D. M., Burger, S., & Munneke, A. (2015). *The in-between machine: The unique value proposition of a robot or why we are modelling the wrong things.* International Conference on Agents and Artificial Intelligence, ICAART, Lissabon, Portugal.

Inglis, S. C., Clark, R. A., Dierckx, R., Prieto-Merino, D., & Cleland, J. G. (2015). Structured telephone support or non-invasive telemonitoring for patients with heart failure. *The Cochrane Library,* (10), CD007228.

Jibo, Inc. (n.d.). Retrieved from https://www.jibo.com/sites/www.jibo.com/files/Jibo-press-kit.zip

Joy for All Pets. (n.d.). Retrieved from http://joyforall.hasbro.com

Kidd, C. D., & Breazeal, C. (2004). *Effect of a robot on user perception.* In Proceedings of the IEEE/RSJ International Conference on Intelligent Robots and Systems (pp. 3559–3564). Sendai, Japan: IEEE.

King, A. C., Bickmore, T. W., Campero, M. I., Pruitt, L. A., & Yin, J. L. (2013). Employing virtual advisors in preventive care for underserved communities: Results from the COMPASS study. *Journal of Health Communication, 18*(12), 1449–1464.

Lee, J. S., Hurley, M. J., Carew, D., Fisher, R., Kiss, A., & Drummond, N. (2007). A randomized clinical trial to assess the impact on an emergency response system on anxiety and health care use among older emergency patients after a fall. *Academic Emergency Medicine, 14*(4), 301–308.

The Lifeline Story. (n.d.). Retrieved from https://www.lifeline.philips.com/about-lifeline/our-story.html

Luckerson, V. (n.d.). Google searches for its future. *Time.* Retrieved from http://time.com/google-now

Machesney, D., Wexler, S. S., Chen, T., & Coppola, J. F. (2014). *Gerontechnology companion: Virtual pets for dementia patients.* Paper presented at IEEE Long Island Systems, Applications and Technology Conference, Long Island, NY.

Marvin, R. (2016, June). How Ray Kurzweil sees the future. *PC Magazine.* Retrieved from http://www.pcmag.com/news/345062/how-ray-kurzweil-sees-the-future

Mehrabian, A., & Epstein, N. (1972). A measure of emotional empathy. *Journal of Personality, 40*(4), 525–543.

Okita, S. Y. (2013). Self–other's perspective taking: The use of therapeutic robot companions as social agents for reducing pain and anxiety in pediatric patients. *Cyberpsychology, Behavior, and Social Networking, 16*(6), 436–441.

Paauwe, R. A., Keyson, D. V., Hoorn, J. F., & Konijn, E. A. (2015). Minimal requirements of realism in social robots—Designing for patients with acquired brain injury. In B. Begole, J. Kim, K. Inkpen, & W. Woo (Eds.), *Proceedings of the 33rd Annual ACM Conference Extended Abstracts on Human Factors in Computing Systems, Seoul, Rep. Korea, April 18–23, 2015* (pp. 2139–2144). New York, NY: ACM. doi:10.1145/2702613.2732875

PARO Therapeutic Robot. (n.d.). Retrieved from http://www.parorobots.com/whitepapers.asp

Perissinotto, C. M., Cenzer, I. S., & Covinsky, K. E. (2012). Loneliness in older persons: A predictor of functional decline and death. *Archives of Internal Medicine, 172*(14), 1078–1084.

Puskar, K., Schlenk, E. A., Callan, J., Bickmore, T., & Sereika, S. (2011). Relational agents as an adjunct in schizophrenia treatment. *Journal of Psychosocial Nursing and Mental Health Services, 49*(8), 22–29.

Redfoot, D., Feinberg, L., & Houser, A. (2013). The aging of the baby boom and the growing care gap: A look at future declines in the availability of family caregivers. *Insight on the Issues*, (85). Retrieved from http://www.aarp.org/content/dam/aarp/research/public_policy_institute/ltc/2013/baby-boom-and-the-growing-care-gap-in-brief-AARP-ppi-ltc.pdf

Shibata, T. (2012). Therapeutic seal robot as biofeedback medical device: Qualitative and quantitative evaluations of robot therapy in dementia care. *Proceedings of the IEEE, 100*(8), 2527–2538.

Shinozawa, K., Naya, F., Yamato, J., & Kogure, K. (2005). Differences in effect of robot and screen agent recommendations on human decision-making. *International Journal of Human-Computer Studies, 62*(2), 267–279.

Sota Home Robot to Care for Japan's Elderly. (2015, July). Retrieved from http://www.roboticstrends.com/article/sota_home_robot_to_care_for_japans_elderly/Household

Teo, A. R., Choi, H., Andrea, S. B., Valenstein, M., Newsom, J. T., Dobscha, S. K., & Zivin, K. (2015). Does mode of contact with different types of social relationships predict depression in older adults? Evidence from a nationally representative survey. *Journal of the American Geriatrics Society, 63*(10), 2014–2022.

Thompson, D., Cullen, K. W., Redondo, M. J., & Anderson, B. (2016). Use of relational agents to improve family communication in Type 1 diabetes: Methods. *JMIR Research Protocols, 5*(3), e151.

Tilley, A. (2015, December). Jibo raises another $16 million to bring its 'family robot' to China and Japan. *Forbes.* Retrieved from http://www.forbes.com/sites/aarontilley/2015/12/09/jibo-raises-another-16-million-to-bring-its-family-robot-to-china-and-japan

Turing, A. M. (1950). Computing machinery and intelligence. *Mind, 59*(236), 433–460.

Vardoulakis, L. P., Ring, L., Barry, B., Sidner, C. L., & Bickmore, T. (2012, September). Designing relational agents as long term social companions for older adults. In Y. Nakano, M. Neff, A. Paiva, & M. Walker (Eds.), *Intelligent Virtual Agents. IVA 2012. Lecture Notes in Computer Science* (Vol. 7502). New York, NY: Springer-Verlag.

Vincent, J. (2014, June). Japanese 'robot with a heart' will care for the elderly and children. *The Independent.* Retrieved from http://www.independent.co.uk/life-style/gadgets-and-tech/softbank-unveils-pepper-japanese-robot-with-a-heart-will-care-for-the-elderly-and-children-9491819.html

Wang, V. (2016). *care.coach: Healing the patient by supporting the person*. Paper presented at National PACE Association Annual Conference, San Francisco, CA. Retrieved from http://npaonline.org/sites/default/files/PDFs/Talking Dogs_Wang.pdf

Watson, A., Bickmore, T., Cange, A., Kulshreshtha, A., & Kvedar, J. (2012). An internet-based virtual coach to promote physical activity adherence in overweight adults: Randomized controlled trial. *Journal of Medical Internet Research, 14*(1), e1.

Wexler, S., et al. (in press). *The use of tablet technology to improve outcomes in hospitalized older adults*. Proceedings of the 21st World Congress of the International Association of Gerontology and Geriatrics, San Francisco, CA.

Wexler, S., & Drury, L. (2017). *The use of an avatar virtual service animal to improve outcomes in hospitalized older adults*. NICHE Conference, Austin, TX. Retrieved from http://conference.nicheprogram.org/wp-content/uploads/2017/04/4_21_2017_Plenary_300_Virtual-Service-Animal-Presentation_POD_S.Wexler_Handout.pdf

Williams, M. V., Li, J., Hansen, L. O., Forth, V., Budnitz, T., Greenwald, J. L., . . . Coleman, E. A. (2014). Project BOOST implementation: Lessons learned. *Southern Medical Journal, 107*(7), 455–465.

Wong, F. K. Y., Chow, S. K. Y., Chan, T. M. F., & Tam, S. K. F. (2014). Comparison of effects between home visits with telephone calls and telephone calls only for transitional discharge support: A randomised controlled trial. *Age and Ageing, 43*(1), 91–97.

Yoshikazu Tsuno. (n.d.). Retrieved from http://www.gettyimages.com/license/482178318

12

Artificial Intelligence and Its Potential to Improve the Health of Older Adults

Gavin W. Hougham, Amir M. Rahimi, Bruce A. McClelland, Nancy J. McMillan, Michael A. Schwemmer, David A. Friedenberg, Jeremy Bellay, Andrew J. Landgraf, and Thomas F. Osborne

Artificial intelligence (AI) is a field of computer science that attempts to understand and simulate features of human intelligence and behavior. Apart from fantastical thinking in antiquity and literature about creating thinking life from inert matter (McCorduck, 2004), the field is almost as old as computer science itself. The idea that it might be possible to make machines that "think" is usually attributed to a small group of creative computer scientists in the 1940s and 1950s, who thought there could be ways of expanding the then-nascent logic and formal reasoning–based computer programming methods to the point where a naïve observer would be unable to determine if a computer or human was at the other end of a conversation. Later theorists argued that what is really needed are computers that solve problems.

Solving problems with AI is not based on *one* method, but whole families of approaches and foundational disciplines. Among the disciplines central to AI are computer science, mathematics, statistics, linguistics, analytic philosophy, psychology, cognitive science, and neuroscience. Some of the important approaches used are statistical classification methods (e.g., naïve Bayes, support vector machines [SVMs], decision trees), machine learning (ML), and natural language processing (NLP). Classification methods are extremely valuable in almost every branch of medicine—for example, distinguishing diseases from each other on the basis of known or "hidden" features, or predicting clinical outcomes of an intervention. ML is a way for computers to build models on the basis of data without being told exactly what kind of model to build. These models can then make predictions outside of the data used to build, or "train," them. NLP focuses on how computers understand, learn from, and sometimes produce, human language; the inherent complex structure of language can be exploited to perform many useful tasks by computers.

In this chapter, we expand on these descriptions and present several areas where AI methods are being used to solve health problems of an aging population. In rough order, we present examples where these methods may be found as part of various technologies designed to help maintain independence, safety, and function. Then we move to systems where AI can aid in clinical diagnosis, clinical decision support, and the use of electronic health record (EHR) and other health information technology (IT) data. Finally, we present some areas where AI is being used to advance discoveries in medicine and pharmaceutical interventions, and end with a coda, hardly fantastical, on how AI approaches may be used to semiautomatically mine large corpora of scientific literature to make new discoveries in aging and gerontology based on complex logical inferences across extremely large numbers of facts.

AI AND TEMPORAL REASONING IN GERONTOLOGY

Decline in cognitive functions can make it more difficult to follow required medication, diet, exercise, and appointment schedules. Traditional routines of prompting, such as arising for work or sitting down for family meals, are often limited for older adults who have left the workforce or suffered the death of a spouse. Lists, analog reminder tools, such as medication organizers, written reminders for follow-up appointments, or home checking of physiological and cognitive indicators, unfortunately tend to rely on the presence of mind to also remember where the lists are, what the medicines do, or how to perform at-home monitoring procedures.

Even without pathological cognitive decline, many patients may still have difficulty adapting to the complexities of rapidly changing health-related information technologies. To further complicate the challenge, comorbid illnesses and disorders often become more common as we age, and these may be treated by ever more and different medicines. Such factors further increase the cognitive load, such that adherence to optimal scheduling of health-related actions can be an even greater challenge. Daily adjustment processes that are manageable for younger generations can sometimes be overwhelming to members of a generation who did not grow up with personal digital appliances, computers, smartphones, or other mobile or networked information devices (Campbell, 2015). Some of the technological challenges that arise in older populations can also be attributed to simple disinterest or frustration with frequent updates, learning new user interfaces, information formats, and constant password changes (University of Alberta, 2007).

People of all ages are encountering environments where infrastructure (buildings, transportation systems, roads) and the technologies of everyday life (cars, refrigerators, televisions) are connected to each other and/or to personal/mobile computing devices. Sometimes, the communication between the objects in this "Internet of Things" goes unnoticed, while in other cases, a person may need to become familiar with yet another interface to control the additional functionality. The expected concomitant increases in cognitive computing and AI (i.e., machines that can do some of our thinking for us) will have to provide ways to compensate for both the increases in system-wide complexity, and for the possible reductions in the abilities of aging individuals to navigate the demands of a changing technological environment.

Prediction From Analysis of EHRs

Emerging federal, state, and local initiatives are aimed at improving both the accessibility and quality of health care. Among the drivers of such initiatives is increasing reliance on EHRs, whose promise to improve the interoperability of patient records among all stakeholders in patient health care has yet to be fulfilled. It is hoped that by automatically recording medical data in standardized formats, ideally in real time as it occurs, medical records will become more amenable to analytics. As an example, recent research from University of New Mexico and Vanderbilt suggests that ML can be applied to EHR data to forecast the future risk of type 2 diabetes mellitus (DM-II; Mani, Chen, Elasy, Clayton, & Denny, 2012; Paxton, Niculescu-Mizil, & Saria, 2013).

The authors used ML and feature selection algorithms (i.e., the process of finding and selecting a set of relevant variables or predictors) to build a diabetes prediction model using information from EHRs. One reason why prediction is so important in diabetes is that for DM-II patients, clinical diagnosis can be delayed 4 to 7 years after onset, and some vascular complications may have already developed by the time diagnosis is made. Hence, the sooner risk is detected, the sooner prevention and intervention strategies can be implemented, thereby potentially reducing morbidity and mortality.

The ML and statistical algorithms applied to the data obtained from the EHRs in this study included naïve Bayes, SVMs, and decision tree classifiers, all of which are supervised ML algorithms (a type of AI) for classification. We say these algorithms are "supervised" because they need to be trained before they can be used, while "unsupervised" methods learn the inherent structure of the data by themselves. Naïve Bayes and SVMs are advantageous in, say, predicting whether a patient has a disease or risk for disease—for example, DM-II—while decision trees "generate clear descriptions of how the machine learning method arrives at a particular prediction" (Mani et al., 2012, p. 609). By combining these and other methods, the investigators demonstrated that "diabetes risk forecasting using data from EHR has the potential to automatically identify high-risk populations for early intervention" (Mani et al., 2012, p. 612), without the need for resource-intensive screening procedures.

Reminder Systems for People With Cognitive Impairments

AI is making significant improvements in human–computer interaction (HCI) systems. For example, AI can enable devices to remind or prompt people to perform activities that may depend more on changing situations or contexts (including cognitive decline), than a fixed calendar. As such, these functions need to be able to perform reasoning about time, which is both aware of necessary or preferred sequences of activities and adaptive to the sorts of factors that can affect people with impaired memory or executive function.

Recent research has demonstrated the benefits of an *adaptive* reminder system based on AI techniques such as *temporal constraint reasoning* and *reinforcement learning* (RL; Rudary, Singh, & Pollack, 2004). Unlike static reminders, such as calendars and alarms, which are triggered by a discrete event such as a date or time, adaptive reminders take into consideration external factors and influences that may be more dynamic. Temporal constraint reasoning is a well-known AI technique for modeling time events—that is, determining when something happens (an event) or holds (an event state)—along with the logical temporal relations, such as sequence (ordering), duration, or conditions between these temporal references (Dechter, Meiri, & Pearl, 1991). With RL, the system learns how to map situations to actions by means of trial-and-error search for certain indicators and delayed "reward" (where the reward, for an ML system, is a numerical value signaling success; Sutton & Barto, 1998). The ability to reason about dynamic events in time, based on these two AI techniques (RL and temporal constraint), can produce an assistive technology for "thinking" that is personalized and adaptive to both short- and long-term changes in users (Barták, Morris, & Venable, 2014). Such a system can support people with impaired memory and/or executive function, by providing personalized reminders of functional daily activities, with a goal of improved self-sufficiency and improved user compliance with beneficial activities. These activities could be as simple as taking a daily pill, to more complex activities such as scheduling a doctor's appointment requiring a period of previsit fasting, arranging for transportation while accounting for different travel times depending on the time of the day, and finally executing the plan with all its real-world potential for hassles and contingencies.

The incorporation of RL in the user interface helps to personalize the reminder functions of the system by inducing an "interaction policy" that considers such factors as time of day, timing, and nature of previous interactions, or even the user's mood. The system must understand which actions are legitimate for reminding the subject about at a given time, and this can depend on the history of the user's activity in the context of a prescribed daily schedule or plan. In cases where there are many inputs into this decision making, this can be computationally complex. To reduce the number of action choices and thus permit the system to provide appropriate reminders within the context of the user's history, plans, and goals of care, constraint-based temporal reasoning is used to prune and optimize the set of best actions to recommend for the user. In these systems, the recommendations could go directly to the subject person (e.g., an impaired older adult) as a reminder, a human caregiver who could reflect and act upon that recommendation on behalf of the subject person, or even another computer system that could check back into the subject's EHR for verification and initiate action on its own (say, dispense a pill from a countertop appliance and vocalize a command to swallow the pill).

Constraint-Based Temporal Reasoning: Real-Time Situation Recognition and Monitoring

Describing, predicting, and planning actions or events is a fundamental aspect of intelligent behavior, whether that of humans or so-called cognitive or AI agents—that is, "software artifacts that exhibit intelligent behavior in complex domains over extended periods of time" (Langley, 2004). The ability to reason about time—not only the *amount* of time available or required for an action or response, but also the *ordering* and *flow* of sequences of such actions—is critical for modeling these sorts of AI agents. When a temporal factor can affect the performance of some monitoring or assistive agent, determining the correct action to be taken at the correct time implies that the time constraints should neither be overconstrained (resulting in no solutions or actions) nor underconstrained (having too many possible solutions or actions). When agents are designed to monitor events in real time—such as the onset of a medical condition, a change in behavior that may signal mounting distress, or even a life-threatening crisis—timeliness is of utmost importance. The appropriate information (or decision) must be presented in time to be *useful* (Chakravarty & Shahar, 1999), which points again to how critical it will be for some systems to have access to the full, rich resource of EHR data in real or close to real time.

In the health care environment, there is also often an added complication, in that the expression of temporal data, such as time points or intervals, may be imprecise, relative, or only conveyable by "temporal abstractions" that must be inferred from statements about events that are known or supposed to occur at a certain time and/or in a certain order (e.g., "before," "then," "during," or "after"). This is especially the case when the inputs are in the form of natural language or so-called unstructured text (patient or physician notes, narrative sections of medical records, etc.).

Processes to extract and represent data from natural language text, which is claimed to be the form in which most usable data are found, are becoming increasingly viable, but in the domain of health care, proper assignment of the temporal aspects of medical reporting, scheduling, and planning described earlier remains a difficult problem. Formalisms for representing time and temporal ordering, such as James Allen's *temporal logic* (Allen, 1983), have been available since the early days of AI, yet it remains a challenge to unambiguously represent mentions of time in unstructured text and infer their relationships to appropriate events to meet the test of *usefulness*. This is due, in part, to the difficulty of appropriately categorizing the broad array of methods for discussing time in human language. On the one hand, text may include specific temporal phrases or explicit mentions of a time point, duration, or event state (e.g., "childhood"). At the same time, references to time may also rely on metaphors, fuzzy phrases, shifts in verb tense, or indirect back references to other time mentions, which may be located in other documents. They may also obliquely reference calendared holidays (e.g., "it was right before New Year's Day") or world events (e.g., "just after we got into WWII").

This is all difficult to do in unstructured data, such as clinical notes, the transcript of a recorded conversation, or even an audio file itself. These can contain words, but also numbers, dates, images, and other types of data. The natural rules of language can help AI systems understand the meaning of such data—especially the text portions—but the ambiguities and poetry of language, the use of shorthand expressions, missing words, or sloppy syntax all need to be inferred by an AI system trying to make sense of unstructured data. In structured or semistructured data, many of these ambiguities are removed by the organized use of higher level rules that impose order on the data. These types of data are often found in databases that are already "tagged" or identified in some predictable ways. An example of this can be seen in your bank account statement; everything in such a statement came directly from a highly structured (and audited) database. Little needs to be inferred in such systems (Friedman & Hripcsak, 1999).

Recent and ongoing AI-related projects, such as the Clinical Narrative Temporal Relation Ontology (CNTRO; Tao, Wei, Savova, & Chute, 2010), which is designed for representing, annotating, and inferring temporal relations and constraints for clinical events in EHRs, are providing improved solutions for overcoming some of these long-standing problems related to the expression of time, whether found in structured or unstructured data.

Logic-Based Representation, Reasoning, and ML for Event Recognition

Events constitute the central discussion point of most textual narratives. In health care applications, identification and categorization of events into possibly multiple appropriate classes can be important goals of AI agents or systems that support the provision of care in a timely manner and enhance decision making that may depend on prior events and current temporal contextual factors.

However, the mere definition of an event can be difficult to establish, in part because the boundaries around what constitutes an event may be fuzzy, or depend, to some extent, on point of view and the purpose behind the need to identify something as an *event*. Among the obstacles to performing automatic event recognition is how to represent events in a way that facilitates reasoning about time—both within an event (subevents within events) and sequences of events. According to Artikis, Paliouras, Portet, and Skarlatidis (2010), the advantages of logic-based representation of event structures are that they "exhibit a formal, declarative semantics," they are efficient and scalable, and, most importantly, are "supported by machine learning tools automating the construction refinement of event structures" (Artikis et al., 2010).

Logic-based temporal representation schemes involve terms that may be related to specific time points or to other propositional terms. In these systems, sequences of time-stamped low-level events (LLE) are recognized as patterns revealing more generalized, high-level events (HLE). The advantage of logic-based over non–logic-based event recognition systems is that the former are very efficient and scalable, and this benefit can be critical in health care situations. One such system is the Chronicle Recognition System (CRS; Dousson & Le Maigat, 2007).

In the CRS approach, time is organized as a discrete set of time points (i.e., instants), which are chronologically ordered, while other attributes for these instants or sequences or intervals can indicate persistence, absence, or repetition of some event. Temporal features of events may be seen as either instantaneous or durative (see earlier discussion of temporal constraints). An HLE, which effectively constitutes a broader or inclusive event, can be defined by the graph of, or the relationships between, two or more LLEs. Such graphs form a temporal constraint network (Rina Dechter, 1991). For example, an HLE indicating the possible consequence of low patient compliance with a drug regimen—which may be the result of memory loss or many other factors—might be defined by a graph of specific LLEs such as specific failures (e.g., to obtain or take medicine, or to ignore refill reminders). At the same time, the HLE must be defined to take into consideration the fact that some optional or nonessential LLEs might not occur, or might not be recognized to have occurred, yet this would not invalidate the conclusion regarding patient compliance.

Mapping patterns of LLEs into more abstract HLEs must take into consideration not only temporal factors and constraints, but also whether a given LLE is always obligatory. For example, if the HLE under consideration is something like "intracranial hemorrhage" (ICH), then we would expect that to be made up of a number of LLEs, at the very least a cascade of symptoms including, say, "headache." But do all headaches count as LLEs within the pattern for the broader ICH event? That is, can headaches occur within the graph of events that define ICH that are not actually related to the hemorrhagic event? If so, what are their distinguishing features? Do they have to be of a certain locus or type?

AI TO SUPPORT PATIENT FUNCTIONAL INDEPENDENCE

Advances in public health, nutrition, and medicine have allowed people to live longer, and, as a result, populations around the world are aging (Beard et al., 2012). Many older adults remain healthy and productive. Unfortunately, for many in this population, physical impairments hinder the performance of even the most basic tasks without assistance. Therefore, the loss of independence that comes with aging is a growing concern. A study in the United Kingdom by the Disabled Living Foundation (2009) revealed that more people worry about losing their independence (49%) than dying (29%) as they grow older.

Patients who suffer focal motor and sensory deficits may have higher brain functions intact. Brain–machine interface (BMI) systems seek to leverage intact brain function to aid physically impaired patients by establishing direct functional connections between certain brain areas and assistive devices that restore motor and sensory function (Aflalo et al., 2015; Bansal, Truccolo, Vargas-Irwin, & Donoghue, 2012; Chapin, Moxon, Markowitz, & Nicolelis, 1999; Hochberg et al., 2012; Kennedy & Bakay, 1998; Santhanam, Ryu, Yu, Afshar, & Shenoy, 2006; Serruya, Hatsopoulos, Paninski, Fellows, & Donoghue, 2002; Taylor, Tillery, & Schwartz, 2002; Velliste, Perel, Spalding, Whitford, & Schwartz, 2008). For example, those paralyzed through either a spinal cord injury or a neurodegenerative condition could regain at least partial mobility owing to a BMI that utilizes their brain activity to control a motorized wheelchair or a robotic limb (Ramli, Arof, Ibrahim, Mokhtar, & Idris, 2015; Srinivasan, Eden, Mitter, & Brown, 2007). The development of BMI systems has proceeded at a rapid pace in recent years, owing, in part, to advances in AI and ML, which allow action commands to be accurately "decoded," or inferred, from a patient's brain activity. Having the systems utilize brain activity, as opposed to more manual control (e.g., voice commands), can allow the prosthetic to feel more natural to the user. Here, we review the basic concepts behind BMI systems, and highlight several exciting results that demonstrate the potential that BMI systems have in allowing physically impaired older adults to regain functional independence.

Translating Neural Signals Into Movement: Brain–Machine Interfaces

BMI systems establish links between active parts of the nervous system—usually intact brain areas but sometimes peripheral nerves—and prosthetic or assistive devices (Lebedev & Nicolelis, 2006; Nicolelis & Lebedev, 2009; Schwartz, Cui, Weber, & Moran, 2006). These systems utilize physiological signals from certain types of motor or sensory actions, which increase the electrical activity in specific brain regions that are known to be associated with those actions. For example, limb flexion or extension are associated with increased electrical activity of neurons in specific areas of the motor region of the cerebral cortex (Wessberg & Nicolelis, 2004). Although the exact functional mapping between electrical activity in a brain region and a specific action is incredibly complex and sometimes variable, researchers have developed ML algorithms that can successfully approximate this mapping (Lebedev & Nicolelis, 2006; Li et al., 2014; Velliste et al., 2008). These algorithms learn associations between a patient's brain activity and intended actions by fine-tuning internal parameters to best match a training dataset, where both the brain activity and intended movement are known. For example, if the algorithm should predict when a patient opens or closes his or her hand, the training dataset would be constructed through a series of trials in which the patient is asked to either open or close his or her hand. The algorithm's job is to effectively "decode" how brain activity gets translated into an intended action.

BMI systems typically consist of sensors to record the activity in certain brain regions, a method to process the raw recorded signals, a decoding algorithm that translates these signals into intended action commands, and a device, such as a robotic arm, that physically executes these commands. There are a number of options for the type of brain signal to utilize in a BMI system, and these systems fall into two basic categories, noninvasive and invasive.

Noninvasive BMIs

Noninvasive BMIs sample neural signals without penetrating biological tissue. The most common noninvasive method is electroencephalography (EEG), in which sensors are placed along the subject's scalp to record voltage fluctuations resulting from the electrical activity of neurons in the brain (da Silva, 2013). EEG-based BMIs have led to many important innovations, including wheelchair navigation (Galan et al., 2008; Ramli et al., 2015), and even control of a mobile robot (Millan, Renkens, Mourino, & Gerstner, 2004). Galan et al. (2008) developed an EEG-based system to allow patients to continuously control the movement of a motorized wheelchair. Their system combines an intelligent wheelchair that senses the surrounding environment with a simple classification algorithm (a naïve Bayes classifier) that infers the most likely intended wheelchair direction (left, right, or forward) from the user's EEG activity. Some stereotypical motor actions, like raising an arm, may be so common and involve a known temporal sequence of actions that the algorithms can "learn" or guess the intended action faster than other more complex tasks, such as counting on one's fingers. The faster the system can respond, the smoother the result. When two subjects mentally drove a simulated wheelchair displayed on a computer monitor from a starting point to a goal following a prespecified path, both could follow the specified goal paths over 80% of the time after only 1 day of training with the system.

Invasive BMIs

Although EEG signals obtained from sensors placed on the scalp are desirable because they are noninvasive, portable, and easy to acquire in any environment, they suffer from a poor signal-to-noise ratio (Vidaurre, Schlogl, Cabeza, Scherer, & Pfurtscheller, 2007). Hence, much recent BMI work has focused on signals recorded directly from the motor cortex via microelectrode arrays (MEA), surgically implanted on the surface of the brain (Kao, Stavisky,

Sussillo, Nuyujukian, & Shenoy, 2014). BMIs using these direct recordings perform better than noninvasive techniques (Kao et al., 2014; Nuyujukian et al., 2014); however, brain surgery is required to implant an MEA. Intracortical BMIs have demonstrated that nonhuman primates and paralyzed humans can, remarkably, control computers, electronic wheelchairs, and robotic arms through imagined movements (Taylor et al., 2002). Recent work by researchers at Battelle and Ohio State University demonstrated that these same intracortically recorded signals can enable a quadriplegic subject to regain functional control of a paralyzed limb using an external muscle stimulation cuff (Bouton et al., 2016). The study utilized an implanted intracortical MEA to record activity from the subject's motor cortex, and applied novel data processing techniques coupled with complex decoding and classification algorithms (SVMs) to translate neuronal activity into control signals. These signals were then passed to the subject's forearm muscles through a customized high-resolution neuromuscular electrical stimulation system. The system provided isolated finger, hand and wrist movements, and, in one experiment, the subject achieved continuous cortical control of six different wrist and hand motions. It was also demonstrated that the subject was able to complete functional tasks relevant to daily living, like lifting a mug and swiping a credit card.

COMPUTER-AIDED DIAGNOSIS

The use of computer-aided diagnosis (CAD) goes back at least to the early 1980s when systematic work in automated medical image analysis started to take off. The aim of CAD was to assist physicians and other clinicians to diagnose illness or other problems (Doi, 2007). Components of CAD may include image processing, feature extraction, and classification using various computing technologies, including ML (Emaminejad et al., 2016; Imani et al., 2016; Shiraishi, Li, Appelbaum, & Doi, 2011; Syeda-Mahmood et al., 2016). Although images are the most often used primary data source in CAD, with recent advances in AI, image data can be augmented with other types of health data to potentially make CAD more patient specific and accurate. Although CAD without AI has been used by physicians since the 1980s (Suzuki, 2012), adding AI capabilities gives CAD the potential to perform early automated screening for cancer or other types of abnormalities by using medical images from different modalities, such as CT, x-ray, MRI, PET, and ultrasound.

ML, in particular artificial neural networks (ANN) or convolutional neural networks (CNN), have been very successful in solving image-related analysis problems, and have made great strides in medical image analysis. Examples of AI applications for detection and diagnosis of diseases most prevalent in older populations (National Institutes of Health, 2007) are early prediction of dementia, cancer, macular degeneration, and cardiovascular disease. In the following sections, we expand on some of these examples.

Chest Pathology Identification

Chest radiographs display a broad range of complex, important, and sometimes subtle information. Therefore, there is significant interest in developing ML-based diagnosis algorithms to assist radiologists in the evaluation of chest radiographs. Deep neural networks classification approaches are particularly suitable to solve such problems because of their ability to learn multiple layers of concept representation with increasingly more complex levels of abstractions from raw data (images). Deep learning methods require a large set of training data to be most effective; however, such large datasets with structured labeling are often not readily available in the medical field. Despite this challenge, the feasibility of using a deep learning approach based on nonmedical learning shows promise (Bar, Diamant, Wolf, & Greenspan, 2015). For example, a CNN that was trained with ImageNet, which is a well-known large-scale nonmedical image database, was tested on a dataset of only 93 images. The model created by ML achieved accuracies (defined as how well a test is able to distinguish those with a disease from those without it, measured by area under a Receiver Operating Characteristic [ROC] curve) of 0.93 for right pleural effusion detection, 0.89 for enlarged heart detection, and 0.79 for classification between healthy and abnormal chest x-ray, where all pathologies are combined into one large class (Bar et al., 2015). An area of 1.0 represents a perfectly accurate test, so these are all good to excellent results. These perhaps surprising findings demonstrate that deep learning algorithms that are trained with nonmedical image databases could be used for general medical image recognition tasks. Performance on real-world clinical medical images, containing artifacts and natural human physiological variation, is yet to be seen with this type of method.

Cardiovascular Disease

According to the American Heart Association/American Stroke Association, about 66% of cardiovascular disease (CVD) deaths occur in people age 75 years and older. In 2009, the leading cause of death in men and women age 65 years or older were diseases of the heart, followed by cancer, stroke, and chronic lower respiratory disease (CLRD) in women, and CLRD and stroke in men (Sidney, Rosamond, Howard, & Luepker, 2013)

A powerful predictor of cardiovascular events is the amount of calcification in the coronary arteries, which can be used to identify high-risk individuals. In one study, low-dose chest CT images were used to train deep convolutional networks (an AI approach influenced by models of biological processes) for coronary artery calcium scoring and detection of coronary calcification (Lessmann et al., 2016; Syeda-Mahmood et al., 2016). The network was trained using 797 of 1,028 low-dose chest CT scans, and was tested with the remaining 231 scans. The detection sensitivity of coronary calcification per scans of the method was 97.2%. The accuracy of risk category assigned to each subject was 84.4%. The detection rate was in excellent agreement with manually determined cardiovascular risk. Convolutional neural networks are particularly adept in unsupervised feature learning (that is to say, self-learning) as demonstrated in this analysis, without reliance on prior knowledge or human expert feature identification. As such, they adapt well to using low-dose chest CT scans from other studies with different acquisition procedures and study subjects. (In supervised learning, the algorithms learn from labeled examples, whereas in unsupervised approaches, the data are not labeled and the algorithm's job is to uncover structure of the unlabeled data.)

Dementia

Alzheimer's disease (AD) is the most common type of dementia. AD causes debilitating cognitive decline and is most prevalent among older adults. It is estimated that one in three older adults die with Alzheimer's or other forms of dementia, and that these diseases will cost the United States $236 billion in 2016 (Alzheimer's Association, 2016). Furthermore, the number of people living with dementia in 2015 throughout the world was estimated to be 46.3 million. If recent trends hold, the annual number of new cases of Alzheimer's and other dementias is projected to double by 2050 (Hebert, Beckett, Scherr, & Evans, 2001).

Early diagnosis of AD has been of interest to researchers who would like to develop and test medications that may help at early stages of the disease. Early prediction of cognitive decline using MRI and blood-based biomarkers has made significant progress in recent years, using advances in novel ML methods. The Alzheimer's disease neuroimaging initiative (ADNI) is an ongoing, longitudinal, multicenter study that follows changes of cognition, function, brain structure and function, and biomarkers in elderly controls, subjects with mild cognitive impairment, and subjects with AD. Using ADNI data, researchers have examined the potential for predicting AD using different types of biomarkers combined with brain MRI (Madsen et al., 2016). In this analysis, a collection of over 400 potential biomarkers was used, including biomarkers from blood panels, demographics, and the AD-risk gene *APOE*. In addition, brain MRI measures were used, including brain volume, gray matter thickness, and surface area measures. Using unsupervised ML methods, a subset of MRI biomarkers were identified as the strongest predictors of AD. Madson's work suggests that combining brain MRI and other biomarkers (including demographics and genetics) achieved the greatest predictive accuracy compared to any individual biomarker group or combination of biomarkers.

Classification of Anatomical Structures in CT

At a more fundamental level, to compute the in-depth numerical features of medical images needed to train diagnosis and detection algorithms, the best-performing AI systems generally require annotation, or labeling of various organs and anatomical regions. Considering the sheer amount of information in medical images, annotating possibly hundreds of thousands of medical images using human interpretation could present a dauntingly time-consuming task. However, ML approaches can be used to numerically measure and quantify specific visual features. ML has shown promise in automating organ classification using a combination of texture features and a so-called *bag of visual words* approach (Jiménez del Toro, Foncubierta-Rodríguez, Depeursinge, & Müller, 2015). In statistical language analysis, a bag of words approach may be used to describe a document on the basis of the words it contains and the number of times those words occur, without even needing to consider the order with which they occur. It provides a simplified and quantitative "fingerprint" of a document. The technique was extended to visual documents, and hence the term bag of visual words (Jiménez del Toro et al., 2015). In this context, each image is represented by a vector of words that describe features of the image. The visual vocabularies are constructed by clustering extracted features into a fixed number of regions or visual words using a combination of texture feature extraction and ML methods. In effect, with this technique, an anatomical structure can be described in terms of a histogram of visual words. For example, if we constructed a histogram of the features of a bicycle, we would see a certain number of wheels, a certain number of spokes, a certain number of brown seats, chrome handlebars, black pedals, and so forth, which in total uniquely describe the image of the bicycle using a structured set of words. This research suggests that the method can achieve classification accuracies of up to 100% for the lungs and other organs with specific textures.

Macular Degeneration

Permanent vision loss due to age-related macular degeneration (AMD) disorder is a common occurrence in older adults. Besides two-dimensional fundus imaging, three-dimensional imaging optical coherence tomography (OCT) is used for AMD diagnosis. Analysis of the OCT volumetric images are time consuming and difficult, especially at the early stages of the disease when only small changes are visible. Considering that patients with intermediate AMD have a high probability of progressing into advanced stages of the disease, early detection of AMD is crucial to preventing vision loss. Unsupervised ML approaches have shown promise in detecting AMD. To that end, a method based on an unsupervised feature learning approach was developed, capable of processing the complete image, without the need for an accurate presegmentation of the retina (Agurto et al., 2016; Sadek, Sidibé, & Meriaudeau, 2015; Venhuizen et al., 2015). This step was followed by a bag of visual words approach to distinguish retinal OCT volumes containing AMD pathology from healthy control subjects, without relying on segmentation algorithms. Instead of defining custom-built features that are aimed at finding the specific characteristics of AMD pathology, an unsupervised grouping method is applied to find a set of the most differentiating features automatically. These features are subsequently used to generate feature vectors (lists) describing each image, which are then fed into another AI classifier to separate the two classes. Experiments using 384 volume scans show that this method can identify AMD patients, obtaining an almost perfect accuracy (using area under the ROC curve) of 0.98 (Sadek et al., 2015; Venhuizen et al., 2015).

CLINICAL DECISION SUPPORT

Clinicians collect and synthesize data to make diagnostic and treatment decisions. Measurements such as blood pressure and body temperature, which are typically measured only sporadically, as well as the patient's self-reported symptoms are now being supplemented with an ever-expanding array of data. These range from genomic biomarkers to sensors that can continuously monitor an extensive number and variety of vital signs, to data from cell phones and environmental conditions, just to name a few. This explosion in data has led some to declare that this is the "data age" of medicine (Business Report: Data-driven Health Care, 2014). In this new era, properly taking advantage of these data could realize savings upward of $450 billion to the U.S. health care system (Groves, Kayyali, Knott, & Van Kuiken, 2013). However, the availability of all these new data is not without challenges. It can be difficult to sift out meaningful signal from unreliable or unimportant noise in the data (Lazer, Kennedy, King, & Vespignani, 2014). An infamous example is the failure of Google Flu Trends to accurately capture the true number of influenza cases in the winter of 2012 after several successful years of predictions (Butler, 2013). While it is undoubtedly difficult to harness and effectively utilize the vast amounts of data that flow through the Internet, or an enterprise health data network, the promise of better, faster, and more actionable information has led to much excitement and activity in the field of clinical decision support using AI (Clifton, Niehaus, Charlton, & Colopy, 2015; Ghassemi, Celi, & Stone, 2015).

Clinical decision support has potential for application in all fields of medicine. A system capable of efficiently reviewing a patient's digital record could integrate relevant information from a vast array of medical literature to present diagnostic and therapeutic options to clinicians, which may not have otherwise been considered. On a population level, similar analysis may reveal that some types of medical interventions are ineffective, or only effective in very select cohorts. For example, in inpatient hospital care settings such as the intensive care unit (ICU), a number of treatments and interventions have been shown to be either ineffective or even harmful to patients (Ospina-Tascón, Büchele, & Vincent, 2008). Therefore, ICUs have been the focus of much interest in clinical decision support research. There are many methods and tools that can be deployed to extract and use information gleaned from ICU health care data. In the rest of this section, we highlight several successful applications of AI and ML to assist clinicians in patient care.

A common ICU challenge that many have attempted to answer with clinical data is predicting mortality. As an example of the number of different approaches to this problem, a 2011 review of predictive models found almost 100 different studies that used 118 different tools, 34 of which were unique (Siontis, 2011). Many of these models utilize various ways of scoring a patient's condition, such as the Acute Physiology Score (APS), which is part of the Acute Physiology, Age, and Chronic Health Evaluation (APACHE) system (Knaus, Zimmerman, Wagner, Draper, & Lawrence, 1981). A newer score described by Johnson, Kramer, and Clifford (2013) uses a carefully optimized set of features determined by an ML technique called *particle swarm optimization,* which demonstrates similar accuracy while reducing the number of variables that need to be measured.

One use of ML models in clinical decision support may help to predict the onset, or the trajectory of a variety of diseases or clinical states. For example, health care–associated infections are among the most common adverse events by some estimates (de Vries, Ramrattan, Smorenburg, Gouma, & Boermeester,

2008; Leape et al., 1991), affecting approximately 13 in every 1,000 patients in the United States (Klevens et al., 2007). Several teams have built AI-based models to facilitate early detection and intervention for such infections (Ehrentraut, Kvist, Sparrelid, & Dalianis, 2014; McMillan & Friedenberg, 2016). In addition, research is underway to develop a generic model that can monitor several diseases simultaneously (Nori, Kashima, Yamashita, Ikai, & Imanaka, 2015). Combining EHRs with genomics data offers the promise of obtaining early prognostic risk indicators for common diseases (Li et al., 2014). Clustering and classification algorithms can be used to separate patients with similar characteristics into distinct subgroups such that patients in the same group are likely to follow similar clinical trajectories (Doshi-Velez, Ge, & Kohane, 2013; Hougham et al., 2014; Schulam, Wigley, & Saria, 2015).

Common to these systems are large databases of patient data that are used to train AI algorithms. While privacy concerns related to protected health information and other factors have often limited their availability to researchers, public release datasets, such as the MIMIC dataset from MIT (Johnson et al., 2016), are becoming increasingly available. This dataset of deidentified information for over 40,000 patients has been used to inform a wide variety of clinical decision support problems (Celi, Mark, Stone, & Montgomery, 2013; Dejam, Malley, & Feng, 2014; Ghassemi, Marshall, Singh, Stone, & Celi, 2014; Velasquez, Ghassemi, & Szolovits, 2014). Data programming competitions that seek to foster the development of ML models relevant to clinical decision support systems are underway, most notably the $3 million Heritage Health Prize, which called for algorithms to predict hospitalizations from patient data (Brierley, Vogel, & Axelrod, 2011). However, the public release of data for such competitions raises privacy concerns that pose real obstacles to making these datasets available to the research community (El Emam et al., 2012). Other examples of mining large databases to predict patient outcomes are IBM's Watson system applied to predicting cancer (Edwards, 2014), and Express Scripts's algorithm to predict medication compliance.

As clinical decision support systems become more prevalent, the inputs to these systems are also being refined. For example, wearable devices can now provide continuous real-time data to a clinical decision support system. Wearable devices can improve outcomes (Cleverley et al., 2013), but they are still in their infancy (Chen, 2013). One value of these devices is that they can measure vital signs or other indicators at frequent intervals, and the algorithms that process these signals can, therefore, more rapidly alert changes in patient status (Welch, Moon, & McCombie, 2012). And yet, many challenges remain to wide adoption of this technology, including issues of reliability, interoperability with other clinical systems, and a financing model.

MACHINE ASSISTANCE IN THE USE OF EHRs FOR HEALTH IMPROVEMENT

EHRs offer new possibilities and models for research into health care quality and the effectiveness of health care interventions, as well as the possibility of improvements in care at the individual patient level (Hripcsak & Albers, 2013). The increasing availability of such detailed health data on a large scale seems to be the perfect match for emerging AI technologies. Several problems are obvious. First, EHRs are designed for clinical use, and the demands of secondary research use (such as health outcomes research) do not always mesh with the data available in an EHR. Second, the clinical implementation of AI technologies within EHR environments will require high levels of accuracy and interpretability before such systems are likely to be accepted by health providers. Third, much of the most important clinical information is contained in unstructured clinician notes. However, machine intelligence is already being deployed in epidemiological and clinical applications of EHRs and holds great promise.

EHRs as Sources of Data

EHRs have become nearly ubiquitous in the United States's health care system. Adoption by hospitals of the Basic With Clinician Notes EHR standard—an Office of the National Coordinator (ONC) standard—has increased from 9.4% in 2008 to 83% in 2015, and 96% of hospitals now use some type of EHR (Henry et al., 2015). Importantly, the Basic With Clinician Notes standard contains text fields for physician and nurse assessments, as well as lab, radiology, and diagnostic test results. The Comprehensive EHR standard includes actual radiological images. However, only 40% of hospitals have adopted this standard. Thus, a large percentage of current inpatient visits are being documented on relatively incomplete EHR platforms. Some medical providers have access to even more sophisticated EHR enterprise systems, which contain near real-time data essential for advancing the state of clinical monitoring and prediction. Of course, the relatively recent adoption of EHR systems means that many patient histories have not been fully incorporated into their EHR. The most common practice among providers has been to consider the patient as new when switching to an EHR system, and requiring them to fill out a comprehensive medical history that might otherwise remain buried in paper-based medical charts. Other approaches have included scanning previous records to maintain "pictures" of old records, or the use of optical character recognition to digitize the clinical content of paper records. Apart from potential discontinuities involved for clinicians who may need access to the complete historical record, variations in these practices can also lead to difficulties for clinical studies where access to historical data is required. Therefore, bringing uniformity to EHR data is an important goal toward complete use of all sources of patient-level data.

There are several different ways clinical information can be systematically coded in records. The United States has recently begun moving to ICD-10 (Centers for Medicare & Medicaid Services, 2016) for inpatient reporting, with variation ICD-10-CM for diagnostic reporting and ICD-10-PCS for inpatient procedures. ICD-10 houses 68,000 clinical concepts and represents a great increase in resolution compared with its predecessor ICD-9, which only had 13,000. However, there are several other coding systems used in different contexts. The Healthcare Common Procedure Coding System (HCPCS) contains current procedural terminology (CPT) codes that are used to report medical procedures and professional services in outpatient settings, including physician visits to inpatients. In addition, Systematized Nomenclature of Medicine–Clinical Terminology (SNOMED-CT) is used for encoding physicians' clinical description of the patient, that is, the "problem list" portion of the record. SNOMED-CT dwarfs even ICD-10 in terms of concepts, and is designed for detailed interoperable descriptions of observations and diagnoses. Finally, there are yet other clinical terminologies such as the Logical Observation Identifiers Names and Codes (LOINC), which describes laboratory orders and test results, and RxNORM, which describes prescription drugs.

While all claims payments are required to use one set of codes, ICD-9, ICD-10, or CPT, clinical narrative is documented in SNOMED-CT, LOINC, or RxNORM. However, unlike billing, the assignment of clinical narrative tags is not structurally incentivized. Thus, the use of clinical vocabularies can vary greatly even within the same system. Additionally, as ICD-10, CPT, and other codes used for billing are sometimes input by support staff members far removed from patients, there may be biases and issues with the reliability of the data. Thus, while EHRs continue to promise to serve as a great data source for novel machine-assisted methods to improve health care, the first task of AI is, at least in part, to aid in the process of making the structured data from EHRs accessible, accurate, and reliable. Tackling unstructured data in EHRs is an even bigger challenge.

Data Mining of Patient Histories

Assuming that EHRs can be obtained for research purposes, there are a number of possibilities for data mining and predictive analytics: (a) *claim codes* (such as ICD-10 or CPT)—as noted earlier, these are nearly always present;

(b) *clinical narrative codes* (such as SNOMED-CT)—sometimes present, could be manually assigned or assigned by an NLP algorithm; (c) *clinical notes*—text provided by physicians and nurses, this is sometimes free text or sometimes semistructured; (d) *clinical data*—radiological images, laboratory test values, and other sensor data—currently, these types of data are not typically available directly in most EHRs, but are included in the ONC's "Comprehensive EHR standard."

NLP of Unstructured Text

Clinical notes are of particular interest because they contain clinical descriptions that are often not included in structured billing codes, and, as noted earlier, the use of clinical narrative codes are often inconsistent or subtly reflective of institutional rather than patient care goals (Ruiter, Liaschenko, & Angus, 2016). These inconsistencies and lack of clinical detail give even more value to free-text notes. For example, something as basic as precise blood pressure values may be recorded in clinical notes but not recorded in the diagnostic and procedure codes necessary for billing. NLP, the use of computer algorithms to map human language into another usable form, has long been looked to for help in automatically decoding clinical notes. However, applying NLP to clinical notes has turned out to be an especially difficult task because clinical notes often do not use standard English (in English-speaking locales), and clinicians are notorious for using nonstandard terms, abbreviations, and acronyms. In addition, clinicians have a variety of ways of describing the same thing, adding to the complexity (Elhadad, Pradhan, Chapman, Manandhar, & Savova, 2015; Pathak et al., 2015). There is a great deal more information in clinical notes than simple categorical diagnoses. As noted earlier, for example, temporality in clinical narrative is important in determining causality, and has been an active area of research (Tissot et al., 2015). NLP pipelines that incorporate multiple NLP technologies have been developed for the express purpose of annotating clinical notes, the Mayo Clinic's clinical Text Analysis and Knowledge Extraction System (cTAKES) being an excellent example (Savova et al., 2010). It is important to note that while the robustness of NLP methods for epidemiological purposes has made considerable headway, their use in tagging for use in the clinical setting is still suspect; a wrong assignment may flag a patient for incorrect treatment. As such, EHR providers and informed clinicians are suspicious of wholesale implementation of NLP for automated clinical coding. Finally, while NLP for clinical notes has not benefited from deep learning approaches on a mass scale (Elhadad et al., 2015), this is probably just a matter of time as methods improve, and the promise for binding coding and clinical text to other data types becomes clearer.

Images and Sensor Data

In addition to codes and free text, EHRs can contain links or reference to images and other kinds of sensor data. Coincidentally, recent technologies for image processing and recognition have improved markedly, largely through the implementation of deep learning approaches that use many layered neural networks (a class of statistical models that are part of AI) that process images at multiple levels of detail (LeCun, Bengio, & Hinton, 2015). These technologies have not only improved machine image processing, but, on some tasks, exceeded human performance in image classification (He, Zhang, Ren, & Sun, 2015). Additionally, by combining image processing and NLP technologies, the text associated with images can be leveraged to identify objects or pathology within the images, and indeed the images can subsequently even be used to produce associated descriptive text (Karpathy & Fei-Fei, 2015). Efforts to use deep learning for medical imaging have been limited in comparison with other applications owing to the relative difficulty of obtaining training data. However, EHRs could potentially provide massive training datasets for these algorithms. In combination, these technologies not only promise to aid radiologists in image analysis, but could potentially advance research in challenging problems such as diagnosis of neurodegenerative conditions such as Parkinson's and Alzheimer's diseases.

Deep learning can be applied to a variety of data types made available through EHRs, including data derived from hospital tests and monitoring, or increasingly common outpatient sensor devices. Perhaps most importantly, DNA sequences are only now being analyzed with deep learning techniques (Alipanahi, Delong, Weirauch, & Frey, 2015). The ability to access large-scale datasets through EHRs could, as in the case of imaging, allow for the training of powerful new algorithms, and uncover previously unknown genotypes associated with diseases, treatment optimization, and health outcomes.

One important drawback of deep learning (and most image processing approaches) is that the algorithms are often uninterpretable. For example, while image processing algorithms can be better than humans at some image recognition, how the algorithm comes to a conclusion may be even more elusive than understanding how a human would accomplish the same task. Humans are often capable of describing why they have come to a particular conclusion, but this is surprisingly beyond the current ability of deep learning techniques. Thus, while an algorithm may exceed human capability in raw computational power, cleverness, and ability to identify faint signal patterns indicating likely disease or other outcome of interest, at present, it is often hard to understand why the algorithm worked the way it did in any specific instance. This tension between wanting machines that solve problems (without understanding how they work) and machines that mimic how we think (understanding them, but not fully utilizing their capabilities) will persist for the foreseeable future.

Current Use of EHRs for Treatment Insight and Clinical Support

The availability of EHRs and the rich data they contain has obvious implications for systematic review, which is the bedrock of evidence-based practice (EBP). Historically, the gold standard for EBP has been randomized controlled clinical trials. For a given medical intervention or practice, such studies are collected and compiled into a systematic review. However, these reviews are time consuming, can take over a decade to convert into practice (Morris, Wooding, & Grant, 2011), and do not necessarily cover the populations that a clinician will encounter in practice. EHRs, of course, are not the product of directed studies, but offer access to the clinical information of massive and diverse populations. One key difficulty in using EHRs for the analysis of treatment effectiveness is the "semantic distance" between labels available in an EHR (such as ICD-10 billing codes), and the specific treatment of interest in the study (Workman & Stoddart, 2012). For example, diabetes can be defined by various specific lab results, but no one of those may be why a given patient is listed with a diabetes ICD-10 in their billing information. However, for certain topics such as acute myocardial infarction, EHRs have already proved useful, giving access to larger and more diverse populations than would likely be available from randomized controlled studies (Rubbo et al., 2015). In addition, deep learning approaches are beginning to be used for preprocessing EHRs to recognize clinical concepts and help close the "semantic distance" between research concepts and clinical concepts (Miotto, Li, Kidd, & Dudley, 2016).

EHRs coupled with machine-supported decision making also has promise in the clinical setting. Enterprise EHR systems that allow real-time updates can be used for the early detection of common inpatient hazards such as acute kidney injury (Goldstein et al., 2013; Kirkendall et al., 2014) and sepsis (Amland & Hahn-Cover, 2016). Importantly, these initial approaches have used detailed clinical models that depend on the real-time capabilities of an enterprise EHR system (i.e., a large-scale system designed to integrate many components in a complex infrastructure), and, therefore, are not necessarily satisfied by the interoperability and other requirements laid out in even the Comprehensive EHR standard.

GENOMICS AND AI IN CANCER RESEARCH

Cancer is currently the second leading cause of death in the United States, and it is expected to surpass heart disease as the leading cause of death in the next few years. From data collected from 2010 to 2012, the lifetime risk of developing cancer was found to be 43% for men and 38% for women. Cancer incidence has been relatively constant over the last two decades. However, cancer mortality has been on a steady decline across that period (22% between 1991 and 2011), thanks, in large part, to fewer Americans smoking, advances in prevention, earlier detection, and new treatment approaches (Siegel, Miller, & Jemal, 2015). Among these advances in prevention, detection, and treatment are approaches based on genomics.

Cancer usually develops in older people; 86% of all cancers in the United States are diagnosed in people 50 years of age or older (Society, 2016), and all metastatic tumors are caused by abnormalities in DNA leading to uncontrolled growth and spread of abnormal cells. These abnormalities typically occur during DNA replication, an ongoing process in all living organisms; errors during the replication process, called *somatic mutations*, result in progressive changes in DNA throughout life (Futreal et al., 2001). This ongoing process of progressive, subtle DNA change is one physiological explanation of why cancers occur more commonly in older adults (Liu, Wylie, Andrews, & Tollefsbol, 2003).

The study of the genetics (genes, gene variation, and heredity) and genomics (sequencing, assembling, and analyzing the function and structure of the genome) of cancer has shifted modern scientific opinion on the contribution of genetic susceptibility to cancer. In the 1960s, '70s, and '80s, the origin of cancer was perceived to be primarily the result of environmental exposure to mutagens. However, more recent studies emphasize genetics as an important predisposing risk factor for cancer (Futreal et al., 2001). For example, one recent study estimates that 50% of the female population has a breast cancer risk of 3% or lower and accounts for only 12% of all breast cancers; conversely, 12% of the population has a breast cancer risk of 10% or higher and accounts for 50% of all breast cancers (Pharoah et al., 2002). Additionally, recent research suggests that a predisposition to cancer owing to a combination of weak genetic variants accounts for a larger percentage of population cancer risk, than the risk from inherited cancers that track closely to individual, rare mutated alleles (Balmain, Gray, & Ponder, 2003).

Given the scope of cancer as a public health problem disproportionately impacting older adults, and the current understanding of the contribution of genetics to cancer susceptibility and survivability, understanding modern genomic cancer research and how AI approaches are being adopted is clearly a priority for those focused on our aging population.

The Role of Analytics and ML in Genomic Cancer Research

Science has long established DNA as the blueprint for living organisms (Croce, 2008). Some background on DNA and the processes and mechanisms associated with its replication and function are necessary to understand the critical role that statistical and ML methods currently play, and will continue to play, in decoding the relationships between specific genetic mutations and cancer. The ability to decode these relationships is fundamental to understanding individual cancer risk and recommending appropriate prevention and treatment options for specific individuals and cancer types (Balmain et al., 2003).

A complete copy of DNA resides within the nucleus of each cell. Over time, cells grow and then divide. To divide, a duplicate copy of DNA must be created in the nucleus so that after division, both cells will have a complete copy of DNA. This natural replication process is where many of the mutations that can ultimately lead to cancer are introduced. Cell biologists, biochemists, and other scientists have produced a rich understanding of how DNA is decoded within the cell and functionally utilized. Human DNA encodes 20,000 to 25,000 genes (International Human Genome Sequencing Consortium, 2004). Genes are segments of DNA that describe how a trait is expressed. Cancer is caused by alterations in oncogenes, tumor-suppressor genes, and microRNA genes, all of which lead to abnormal cells and uncontrolled cell growth. Oncogenes control cell proliferation, apoptosis, or both. MicroRNA regulates the expression of other genes (Croce, 2008). Genes are expressed through a process called *transcription*, which produces RNA, a more portable, but less stable, copy of a DNA segment. With current technology, researchers have developed approaches to measuring gene expression for a targeted set of genes, by assessing relative or semiquantitative amounts of RNA, including high-density microarray, low-density microarray, and real-time polymerase chain reaction (PCR) (Chung, Levy, Chaurand, & Carbone, 2007).

DNA itself is composed of sequences of just four nucleotides, adenine (A), guanine (G), cytosine (C), and thymine (T). However, in 2004, the human genome sequence (Build 35) was announced to contain 2.85 billion nucleotide pairs (International Human Genome Sequencing Consortium, 2004). The sheer size of the human genome provides the first indication of why ML is growing in importance as a cancer research tool; determining which mutations or combinations of mutations are associated with specific cancers is a task of sorting through a large number of mutations. This is a task to which ML is well suited. As technology advances, and the time and cost to produce whole genome sequences for large numbers of individuals progresses, statistical and ML approaches to detect the effects of vast numbers of mutations and permutations of mutations will be required.

Examples of ML in Genomic Cancer Research

A significant number of research publications have used ML techniques to assess cancer susceptibility, recurrence, and survival (Kourou, Exarchos, Exarchos, Karamouzis, & Fotiadis, 2015). As examples, SVMs, decision trees, and naïve Bayes classifiers have been used on a dataset of 174 breast cancer patients and matched controls to assess breast cancer susceptibility. Predictor variables consisted of 98 single nucleotide polymorphisms (SNPs) spread across 45 genes of potential breast cancer relevance (Listgarten et al., 2004). In this work, three SNPs were identified as significant predictors of breast cancer susceptibility. SVMs performed best among the ML methods considered, achieving a predictive power in distinguishing between breast cancer patients and controls of 69%. The relative locations of these three SNPs, on different genes spread widely across the genome, provides additional evidence for the theory that cancer results from a combination of weak genetic variants.

To better explain the next example, a brief discussion of how the terms *supervised, semisupervised,* and *unsupervised* are used in the vernacular of classification models and algorithms is provided. The words supervised, unsupervised, and semisupervised all refer to whether the response or dependent variable is known in the training dataset. In supervised methods, the category is known for all the observations; for unsupervised methods, the category is not known for any of the observations; semisupervised methods are used when the category is known for some of the observations, but not all. Semisupervised methods assume that there is information in the structure of the explanatory variables in the uncategorized observations, helpful to building the model or algorithm for classifying observations. The data in the problems in the earlier paragraphs consist of explanatory or independent variables (the SNPs in the preceding example), and a response or dependent variable that encodes the category to which each observation belongs (breast cancer patient or control in the preceding example). The purpose of classification models and algorithms built on data such as these is to learn the relationship between the explanatory variables and the response, such that for future or new observations, predictions of the response can be produced from the explanatory variables alone, preferably with known confidence in the prediction (the algorithms in the previous example used SNPs to categorize observations into breast cancer patients or controls).

In the next example, data related to invasive breast cancer samples and colorectal cancer patients from the Gene Expression Omnibus (GEO) database have been used to predict cancer recurrence (Park, Ahn, Kim, & Park, 2014). Gene expression and protein interaction data were used to predict recurrence using a semisupervised graph regularization approach (discussed in detail subsequently). A semisupervised approach was used in this study because recurrence status was unknown for a percentage of both breast and colorectal cancers. Explaining graph regularization is beyond the scope of this chapter. However, one can think of this method as using the explanatory variables to construct weighted links among all the observations, both categorized and uncategorized, and assigning categories to the uncategorized observations on the basis of link-weighted voting of the categorized observations. Key to this method is choice of the function chosen to determine link weights; the authors chose to threshold the well-known Pearson correlation coefficient to establish their weights. The Pearson correlation coefficient is the standard correlation calculation used for real-valued, continuous variables. Thus, the link weight is based on the gene correlation between cancer patient observations. Results from the semisupervised graph regularization approach were compared with supervised SVM, naïve Bayes, and other classifiers; the semisupervised method exhibited performance benefits over the supervised ML approaches in these GEO database examples.

As a final example of how ML methods are revolutionizing cancer prognosis, an SVM-based technique was used to select a 50-gene signature predicting breast cancer survival from microarray-based gene expression data that demonstrated a 21% improvement in overall accuracy, compared with a previously developed 70-gene panel. High dimensional microarray data from 295 breast cancer patients were used to develop the gene panel. This 50-gene signature achieved an accuracy of 0.97, a sensitivity of 0.99, and a specificity of 0.93 on the training data (Xu, Zhang, Zou, Wang, & Li, 2012). Further, this tool was shown to effectively predict metastases and distinguish which patients should receive adjuvant therapy. Improved prognosis tools such as this 50-gene panel can reduce the number of patients who unnecessarily undergo adjuvant systemic therapy.

SMART MEDICATION DEVELOPMENT AND OPTIMIZATION

There are many important recent advances in medication delivery such as targeted drug delivery for cancer patients, where medications are directed specifically at a tumor (Douglas, Bachelet, & Church, 2012; Mills & Needham, 1999; Roza, Hakim, van Poppel, & Joniau, 2013).

AI is also being utilized to optimize drug delivery methods. For example, in prescribing medications, it is often challenging to determine the optimal drug concentration and length of time to effectively treat the disease with as few side effects as possible. To this end, Li, Lenaghan, and Zhang (2012) demonstrated one example of using ML methods to address this problem for infectious diseases, using in vitro experiments with *Giardia lamblia*, a protozoan parasite. They predicted with 73% accuracy the effectiveness of a drug dose given only four test combinations of drug concentration and pathogen states, and the accuracy of their prediction rose to over 97% with nine data points. This data-driven approach is advantageous in that it requires very little physician supervision, and can adapt to changes in the pathogen population.

Smart Drug Development

The amount of data collected on the effects of chemical compounds has been dramatically increasing by high-throughput and high-content screening. With so many compounds to control for when screening for a given target, a very large number of experiments would be required to make complete sense of the data. For example, if there are just 20 compounds to control for, testing each unique combination of the 20 compounds would result in over a million experiments (to be exact, it is 2 to the 20th power, or 1,048,576). In addition, a given drug may have variable effects depending on factors related to the individual, such as age, comorbidities, genetics, and even the environment, which increases the number of possible scenarios even further. Current practice requires scientists to choose a subset of experiments to run, which they think will provide the most information at a reasonable cost. This process has many downsides, including the difficulty of the scientists in making predictions in the presence of potentially complex interactions.

Murphy (2011) summarizes the approach of active learning to aid in drug development. In active learning, a predictive model is first built, which should incorporate complex interactions, and then that model is used to select new experiments to run. For example, a model may be built to predict the phenotype, given a perturbagen, target, and cell type. New experiments are only designed to improve the model (e.g., where the model is very uncertain of the phenotype response), not experiments where the outcome is highly predictable. This process leads to the improved ability to predict the phenotypes for unseen combinations of perturbagen, target, and cell type. Incorporating even more AI, Naik, Kangas, Sullivan, and Murphy (2016) expanded on the use of active learning for selecting the next experiment. In addition to selecting the experiment with AI, they developed a robotic system to run experiments, which determined the effects of chemical compounds on subcellular localization of proteins. The experiments were run and the results were collected without human interaction, with the active learning algorithm guiding the decision of which experiment to try next. Using this approach, the robotic system needed to perform less than a third of the total possible experiments that would have been required with an exhaustive but manual approach. This points to a future where limited human involvement decreases the cost and time necessary for drug development.

While these active learning approaches can help find promising treatments, identifying significant drug–drug interactions is also important. These interactions can cause many adverse effects including increased morbidity and increasing health care costs. There have been studies in the literature to predict drug–drug interactions before they happen. Cheng and Zhao (2014) used an ML approach to do so. They first built a database of drug pairs that were known either to interact or not. Then they calculated the similarity of each of the pairs of drugs using four well-known metrics for drug similarity. Finally, they used these similarity scores as predictors of the presence or absence of a drug–drug interaction in several ML models. Although the research is still early, they found that many of their predictions of drug–drug interactions were supported by the literature, and overall they were able to predict them more accurately than by random chance alone.

AI FOR EXTRACTING NEW KNOWLEDGE FROM THE SCIENTIFIC LITERATURE

Research in aging and related health care fields continues to grow so rapidly that it is becoming harder to analyze and evaluate the various, often disparate, findings and conclusions reported in the literature. No longer will simply retrieving the most relevant documents—a challenge to which the National Library of Medicine, Google, and others have responded admirably—address tomorrow's true knowledge requirements. Often it is not a "document" that is needed, but rather specific and linked pieces of knowledge—assertions and claims and data points, the correct interpretation of which may depend on their relationships to contextual or explanatory knowledge found in multiple, perhaps not obviously related, documents.

NLP was among the first goals of AI, as human knowledge and intelligence itself are transmitted primarily by means of language. While early attempts at automated language understanding were severely constrained by computational resources, today people regularly interact with computers that can "understand" and generate natural language. With regard to complex written documents, however, we are still at a very early stage of being able to perform humanlike reasoning about the content of the documents that constitute the discourse domain of scientific and technical literature.

Computational Linguistics

The interdisciplinary field of computational linguistics tends to be aligned along two fundamental approaches to language comprehension, often referred to as *statistical* and *knowledge based* (Dina Demner-Fushman, 2007). Some sort of ML plays a significant role in each, and indeed each of these two basic models seems to require some reliance on the other to be optimally effective. The former approach emphasizes statistical correlations—among words, phrases, concepts, or topics—to discern patterns in spoken or written language, and thereby infer the "aboutness" of a document or discourse by means of *topic modeling*, and recognizing explicit or implicit relationships between concepts or topics. Knowledge-based approaches, on the other hand, apply formal and logical representations of subject matter expertise to capture nuances that cannot be easily discovered by statistics alone.

Extracting Knowledge

For the fields of aging, geriatrics, and gerontology, domain-specific vocabularies or "sublanguages" are sometimes used in the literature to characterize and analyze the details and findings of research in those disciplines. Knowledge-based approaches to understanding text rely on *semantic processing*, often by means of domain ontologies. An ontology in this sense is a "formal naming and definition of the types, properties, and interrelationships of the entities that really or fundamentally exist for a particular domain of discourse" ("Ontology," 2017). The advantage of ontologies for understanding scientific literature is that they can define the necessary logical characteristics of the relationships between the different sorts of entities discussed in the literature of that domain. By encoding scientific and other contextual knowledge in an ontology, knowledge bases can be automatically constructed that tie facts and assertions together, supporting queries that may require *inferential* (especially deductive) *reasoning* to answer questions about the research.

Depending on how the output of *semantic tagging* is structured, the knowledge extracted from literature can be visualized in graph form, which permits examination of linkages and gaps in the knowledge obtainable from the literature. In addition to uses such as summarizing findings from mass corpora of literature (i.e., a structured literature review), this type of approach may also yield discoveries and testable hypotheses by way of chaining large numbers of logical kernels of reported findings to conclusions not yet published (Gubiani, Petrič, Fabbretti, & Urbančič, 2015).

Furthermore, as this kind of processing generates assertions extracted from text in a common and logical form, the resulting knowledge can be used to support the meta-analytic goals of systematic review. Among the complications of meta-analysis is the requirement for a common statistical measure among studies under review. Qualitative and even quantitative differences in methodologies, approaches, and results are often discussed in natural language. While meta-analysis is a statistical process, the preprocessing required to normalize findings and associate them with similar conditions can be streamlined by means of knowledge representation based on NLP.

Advances in these areas of AI, ML, and computational linguistics will eventually also enable high-quality, foreign-language understanding, which could be very valuable when mining the geriatrics and gerontology literatures of other aging nations. Other research programs will also likely benefit, such as social-network-analysis–driven historical trajectories of knowledge growth through time, and "deep scientometrics" to better understand the paths and contexts of aging research and discovery.

CONCLUSION

We have introduced and illustrated some of the ways that AI can improve the health and well-being of older adults. The technologies of AI are maturing and hold great promise in many areas, from managing the timing and sequencing of events in the care of older persons—for example, in smart medication reminder or other care management systems—to streamlining and hastening the development of medications, and how to use them by using computational methods of more accurately calculating appropriate medication dosage. For clinical providers, AI's abilities to mine vast amounts of data hold great promise to quickly find and synthesize new knowledge, improve decision support systems, assist physicians with the detection of disease, and manage multiple incongruent patient health record information systems. Brain–machine interfaces will be an area of ongoing development because of its potential to help return motor function to neurologically impaired older adults. Similarly, as adjunct "thinkers" to cognitively impaired persons and their caregivers,

AI-driven cognitive agents will be another active area of research and development. Although there are many issues to be resolved in the coming years (such as those outlined in Chapter 1), continuing advances suggest that these technologies will, one day, become clinically viable, and maybe even routine, options to allow persons with impairments to retain or regain some degree of independence. However, the biggest challenges to taking the fruits of these endeavors to scale in service of aging populations have less to do with the limits of science, engineering, and medicine, and more to do with finding safe and sustainable ways to implement them in real-world settings.

REFERENCES

Aflalo, T., Kellis, S., Klaes, C., Lee, B., Shi, Y., Pejsa, K., . . . Andersen, R. A. (2015). Decoding motor imagery from the posterior parietal cortex of a tetraplegic human. *Science, 348*(6237), 906–910. doi:10.1126/science.aaa5417

Agurto, C., Nemeth, S., Zamora, G., Vahtel, M., Soliz, P., & Barriga, S. (2016). *Comprehensive eye evaluation algorithm*. Paper presented at the Medical Imaging 2016: Computer-Aided Diagnosis. doi:10.1117/12.2217130

Alipanahi, B., Delong, A., Weirauch, M. T., & Frey, B. J. (2015). Predicting the sequence specificities of DNA- and RNA-binding proteins by deep learning. *Nature Biotechnology, 33*, 831–838. doi:10.1038/nbt.3300

Allen, J. (1983). Maintaining knowledge about temporal intervals. *Communications of the ACM, 26*(11), 12.

Alzheimer's Association. (2016). *2016 Alzheimer's disease facts and figures* (pp. 1–84). Chicago, IL: Alzheimer's Association

American Cancer Society. (2016). *Cancer facts & figures 2016*. Atlanta, GA: Author.

Amland, R. C., & Hahn-Cover, K. E. (2016). Clinical decision support for early recognition of sepsis. *American Journal of Medical Quality, 31*, 103–110.

Artikis, A., Paliouras, G., Portet, F., & Skarlatidis, A. (2010). *Logic-based representation, reasoning and machine learning for event recognition*. Paper presented at the Proceedings of the Fourth ACM International Conference on Distributed Event-Based Systems, Cambridge, United Kingdom.

Balmain, A., Gray, J., & Ponder, B. (2003). The genetics and genomics of cancer. *Nature Genetics, 33*, 238–244.

Bansal, A. K., Truccolo, W., Vargas-Irwin, C. E., & Donoghue, J. P. (2012). Decoding 3D reach and grasp from hybrid signals in motor and premotor cortices: Spikes, multiunit activity, and local field potentials. *Journal of Neurophysiology, 107*(5), 1337–1355. doi: 10.1152/jn.00781.2011

Bar, Y., Diamant, I., Wolf, L., & Greenspan, H. (2015). Deep learning with non-medical training used for chest pathology identification. *Medical Imaging 2015: Computer-Aided Diagnosis, 9414*. doi:10.1117/12.2083124

Barták, R., Morris, R. A., & Venable, K. B. (2014). An introduction to constraint-based temporal reasoning. *Synthesis Lectures on Artificial Intelligence and Machine Learning, 8*(1), 1–121.

Beard, J., Biggs, S., Bloom, D. E., Fried, L. P., Hogan, P. R., Kalache, A., & Olshansky, S. J. (2012). *Global population ageing: Peril or promise?* Program on the Global Demography of Aging. Geneva, Switzerland: World Economic Forum.

Bouton, C. E., Shaikhouni, A., Annetta, N. V., Bockbrader, M. A., Friedenberg, D. A., Nielson, D. M., . . . Rezai, A. R. (2016). Restoring cortical control of functional movement in a human with quadriplegia [Research Support, Non-U.S. Gov't]. *Nature, 533*(7602), 247–250. doi:10.1038/nature17435

Brierley, P., Vogel, D., & Axelrod, R. (2011). Heritage Provider Network Health Prize. Round 1 milestone prize: How we did it—Team 'Market Makers.' Retrieved from https://foreverdata.org/1015/content/milestone2-1.pdf

Business Report: Data-driven Health Care. (2014). *MIT Technology Review, 117*. Retrieved from https://www.technologyreview.com/business-report/data-driven-health-care

Butler, D. (2013). When Google got flu wrong. *Nature, 494*, 155–156. doi:10.1038/494155a

Campbell, O. (2015). Designing for the elderly: Ways older people use digital technology differently. *Smashing Magazine*. Retrieved from https://www.smashingmagazine.com/2015/02/designing-digital-technology-for-the-elderly

Celi, L. A., Mark, R. G., Stone, D. J., & Montgomery, R. A. (2013). "Big data" in the intensive care unit. Closing the data loop. *American Journal of Respiratory and Critical Care Medicine, 187*, 1157–1160. doi:10.1164/rccm.201212-2311ED

Centers for Medicare & Medicaid Services. (2016). ICD-10. Retrieved from https://www.cms.gov/Medicare/Coding/ICD10/index.html

Chakravarty, S., & Shahar, Y. (1999). *Specification and detection of periodic patterns in clinical data*. Paper presented at the Fourth Workshop on Intelligent Data Analysis in Medicine and Pharmacology (IDAMAP-99). Retrieved from http://www.ifs.tuwien.ac.at/~silvia/idamap99/idamap99-03.pdf

Chapin, J. K., Moxon, K. A., Markowitz, R. S., & Nicolelis, M. A. L. (1999). Real-time control of a robot arm using simultaneously recorded neurons in the motor cortex. *Nature Neuroscience, 2*(7), 664–670. doi:10.1038/10223

Chen, E. H. (2013). Appropriate use of telemetry monitoring in hospitalized patients. *Current Emergency and Hospital Medicine Reports, 2*(1), 52–56. doi:10.1007/s40138-013-0030-6

Cheng, F., & Zhao, Z. (2014). Machine learning-based prediction of drug–drug interactions by integrating drug phenotypic, therapeutic, chemical, and genomic properties. *Journal of the American Medical Informatics Association, 21*(e2), e278–e286. doi:10.1136/amiajnl-2013-002512

Chung, C. H., Levy, S., Chaurand, P., & Carbone, D. P. (2007). Genomics and proteomics: Emerging technologies in clinical cancer research. *Critical Reviews in Oncology/Hematology, 61*(1), 1–25. doi:10.1016/j.critrevonc.2006.06.005

Cleverley, K., Mousavi, N., Stronger, L., Ann-Bordun, K., Hall, L., Tam, J. W., . . . Philipp, R. K. (2013). The impact of telemetry on survival of in-hospital cardiac arrests in non-critical care patients. *Resuscitation, 84*(7), 878–882. doi:10.1016/j.resuscitation.2013.01.038

Clifton, D. A., Niehaus, K. E., Charlton, P., & Colopy, G. W. (2015). Health informatics via machine learning for the clinical management of patients. *Yearbook of Medical Informatics, 10*(1), 38–43. doi:10.15265/iy-2015-014

Croce, C. M. (2008). Oncogenes and cancer. *New England Journal of Medicine, 358*(5), 502–511. doi:10.1056/NEJMra072367

da Silva, F. L. (2013). EEG and MEG: Relevance to neuroscience. *Neuron, 80*(5), 1112–1128.

de Vries, E. N., Ramrattan, M. A., Smorenburg, S. M., Gouma, D. J., & Boermeester, M. A. (2008). The incidence and nature of in-hospital adverse events: A systematic review. *Quality and Safety in Health Care, 17*(3), 216–223.

Dechter, R., Meiri, I., & Pearl, J. (1991). Temporal constraint networks. *Artificial Intelligence, 49*(1–3), 61–95.

Dejam, A., Malley, B. E., & Feng, M. (2014). The effect of age and clinical circumstances on the outcome of red blood cell transfusion in the critically ill patients. *Critical Care, 18,* 487. doi:10.1186/s13054-014-0487-z

Dina Demner-Fushman, J. L. (2007). Answering clinical questions with knowledge-based and statistical techniques. *Computational Linguistics, 33*(1), 42.

Doi, K. (2007). Computer-aided diagnosis in medical imaging: Historical review, current status and future potential. *Computerized Medical Imaging and Graphics: The Official Journal of the Computerized Medical Imaging Society, 31*(4–5), 198–211. doi:10.1016/j.compmedimag.2007.02.002

Doshi-Velez, F., Ge, Y., & Kohane, I. (2013). Comorbidity clusters in autism spectrum disorders: An electronic health record time-series analysis. *Pediatrics, 133*(1), e54–e63. doi:10.1542/peds.2013-0819

Douglas, S. M., Bachelet, I., & Church, G. M. (2012). A logic-gated nanorobot for targeted transport of molecular payloads. *Science, 335*(6070), 831–834. doi:10.1126/science.1214081

Dousson, C., & Le Maigat, P. (2007). *Chronicle recognition improvement using temporal focusing and hierarchization*. Paper presented at the IJCAI-07. Retrieved from https://www.aaai.org/Papers/IJCAI/2007/IJCAI07-050.pdf

Edwards, C. (2014). Using patient data for personalized cancer treatments. *Communications of the ACM, 57*. doi:10.1145/2581892

Ehrentraut, C., Kvist, M., Sparrelid, E., & Dalianis, H. (2014, October 6–7). *Detecting healthcare-associated infections in electronic health records: Evaluation of machine learning and preprocessing techniques.* Paper presented at the Sixth International Symposium on Semantic Mining in Biomedicine (SMBM 2014), Aveiro, Portugal.

El Emam, K., Arbuckle, L., Koru, G., Eze, B., Gaudette, L., Neri, E., . . . Gluck, J. (2012). De-identification methods for open health data: The case of the Heritage Health Prize claims dataset. *Journal of Medical Internet Research, 14*(1), e33.

Elhadad, N., Pradhan, S., Chapman, W. W., Manandhar, S., & Savova, G. K. (2015). *SemEval-2015 task 14: Analysis of clinical text.* Paper presented at the Proceedings 9th International Workshop on Semantic Evaluation, Association for Computational Linguistics, Denver, Colorado.

Emaminejad, N., Yan, S., Wang, Y., Qian, W., Guan, Y., & Zheng, B. (2016). *Applying a radiomics approach to predict prognosis of lung cancer patients*. Paper presented at Medical Imaging 2016: Computer-Aided Diagnosis. doi:10.1117/12.2214672

Disabled Living Foundation. (2009). Losing independence is a bigger ageing worry than dying. Retrieved from http://www.dlf.org.uk/blog/losing-independence-bigger-ageing-worry-dying

Friedman, C., & Hripcsak, G. (1999). Natural language processing and its future in medicine. *Academic Medicine, 74*(8), 890–895.

Futreal, P. A., Kasprzyk, A., Birney, E., Mullikin, J. C., Wooster, R., & Stratton, M. R. (2001). Cancer and genomics. *Nature, 409*(6822), 850–852. Retrieved from http://www.nature.com/nature/journal/v409/n6822/full/409850a0.html

Galan, F., Nuttin, M., Lew, E., Ferrez, P. W., Vanacker, G., Philips, J., & Millan Jdel, R. (2008). A brain-actuated wheelchair: Asynchronous and non-invasive brain-computer interfaces for continuous control of robots [Research Support, Non-U.S. Gov't]. *Clinical Neurophysiology, 119*(9), 2159–2169. doi:10.1016/j.clinph.2008.06.001

Ghassemi, M., Celi, L. A., & Stone, D. J. (2015). State of the art review: The data revolution in critical care. *Critical Care, 19*(1), 1–9. doi:10.1186/s13054-015-0801-4

Ghassemi, M., Marshall, J., Singh, N., Stone, D. J., & Celi, L. A. (2014). Leveraging a critical care database: Selective serotonin reuptake inhibitor use prior to ICU admission is associated with increased hospital mortality. *Chest, 145*, 745–752. doi:10.1378/chest.13-1722

Goldstein, S. L., Kirkendall, E., Nguyen, H., Schaffzin, J. K., Bucuvalas, J., Bracke, T., . . . Muething, S. (2013). Electronic health record identification of nephrotoxin exposure and associated acute kidney injury. *Pediatrics, 132*, e756–e767.

Groves, P., Kayyali, B., Knott, D., & Van Kuiken, S. (2013). The 'big data' revolution in healthcare. *McKinsey Quarterly.* Retrieved from http://www.mckinsey.com/industries/healthcare-systems-and-services/our-insights/the-big-data-revolution-in-us-health-care

Gubiani, D., Petrič, I., Fabbretti, E., & Urbančič, T. (2015, October 5). Mining scientific literature about ageing to support better understanding and treatment of degenerative diseases. Paper presented at the Conference on Data Mining and Data Warehouses (SiKDD 2015), Ljubljana, Slovenia.

He, K., Zhang, X., Ren, S., & Sun, J. (2015). *Delving deep into rectifiers: Surpassing human-level performance on ImageNet classification.* Paper presented at the Proceedings of the IEEE International Conference on Computer Vision, Santiago, Chile.

Hebert, L. E., Beckett, L. A., Scherr, P. A., & Evans, D. A. (2001). Annual incidence of Alzheimer disease in the United States projected to the years 2000 through 2050. *Alzheimer Disease and Associated Disorders, 15*(4), 169–173.

Henry, J., Pylypchuck, Y., Searcy, Y., & Patel, V. (2015). Adoption of electronic health record systems among U.S. non-federal acute care hospitals: 2008–2015. *ONC Data Brief,* No. 35. Retrieved from http://dashboard.healthit.gov/evaluations/data-briefs/non-federal-acute-care-hospital-ehr-adoption-2008-2015.php

Hochberg, L. R., Bacher, D., Jarosiewicz, B., Masse, N. Y., Simeral, J. D., Vogel, J., . . . Donoghue, J. P. (2012). Reach and grasp by people with tetraplegia using a neurally controlled robotic arm. *Nature, 485*(7398), 372–375. doi:10.1038/nature11076

Hougham, G. W., Ham, S. A., Ruhnke, G. W., Schulwolf, E., Auerbach, A. D., Schnipper, J. L., . . . Meltzer, D. O. (2014). Sequence patterns in the resolution of clinical instabilities in community-acquired pneumonia and association with outcomes. *Journal of General Internal Medicine, 29*(4), 563–571.

Hripcsak, G., & Albers, D. J. (2013). Next-generation phenotyping of electronic health records. *Journal of the American Medical Informatics Association, 20*(1), 117–121.

Imani, F., Ghavidel, S., Abolmaesumi, P., Khallaghi, S., Gibson, E., Khojaste, A., . . . Mousavi, P. (2016). *Fusion of multi-parametric MRI and temporal ultrasound for characterization of prostate cancer: In vivo feasibility study.* Paper presented at Medical Imaging 2016: Computer-Aided Diagnosis. doi:10.1117/12.2217205

International Human Genome Sequencing Consortium. (2004). Finishing the euchromatic sequence of the human genome. *Nature, 431*(7011), 931–945. doi:10.1038/nature03001

Jiménez del Toro, O. A., Foncubierta-Rodríguez, A., Depeursinge, A., & Müller, H. (2015). *Texture classification of anatomical structures in CT using a context-free machine learning approach.* Paper presented at Medical Imaging 2015: Computer-Aided Diagnosis. doi:10.1117/12.2082273

Johnson, A. E. W., Kramer, A. A., & Clifford, G. D. (2013). A new severity of illness scale using a subset of acute physiology and chronic health evaluation data elements shows comparable predictive accuracy. *Critical Care Medicine, 41*(7), 1711–1718. doi:10.1097/ccm.0b013e31828a24fe

Johnson, A. E. W., Pollard, T. J., Shen, L., Lehman, L.-W. H., Feng, M., Ghassemi, M., . . . Mark, R. G. (2016). MIMIC-III, a freely accessible critical care database. *Scientific Data, 3*, 160035.

Kao, J. C., Stavisky, S. D., Sussillo, D., Nuyujukian, P., & Shenoy, K. V. (2014). Information systems opportunities in brain–machine interface decoders. *Proceedings of the IEEE, 102*(5), 666–682. doi:10.1109/Jproc.2014.2307357

Karpathy, A., & Fei-Fei, L. (2015). *Deep visual-semantic alignments for generating image descriptions.* Paper presented at the Proceedings of the IEEE Conference on Computer Vision and Pattern Recognition, Boston, MA.

Kennedy, P. R., & Bakay, R. A. E. (1998). Restoration of neural output from a paralyzed patient by a direct brain connection. *Neuroreport, 9*(8), 1707–1711. doi:10.1097/00001756-199806010-00007

Kirkendall, E. S., Spires, W. L., Mottes, T. A., Schaffzin, J. K., Barclay, C., & Goldstein, S. L. (2014). Development and performance of electronic acute kidney injury triggers to identify pediatric patients at risk for nephrotoxic medication-associated harm. *Applied Clinical Informatics, 5*, 313–333. doi:10.4338/ACI-2013-12-RA-0102

Klevens, R. M., Edwards, J. R., Richards Jr, C. L., Horan, T. C., Gaynes, R. P., Pollock, D. A., & Cardo, D. M. (2007). Estimating health care-associated infections and deaths in US hospitals, 2002. *Public health reports, 122*, 160–166.

Knaus, W. A., Zimmerman, J. E., Wagner, D. P., Draper, E. A., & Lawrence, D. E. (1981). APACHE—Acute physiology and chronic health evaluation: A physiologically based classification system. *Critical Care Medicine, 9*(8), 591–597. doi:10.1097/00003246-198108000-00008

Kourou, K., Exarchos, T. P., Exarchos, K. P., Karamouzis, M. V., & Fotiadis, D. I. (2015). Machine learning applications in cancer prognosis and prediction. *Computational and Structural Biotechnology Journal, 13*, 8–17. doi:10.1016/j.csbj.2014.11.005

Langley, P. (2004). *Cognitive architectures and the construction of intelligent agents* (p. 82). Paper presented at the Proceedings of the AAAI-2004 Workshop on Intelligent Agent Architectures, Stanford, CA.

Lazer, D., Kennedy, R., King, G., & Vespignani, A. (2014). The parable of Google flu: Traps in big data analysis. *Science, 343*, 1203–1205. doi:10.1126/science.1248506

Leape, L. L., Brennan, T. A., Laird, N., Lawthers, A. G., Localio, A. R., Barnes, B. A., . . . Hiatt, H. (1991). The nature of adverse events in hospitalized patients: Results of the Harvard Medical Practice Study II. *New England Journal of Medicine, 324*(6), 377–384.

Lebedev, M. A., & Nicolelis, M. A. (2006). Brain–machine interfaces: Past, present and future. *Trends in Neurosciences, 29*(9), 536–546.

LeCun, Y., Bengio, Y., & Hinton, G. (2015). Deep learning. *Nature, 521*, 436–444. doi:10.1038/nature14539

Lessmann, N., Isgum, I., Setio, A. A. A., de Vos, B. D., Ciompi, F., de Jong, P. A., . . . van Ginneken, B. (2016). *Deep convolutional neural networks for automatic coronary calcium scoring in a screening study with low-dose chest CT.* Paper presented at Medical Imaging 2016: Computer-Aided Diagnosis. doi:10.1117/12.2216978

Li, L., Ruau, D. J., Patel, C. J., Weber, S. C., Chen, R., Tatonetti, N. P., . . . Butte, A. J. (2014). Disease risk factors identified through shared genetic architecture and electronic medical records. *Science Translational Medicine, 6*(234), 234–257. doi:10.1126/scitranslmed.3007191

Li, Y., Lenaghan, S. C., & Zhang, M. (2012). A data-driven predictive approach for drug delivery using machine learning techniques. *PLOS ONE, 7*(2), e31724. doi:10.1371/journal.pone.0031724

Listgarten, J., Damaraju, S., Poulin, B., Cook, L., Dufour, J., Driga, A., . . . Zanke, B. (2004). Predictive models for breast cancer susceptibility from multiple single nucleotide polymorphisms. *American Association for Cancer Research, 10*(8), 2725–2737. doi:10.1158/1078-0432.CCR-1115-03

Liu, L., Wylie, R. C., Andrews, L. G., & Tollefsbol, T. O. (2003). Aging, cancer and nutrition: The DNA methylation connection. *Mechanisms of Ageing and Development, 124*(10–12), 989–998. doi:10.1016/j.mad.2003.08.001

Madsen, S. K., Ver Steeg, G., Daianu, M., Mezher, A., Jahanshad, N., Nir, T. M., . . . Thompson, P. M. (2016). *Relative value of diverse brain MRI and blood-based biomarkers for predicting cognitive decline in the elderly*. Paper presented at Medical Imaging 2016: Image Processing. doi:10.1117/12.2216964

Mani, S., Chen, Y., Elasy, T., Clayton, W., & Denny, J. (2012). Type 2 diabetes risk forecasting from EMR data using machine learning. *AMIA Annual Symposium Proceedings, 2012*, 606–615.

McCorduck, P. (2004). *Machines who think: A personal inquiry into the history and prospects of artificial intelligence*. Natick, MA: A. K. Peters.

McMillan, N., & Friedenberg, D. (2016). *Enhancing patient outcomes with big data: Two case studies*. Paper presented at the HIMSS, Las Vegas, Nevada. Retrieved from http://www.himssconference.org/sites/himssconference/files/pdf/89.pdf

Millan, J. D., Renkens, F., Mourino, J., & Gerstner, W. (2004). Noninvasive brain-actuated control of a mobile robot by human EEG. *IEEE Transactions on Biomedical Engineering, 51*(6), 1026–1033. doi:10.1109/Tbme.2004.827086

Mills, J. K., & Needham, D. (1999). Targeted drug delivery. *Expert Opinion on Therapeutic Patents, 9*(11), 1499–1513. doi:10.1517/13543776.9.11.1499

Miotto, R., Li, L., Kidd, B. A., & Dudley, J. T. (2016). Deep patient: An unsupervised representation to predict the future of patients from the electronic health records. *Scientific Reports, 6*, 26094. doi:10.1038/srep26094

Morris, Z. S., Wooding, S., & Grant, J. (2011). The answer is 17 years, what is the question: Understanding time lags in translational research. *Journal of the Royal Society of Medicine, 104*, 510–520. doi:10.1258/jrsm.2011.110180

Murphy, R. F. (2011). An active role for machine learning in drug development. *Nature Chemical Biology, 7*(6), 327–330. doi:10.1038/nchembio.576

Naik, A. W., Kangas, J. D., Sullivan, D. P., & Murphy, R. F. (2016). Active machine learning-driven experimentation to determine compound effects on protein patterns. *eLife, 5*. doi:10.7554/elife.10047

National Institute of Health. (2007). 8 Areas of age-related change. *NIH MedlinePlus, 2*, 4.

Nicolelis, M. A., & Lebedev, M. A. (2009). Principles of neural ensemble physiology underlying the operation of brain–machine interfaces. *Nature Reviews Neuroscience, 10*(7), 530–540. doi:10.1038/nrn2653

Nori, N., Kashima, H., Yamashita, K., Ikai, H., & Imanaka, Y. (2015). *Simultaneous modeling of multiple diseases for mortality prediction in acute hospital care*. Paper presented at the Proceedings of the 21th ACM SIGKDD International Conference on Knowledge Discovery and Data Mining, Sydney, Australia.

Nuyujukian, P., Kao, J. C., Fan, J. M., Stavisky, S. D., Ryu, S. I., & Shenoy, K. V. (2014). Performance sustaining intracortical neural prostheses. *Journal of Neural Engineering, 11*(6), 066003.

Ontology. (2017). In *Wikipedia: The Free Encyclopedia*. Retrieved from https://en.wikipedia.org/wiki/Ontology_(information_science)

Ospina-Tascón, G. A., Büchele, G. L., & Vincent, J.-L. (2008). Multicenter, randomized, controlled trials evaluating mortality in intensive care: doomed to fail? *Critical Care Medicine, 36*(4), 1311–1322.

Park, C., Ahn, J., Kim, H., & Park, S. (2014). Integrative gene network construction to analyze cancer recurrence using semi-supervised learning. *PLOS ONE, 9*(1), e86309. doi:10.1371/journal.pone.0086309

Pathak, P., Patel, P., Panchal, V., Soni, S., Dani, K., Choudhary, N., & Patel, A. (2015). *ezDI: A supervised NLP system for clinical narrative analysis* (pp. 412–416). Proceedings of the 9th International Workshop on Semantic Evaluation (SemEval 2015), Denver, Colorado.

Paxton, C., Niculescu-Mizil, A., & Saria, S. (2013). Developing predictive models using electronic medical records: Challenges and pitfalls. *AMIA Annual Symposium Proceedings, 2013*, 1109–1115.

Pharoah, P. D. P., Antoniou, A., Bobrow, M., Zimmern, R. L., Easton, D. F., & Ponder, B. A. J. (2002). Polygenic susceptibility to breast cancer and implications for prevention. *Nature Genetics, 31*(1), 33–36.

Ramli, R., Arof, H., Ibrahim, F., Mokhtar, N., & Idris, M. Y. I. (2015). Using finite state machine and a hybrid of EEG signal and EOG artifacts for an asynchronous wheelchair navigation. *Expert Systems With Applications, 42*(5), 2451–2463. doi:10.1016/j.eswa.2014.10.052

Rina Dechter, I. M., & Judea Pearl. (1991). Temporal constraint networks. *Artificial Intelligence, 49*, 35.

Roza, T., Hakim, L., van Poppel, H., & Joniau, S. (2013). Bone-targeted therapies for elderly patients with renal cell carcinoma: Current and future directions. *Drugs Aging, 30*(11), 877–886. doi:10.1007/s40266-013-0117-5

Rubbo, B., Fitzpatrick, N. K., Denaxas, S., Daskalopoulou, M., Yu, N., Patel, R. S., & Hemingway, H. (2015). Use of electronic health records to ascertain, validate and phenotype acute myocardial infarction: A systematic review and recommendations. *International Journal of Cardiology, 187*, 705–711. doi:10.1016/j.ijcard.2015.03.075

Rudary, M., Singh, S., & Pollack, M. E. (2004). *Adaptive cognitive orthotics: Combining reinforcement learning and constraint-based temporal reasoning*. Paper presented at the Proceedings of the Twenty-First International Conference on Machine learning, Banff, Alberta, Canada.

Ruiter, H. P., Liaschenko, J., & Angus, J. (2016). Problems with the electronic health record. *Nursing Philosophy, 17*(1), 49–58.

Sadek, I., Sidibé, D., & Meriaudeau, F. (2015). *Automatic discrimination of color retinal images using the bag of words approach*. Paper presented at Medical Imaging 2015: Computer-Aided Diagnosis. doi:10.1117/12.2075824

Santhanam, G., Ryu, S. I., Yu, B. M., Afshar, A., & Shenoy, K. V. (2006). A high-performance brain-computer interface. *Nature, 442*(7099), 195–198. doi:10.1038/nature04968

Savova, G. K., Masanz, J. J., Ogren, P. V., Zheng, J., Sohn, S., Kipper-Schuler, K. C., & Chute, C. G. (2010). Mayo clinical Text Analysis and Knowledge Extraction System (cTAKES): Architecture, component evaluation and applications. *Journal of the American Medical Informatics Association, 17*, 507–513. doi:10.1136/jamia.2009.001560

Schulam, P., Wigley, F., & Saria, S. (2015). *Clustering longitudinal clinical marker trajectories from electronic health data: Applications to phenotyping and endotype discovery* (pp. 2956–2964). Paper presented at the Proceedings of the 29th AAAI Conference on Artificial Intelligence. Retrieved from https://www.aaai.org/ocs/index.php/AAAI/AAAI15/paper/view/10015/9966

Schwartz, A. B., Cui, X. T., Weber, D. J., & Moran, D. W. (2006). Brain-controlled interfaces: Movement restoration with neural prosthetics. *Neuron, 52*(1), 205–220. doi:10.1016/j.neuron.2006.09.019

Serruya, M. D., Hatsopoulos, N. G., Paninski, L., Fellows, M. R., & Donoghue, J. P. (2002). Instant neural control of a movement signal. *Nature, 416*(6877), 141–142. doi:10.1038/416141a

Shiraishi, J., Li, Q., Appelbaum, D., & Doi, K. (2011). Computer-aided diagnosis and artificial intelligence in clinical imaging. *Seminars in Nuclear Medicine, 41*(6), 449–462. doi:10.1053/j.semnuclmed.2011.06.004

Sidney, S., Rosamond, W., Howard, V., & Luepker, R. (2013). Heart disease and stroke statistics—2013 update. *Circulation, 127*(1), 4. doi:10.1161/CIRCULATIONAHA.112.155911

Siegel, R. L., Miller, K. D., & Jemal, A. (2015). Cancer statistics, 2015. *CA: A Cancer Journal for Clinicians, 65*(1), 5–29. doi:10.3322/caac.21254

Siontis, G. C. M. (2011). Predicting death. *Archives of Internal Medicine, 171*(19), 1721. doi:10.1001/archinternmed.2011.334

Srinivasan, L., Eden, U. T., Mitter, S. K., & Brown, E. N. (2007). General-purpose filter design for neural prosthetic devices. *Journal of Neurophysiology, 98*(4), 2456–2475. doi:10.1152/jn.01118.2006

Sutton, R. S., & Barto, A. G. (1998). *Reinforcement learning: An introduction* (Vol. 1). Cambridge, MA: MIT Press.

Suzuki, K. (2012). Pixel-based machine learning in medical imaging. *Journal of Biomedical Imaging, 2012*, 1–18. doi:10.1155/2012/792079

Syeda-Mahmood, T., Walach, E., Beymer, D., Gilboa-Solomon, F., Moradi, M., Kisilev, P., . . . Hashoul, S. (2016). *Medical sieve: A cognitive assistant for radiologists and cardiologists.* Paper presented at Medical Imaging 2016: Computer-Aided Diagnosis. doi:10.1117/12.2217382

Tao, C., Wei, W., Savova, G., & Chute, C. (2010). *A semantic web ontology for temporal relation inferencing in clinical narratives.* Paper presented at the Proceedings of the American Medical Informatics Association (AMIA) 2010 Annual Symposium, Washington, DC.

Taylor, D. M., Tillery, S. I. H., & Schwartz, A. B. (2002). Direct cortical control of 3D neuroprosthetic devices. *Science, 296*(5574), 1829–1832. doi:10.1126/science.1070291

Tissot, H., dos Santos, C. F. H., Gorrell, G., Roberts, A., Derczynski, L., & Del Fabro, M. D. (2015). *UFPRSheffield: Contrasting rule-based and support vector machine approaches to time expression identification in clinical TempEval* (p. 835). Proceedings of the 9th International Workshop on Semantic Evaluation (SemEval 2015), Denver, Colorado.

University of Alberta. (2007, 17 March). Why computers frustrate older adults. *ScienceDaily*. Retrieved from https://www.sciencedaily.com/releases/2007/03/070316140944.htm

Velasquez, A., Ghassemi, M., & Szolovits, P. (2014). Long-term outcomes of minor troponin elevations in the intensive care unit. *Anaesthesia and Intensive Care, 42*, 356–364.

Velliste, M., Perel, S., Spalding, M. C., Whitford, A. S., & Schwartz, A. B. (2008). Cortical control of a prosthetic arm for self-feeding. *Nature, 453*(7198), 1098–1101. doi:10.1038/nature06996

Venhuizen, F. G., van Ginneken, B., Bloemen, B., van Grinsven, M. J. J. P., Philipsen, R., Hoyng, C., . . . Sánchez, C. I. (2015). *Automated age-related macular degeneration classification in OCT using unsupervised feature learning.* Paper presented at Medical Imaging 2015: Computer-Aided Diagnosis. doi:10.1117/12.2081521

Vidaurre, C., Schlogl, A., Cabeza, R., Scherer, R., & Pfurtscheller, G. (2007). Study of on-line adaptive discriminant analysis for EEG-based brain computer interfaces. *IEEE Transactions on Biomedical Engineering, 54*(3), 550–556. doi:10.1109/TBME.2006.888836

Welch, J., Moon, J., & McCombie, S. (2012). Early detection of the deteriorating patient: The case for a multi-parameter patient-worn monitor. *Biomedical Instrumentation & Technology, 46*(s2), 57–64. doi:10.2345/0899-8205-46.s2.57

Wessberg, J., & Nicolelis, M. A. L. (2004). Optimizing a linear algorithm for real-time robotic control using chronic cortical ensemble recordings in monkeys. *Journal of Cognitive Neuroscience, 16*(6), 1022–1035. doi:10.1162/0898929041502652

Workman, T. E., & Stoddart, J. M. (2012). Rethinking information delivery: Using a natural language processing application for point-of-care data discovery [Evaluation Studies Research Support, N.I.H., Extramural]. *Journal of the Medical Library Association, 100*(2), 113–120. doi:10.3163/1536-5050.100.2.009

Xu, X., Zhang, Y., Zou, L., Wang, M., & Li, A. (2012). *A gene signature for breast cancer prognosis using support vector machine.* Paper presented at the 5th International Conference on Biomedical Engineering and Informatics (BMEI), Chongqing, China.

13

Advances in Health Education Technology

Ashley Reynolds, Thomas F. Osborne, John Waggoner, Renee Melton, Ramin Motarjemi, Jürgen P. Schulze, and Diane Chau

The passing of knowledge from one to another is a practice as old as time. For millennia, educated scholars have communicated their knowledge to students. While this transmission of information is not new, the mechanisms by which this information is transferred have changed drastically. Rapid advances in immersive technologies like virtual reality (VR), or augmented reality (AR), are beginning to transform experiential learning in ways that allow for failure without risking patient safety. From online digital classrooms to mobile applications and smartphones, technology is changing how health education is being delivered to both clinical professionals and patients.

In the context of health education, the process of learning involves practice, observation, modeling, peer support, and didactic experiences. One of the cornerstones of clinical professional education is experiential learning through practical experience. For example, medical, nursing, pharmacy, and dietary professions each require clinical practice as part of their curricula. Learning through practice allows students to attempt tasks to refine their execution, solidify comprehension, and reduce fear when attempting newly acquired or unfamiliar skills. However, this model can pose some risk for patients when applied in a clinical setting. Attempting complex procedures on living patients can be daunting, with the margin of error small. Traditionally, health education programs have focused on classroom, patient teaching, and clinical experiences to educate professionals and patients alike.

Patients also learn through practice. For example, self-care activities such as self-catheterization, insulin injection, or ostomy care are often foreign and uncomfortable, yet these skills are necessary to maintain health or manage chronic illnesses. Health education technologies represent opportunities to teach these skills in a risk-free environment, thereby reducing or eliminating patient fears when learning unfamiliar tasks.

Health education technology has advanced from basic informational websites to fully immersive interactive systems which can now provide dynamic learning experiences, social interactivity, and realistic, automated scenarios that mimic clinical events with live patients. These improvements can be attributed to increased processing power of computing tools, proliferation of high-speed Internet connectivity, and innovative new tools such as VR devices. According to Thibault (2015), when technology is used correctly in health education, it facilitates learning while freeing the learner to engage in teamwork and patient-care skill mastery. In this chapter, we explore why technology is needed in health education, review examples of different types of technology in use today, and examine how these tools may be used to support training of clinical professionals as well as educating patients.

WHY IS HEALTH TECHNOLOGY NEEDED?

There are many factors influencing the need for technology-supported education. For example, many clinical professions like pharmacy (Patry & Eiland, 2007), nursing (American Association of Colleges of Nursing, 2015), and medicine and allied health (Moskowitz, 2007) are suffering from clinical faculty shortages, making it difficult to enroll students in these programs. While the reasons for these shortages are varied, they are not the focus of this chapter. Nevertheless, these shortages have motivated educational institutions to find ways to deliver clinical professional education in the most efficient way possible.

Furthermore, the clinical workforce is changing. Younger professionals seeking education and entering the workforce have grown up with technology at the center of their lives. These generational differences mean that digital native learners place a higher emphasis on technology, and are more comfortable using it (Reynolds, 2013; Satterfield, 2015). They expect cutting-edge educational programs to include innovative technologies.

The environment in health care has also become increasingly technical. Medical devices, computerized charting, at-home monitoring, and other tools are changing how professionals deliver care to patients. Clinical professionals entering the workforce need to be prepared to operate, understand, and interact with highly complex digital systems in order to provide care. As more care is being shifted outside of the hospital setting, technology is needed to support patient self-monitoring and management. In-hospital educational systems begin teaching patients from the moment they are admitted and, in some instances, can include ongoing monitoring and technology-mediated educational support once discharged. For example, transitional care programs that focus on preventing readmissions postdischarge often include self-monitoring technologies and educational tools using wearable or connected devices, videoconferencing, and tablet computers.

EXAMPLES OF TECHNOLOGY IN HEALTH EDUCATION

Learning Management Systems

The ability to efficiently share information is a critical component to the prosperity of any health care organization. An important component to this success is having an effective infrastructure for learning to facilitate patient empowerment, provider competence, and career development. Furthermore, there are also mandated requirements for the appropriate delivery, documentation, and tracking of specific types of educational material ranging from professional medical licensing to government-compliance training and patient-informed consent. Managing these course records can be a significant administrative burden and risk, if done manually. Therefore, efficient scalable electronic solutions for education management have become a key strategic initiative for numerous health care organizations. More specifically, e-learning provides opportunities uniquely suited to address the concerns of geriatrics educators, such as the trend to move teaching venues to decentralized community settings, competency-based education requirements, and the need to train at a time when geriatric health care professionals have limited time available to share knowledge (Ruiz, Teasdale, Hajjar, Shaughnessy, & Mintzer, 2007).

Many people in health care perceive e-learning as a complement to traditional forms of medical education (Cook et al., 2008; Ruiz, Mintzer, & Leipzig, 2006). However, research suggests that the effectiveness of computer-based teaching is at least equivalent to lecture-based medical education (Davis et al., 2007). Furthermore, recent research suggests that an electronic-based informed consent may actually improve patient understanding compared to paper-based consent processes (Rothwell et al., 2014).

There are a variety of electronic solutions available to meet an organization's educational needs. Some institutions have decided to utilize a mix of existing applications typically intended for other purposes, such as email, desktop folders, online meeting tools, and spreadsheet software. However, the lack of interoperability and automation with this type of strategy results in the need for dedicated resources to manually upload and track information, which quickly becomes an unmanageable burden for even small organizations. As a result, an entire industry of dedicated software applications has emerged for e-learning. One of the most common tools used in e-learning today is the learning management system (LMS; García-Peñalvo & Alier Forment, 2014).

What Is an LMS?

An LMS is a centralized software infrastructure that delivers and manages training and learning modules. Part of this management involves handling the registration, scheduling, and tracking of electronic classes in an automated or semiautomated way. With an LMS, course test questions can be integrated into modules and automatically documented to meet the continuing education requirements of accreditation boards. Most LMSs also have an analytics component that can provide insight into the performance of an individual, group, or even the course itself (Abdullateef, Elias, Mohamed, Zaidan, & Zaidan, 2016).

Advantages of an LMS

The automated features of an LMS provide scalable efficiencies and advantages compared to traditional educational management workflows. This is relevant for any industry, but is particularly significant in health care owing to the high volume of training and compliance requirements. The ability to efficiently track governmentally mandated health care–compliance requirements is an important feature of an LMS. In a typical LMS, courses may be available for self-registration or may be prescheduled for individual, group, or subgroup delivery. Alert thresholds can be adjusted to remind learners or managers about overdue modules, and certificates can be automatically issued after the satisfactory completion of training. Importantly, the on-demand availability and self-guided services of the web-based courses made available through an LMS add convenience to the busy schedules of medical professionals. Most LMSs provide learners and administrators with custom dashboards that arrange relevant content by requirements, topics, or subjects. Some dashboards may also have integrated calendars and timelines to further enhance the user experience. Ideally, entering a new hire's information into the system will automatically trigger a set of training modules to be delivered to an individual that is specific to the individual's role within the company. Web-based learning has been shown to be an effective method of training medical professionals regardless of their age, education, or prior computer experience; an LMS provides the infrastructure for efficient delivery of e-learning to an entire organization (Atreja et al., 2008; Ellis, 2009).

Available LMS Options

Although the LMS market is relatively new, there are currently hundreds of LMSs available to choose from. Deciding on the most appropriate and cost-effective solution for the specific needs of a health care organization depends on understanding the institutional goals, available resources, and target audience(s). In general, user experience and reliability of a product are typically among the most important factors (Zaharias & Pappas, 2016). The following are additional options to consider from the perspectives of several different key stakeholders.

From a learner's perspective, the ability to provide feedback about a course or software has been correlated with improved outcomes in health education (Cook, Levinson, et al., 2010). There are some LMSs that have more advanced collaborative functionalities that provide platforms for online interaction with course creators, coaches, and learners. Regardless of the content and delivery method, an optional single-sign-on (SSO) feature that integrates with existing security credentials eliminates the need for additional login prompts, or the need for an employee to remember a different set of passwords and user names. Being able to access content on mobile devices is an additional convenience for learners, but not currently available with many LMSs (Dahlstrom, Brooks, & Bichsel, 2014).

It is important to find an LMS solution that matches the needs and technical abilities of the expected course creators at an institution. Many traditional LMSs require educational material to be incorporated from different software, such as videos or slide presentations. It is, therefore, critical to confirm that the components to be utilized are compatible and that the process of creating a course is streamlined to promote efficiency and user adoption. However, there is a growing trend for systems to provide authoring tools and templates that allow the creation and modification of content completely within the same LMS solution. Some LMS vendors also have premade content in their database that may be available to satisfy specific requirements. The ability to integrate course material from third-party courseware is also an important factor that can significantly decrease the burden of creating specific, mandated courses.

For marketing and sales, the ability to integrate an LMS within a corporate website may be particularly important if there is a desire to connect with patients and nonemployee partners. Furthermore, making valuable educational content available on an external website can promote an organization's brand equity, or be combined with an e-commerce module to create an additional revenue stream. The additional web traffic to the LMS component of a corporate website is also expected to increase the search engine optimization (SEO) ranking of that website. However, the ability to integrate with an external website platform is not available with many LMSs. Branding the LMS vendor solution to appear as an integrated part of the electronic health care platform is an additional optional feature with variable penetrance in the LMS market.

The majority of the previously mentioned features are important for consideration by technical and support staff who are typically also charged with the task of implementation, integration, configuration, and disaster recovery planning of an LMS, as well as initial training of the end users (Ellis & Calvo, 2007). The ability to effectively establish and manage the user permissions and security of the LMS are also important technical factors.

Additional technical considerations include the foundational infrastructure of the solution. For example, LMSs may be installed on in-house servers (on premises), or may be accessible through remote vendor servers as a Cloud "Software as a Service" (SAAS) solution. In general, an SAAS solution is a less expensive option, in part because implementation, maintenance, and information technology (IT) support are typically provided externally by the vendor. However, an on-premises LMS is generally more customizable, and may, therefore, be easier to integrate with other locally hosted software products. A third-party maintenance model takes elements of both options: the software is installed on-premises but the maintenance and upgrades are managed by the LMS vendor (Ellis, 2009).

If there is a desire to incorporate video content into educational courses, there are additional technical considerations. Video can be obtained from a variety of sources ranging from smartphones, online meeting tools, and dedicated software. Specific software can be used to record computer screens with audio narration (often referred to as *screencasts* or *video screen capture*). Screencasts can be an effective and efficient way to train employees on the use of specific desktop software, onboarding, and career development. However, regardless of the video solution utilized, it is important to ensure that the content can be efficiently managed and the specific video format can be integrated with the LMS vendor solution being utilized.

An LMS has the potential to efficiently deliver a variety of critical health care educational material to a wide range of consumers. Therefore, from a leadership and management perspective, it is critical to establish a centralized strategy and organized plan for success. The different needs and insights of individuals and departments must be fully understood to prevent the formation of a disconnected and fractured platform that is difficult to navigate and maintain. Dedicated requirement gathering will help to inform an organized project and governance plan to account for the specific perspectives of expected stakeholders such as clinical, legal, compliance, and human resource (HR) departments.

Augmented Reality and Virtual Reality

Virtual and augmented realities have moved from the gaming world into health and medical education. In VR, the user experiences a completely computer-simulated environment. Most video games utilize elements of VR technology. By contrast, AR allows users to interact live with technology-enhanced versions of reality, which have been married with digital media, imposing objects into the real world. Both can engage multiple senses and include sound, digital video, or graphics, as well as engaging the sense of touch through haptic response.

Experimentation with primitive versions of VR began in the first half of the 20th century through three-dimensional (3D) imagery and video, early flight simulators, and primitive headset displays. The term *virtual reality* was coined in the 1980s by researcher Jaron Lanier, who went on to develop early versions of VR head-mounted displays, goggles, and gloves, according to the Virtual Reality Society (2016). In addition, over the past 30 years, true AR has also made its way into mainstream culture, from virtual lines marking first downs during live NFL games, to interactive displays used by soldiers and astronauts.

User interaction with modern VR and AR occurs through a variety of modalities. VR products, having been in the marketplace for over 30 years, offer a wider variety of options. Head-mounted displays with 3D controllers, such as the Oculus Rift (2016) or the HTC Vive, or cell phone–based viewers, such as the Samsung Gear VR, are newer and provide a more immersive experience. Video gaming systems create virtual worlds through digital media, sound, and haptic feedback. Numerous products are scaled, or created for, smaller screens of smartphones and tablets for greater reach, access, and portability.

AR products for the consumer are relatively new to the marketplace. Products such as Microsoft HoloLens glasses (Microsoft Corporation, 2016) project holographic images, overlaying the real world, allowing users to interact with both at the same time. Also, in 2016, smartphones and tablets have joined the AR world. Pokémon GO, which became wildly popular in mid-2016, but not originally intended for this purpose, is an example of how AR could improve health, in this case, by increasing physical activity. Utilizing a mobile phone's global positioning system (GPS) and camera functionality, users of Pokémon GO must move about to capture and interact with digital creatures.

One area in which AR has great potential for broad commercial success is remote training on medical devices. For example, researchers at University of California, San Diego (UCSD), are studying innovative uses of VR (Oh et al., 2016). They have built a prototype of a remote training system for a wound care device, the WoundVac. The instructor uses a VR setup, in our case an HTC Vive system, to see what the student can see, who has a real WoundVac system they are learning how to use. To allow the instructor to help the student use the WoundVac, the student can see the instructor's hands, as well as 3D annotations, through a HoloLens. The two systems are connected over the regular Internet—no dedicated network connection is required. The system allows the training on complex medical devices much like when instructor and student are in the same location. This can allow experienced instructors to give one-on-one training to many more students than they could if they were to physically travel to each student's location. Figure 13.1 illustrates the concept of how the student can see the instructor's hands, as well as a virtual copy of the main WoundVac unit which the instructor moved to a new location to make room for connecting the vacuum hose to it.

Over the past few years, the uses of AR and VR have found success in health care applications, both in training health care professionals and imparting or improving patient skills. Through both media, patients and students alike can experience situations, providing for desensitization or practice with varying behaviors in a safe environment (García-Betances, Fico, Salvi, Ottaviano, & Arredondo, 2015).

Explosive growth is expected with AR taking a great role according to the Virtual Reality Society (2016). An international organization, the VR/AR Association, has been created "to foster collaboration between innovative companies and people in the virtual reality and augmented reality ecosystem that accelerates growth, fosters research and education, helps develop

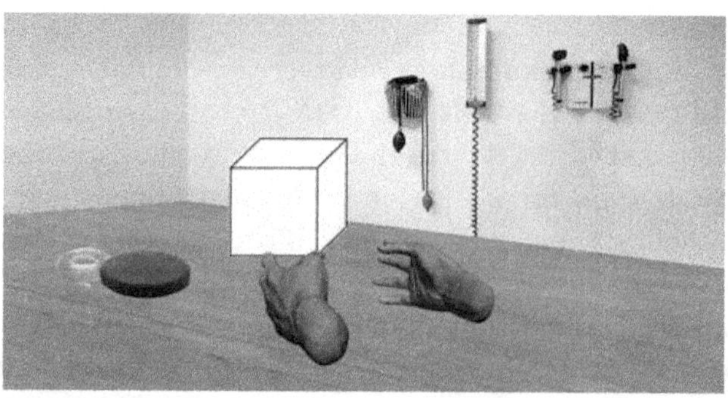

FIGURE 13.1 Wound vacuum (represented as white box) as seen by student, with instructor's virtual hand.

industry standards, connects member organizations and promotes the services of member companies" (VR/AR Association, 2016), including a committee wholly focused on digital health, medical education, health care, and education.

VR/AR in Health Professional Education

Medical applications allow for skill building in fields ranging from virtual surgery and dentistry training, to in-field assistance devices for phlebotomy, such as illuminating vein maps on skin surface. Ferguson, Davidson, Scott, Jackson, and Hickman (2015) examined the opportunities AR and VR bring to nursing education and training, such as virtual classrooms or video game training, and recommended these be integrated as teaching and learning strategies. Given the pervasiveness of smartphones, integration of VR/AR in provider training is almost a necessity to disseminate low-cost health care solutions (Ferguson et al., 2015; García-Betances et al., 2015). Mobility of phones allows the classroom to go with the student (or patient; McMahon, Cihak, Gibbons, Fussell, & Mathison, 2013).

In dietetics education, several VR simulation platforms are being utilized, which focus on skill building from nutrition evaluation, patient interactions (interviewing and counseling), to nutrition support. Not only do these methods exercise critical thinking skills and problem solving in the student, they also serve as evaluation of student progress and readiness (Camacho, 2014; Davis, 2015).

VR/AR in Patient Education

Patient care and treatment options in VR and AR are ubiquitous, with existing solutions aimed at improving, enhancing, or even replacing traditional therapies and text-heavy patient education. VR affords users the ability to develop and practice self-regulation skills necessary for success in managing health conditions, ultimately improving adherence, and provide ongoing support (Coons, Roehrig, & Spring, 2011). Examples are in ophthalmology using 3D digital education, mental health by promoting relaxation and meditation, and nutrition by promoting weight loss and healthy food choices. Recent data suggest that these tools are effective at improving patient behaviors. To illustrate, researchers found a VR-based weight loss intervention to be as effective in producing weight change as face-to-face intervention, and more effective in improving indicators of behavior change and self-efficacy (Behm-Morawitz, Lewallen, & Choi, 2016; Johnston, Massey, & DeVaneaux, 2012). In children, multiple health behavior changes were realized using virtual pets to increase physical activity and fruit and vegetable intake (Ahn, Johnsen, Moore, & Ball, 2016; Ahn, Johnsen, Robertson, & Basu, 2015).

An AR mobile intervention was developed by a Mexican research group to reduce sugar intake, and combat common challenges in understanding food labels for highly processed, sweetened beverages (Escárcega-Centeno, Hérnandez-Briones, Ochoa-Ortiz, & Gutiérrez-Gómez, 2015). Use of VR avatars showing weight gain related to soda consumption allowed users to experience effects virtually, positively altered user perception and soft drink consumption, and was more successful than traditional educational handouts (Ahn, 2016).

García-Betances, Jiménez-Mixco, Arredondo, and Cabrera-Umpiérrez (2014) recognized VR and AR therapies as game changers in the field of dementia. Several studies showed significant improvements in poststroke and Alzheimer's dementia patients (gait, balance, and motor function) with a variety of VR interventions, varying from custom design to commercially available, such as Wii-Fit, when compared to traditional therapies (Allain et al., 2014; Imam & Jarus, 2014; Luque-Moreno et al., 2015; Padala et al., 2012; Tsoupikova et al., 2015). Fully immersive 3D therapies hold advantages over 2D environments given the increased sensory resources required (S. M. Slobounov, Ray, Johnson, E. Slobounov, & Newell, 2015). Other medical interventions identified as successfully benefiting from VR/AR exposure include pain mitigation (Trost & Parsons, 2014), and teaching food allergy management to individuals with intellectual disabilities (McMahon et al., 2013).

While research supports the use of VR and AR in various settings, there are challenges. The upfront development costs can be high in custom implementations. Furthermore, there is concern that fully immersive technologies may deliver an overwhelming amount of information to the user, rendering them less effective. Finally, some individuals may be susceptible to cyber sickness, similar to motion sickness, and unable to benefit (Keshavarz, Riecke, Hettinger, & Campos, 2015).

The potential for AR to enhance geriatrics education is vast, given its ability to now create those complex interdisciplinary teams, the nursing home scenarios, the locked dementia units, the wound care complexities. If we applied AR over existing simulation, we have the potential to create the home safety environments that a geriatrician needs to perform functional assessments.

TECHNOLOGY IN GERIATRIC MEDICAL EDUCATION

Although technological advances continue to reshape global social, economic, and scientific landscapes, few technological solutions currently address the growing need for physicians serving in geriatric medicine in the United States. Recent proposals by Golden, Silverman, and Issenberg (2015) to increase geriatrician numbers suggested abbreviated specialized training programs similar to those of nurse practitioners, or offering financial incentives to attract more qualified residents to the field; however, these ideas require further expansion and refinement to clearly identify ways in which the stated goals could reasonably be achieved. One step in the right direction involves harnessing technology to fundamentally transform existing medical–educational paradigms, particularly for aspiring physicians seeking service in geriatric medicine.

The Institute of Medicine's *Retooling for an Aging America* (Institute of Medicine of the National Academies, 2007) addressed rising health care costs associated with aging populations and physician shortages, endorsing a philosophy of "retooling" collective approaches to devise innovative solutions and growth of the geriatric population's health care workforce. The institute's paper established guiding principles upon which current notions of educational reform and allocation of resources to implement novel educational technologies among allopathic and osteopathic medical training programs in the United States have been built. Drake's (2013) "Retrospective and Prospective Look at Medical Education," for example, reviewed ongoing changes in approaches to teaching the anatomical sciences in medical school today. His paper encouraged university administrators and program directors to embrace creativity and focus on devising curricula geared toward active learning and longitudinal approaches. To accomplish these objectives, we must carefully examine traditional undergraduate and graduate medical training programs, and seek ways to implement high-tech, self-paced, competency-based educational paradigms. Such shifts in medical education would also accelerate professional qualification and significantly reduce financial burdens for trainees, ultimately helping to incentivize and meet the rising demand for geriatricians.

SLOW TO CHANGE

While ostensibly, medical education is likely to benefit from the implementation of new technologies, medical organizations can be slow to embrace innovation, with hospital and university-based systems resisting the costs and institutional difficulties associated with implementing new technologies. Current models of undergraduate medical education remain largely based on 4-year models first developed at Johns Hopkins in the 1870s and championed by Abraham Flexner in 1910, as part of his landmark critique that spurred the first radical curricular reforms in the United States. As Ludmerer

(2010) pointed out in his "Understanding the Flexner Report," many of Flexner's reforms are still current today; however, Flexner would likely endorse efforts to reform his own system, so long as those reforms were in the best interests of the students, the medical profession, and the general public good.

Confronting an increasingly complex and rapidly expanding body of scientific discovery and peer-reviewed literature, medical schools and residency-training programs have begun to embrace certain types of technology to facilitate pedagogical, informational, clinical, and heuristic aspects of training; however, the overarching structure of medical education remains largely unchanged over the past 100 years. Moving to embrace and implement novel technologies could provide revolutionary changes required to provoke a 21st-century Flexnerian reform, and address critical shortages in primary and geriatric medicine faced today.

In addition to costs and administrative challenges associated with institutional reforms, the emphasis on standardization and accreditation processes, emergence of profitable tuition-payment schedules for universities and graduate-education funding, and difficulties replacing regimented time-based curricula also contribute to the hesitancy to broadly change medical education. The Carnegie Foundation's 2010 modernization of the Flexner Report, *Educating Physicians: A Call for Reform of Medical Schools and Residency Programs* (Cooke, Irby, & Obrien, 2010), made medical educational reform a hot topic once again within the academic literature. The authors of the Carnegie report called for changes along the lines of greater integration of academics with clinical experiences, individualization of the learning process, trainee commitment to excellence, and professional-identity development in medical educational systems. Although technology is mentioned as a way to help bridge the gap between academics and the clinic, technological innovation in today's medical training pipeline could help to accomplish each of these four objectives. Medical education offers an environment ripe for technological change, one in which innovational risks can be taken to improve and streamline training processes.

CURRENT TECHNOLOGY IN MEDICAL EDUCATION

Typical geriatricians spend 4 years completing an undergraduate degree, 4 years in medical school, 3 years in an internal or family medicine residency program, and 1 or 2 years in a geriatrics fellowship. Geriatric medicine physicians spend at least 12 years pursuing the necessary academic training to obtain board certification and eventually begin clinical practice. With respect to other phases of medical training, geriatrics fellowships around the country also do not frequently utilize simulation-based or other technological means to enhance educational outcomes, instead opting for additional patient-based contacts and logging hours on the inpatient wards or visiting numerous outpatient clinics. This approach is at odds with the many suggestions for technological reform in today's medical educational pipeline, as it focuses on chronological benchmarks rather than competency—or skills-based protocols for graduation. Geriatric training often requires hands-on training with cognitively impaired patients, their families, large interprofessional teams that are difficult to create through a simulation lab as the settings do not occur or mimic adult day health centers, skilled nursing homes, dementia locked wards where many geriatricians practice. The single manikin simulation does not present the functional limitation assessments most geriatricians need to perform in assessments of gait, truncal stability, and activities of daily living skills. The large interdisciplinary teams create challenges and training inefficiencies in geriatric training.

Taking a look at medical education today, some medical schools began experimenting with accelerated curricula for students entering primary care specialties. Medical education is considered a nonterminal degree, meaning a physician after graduation with an MD cannot practice medicine without added clinical internship or residency training. Thus, the basic 4 years of medical education within medical schools is termed *undergraduate medical education* (UME), whereas the added clinical internship, residencies, and fellowships are termed *graduate medical education* (GME). The vast majority of undergraduate medical programs still follow the traditional 2+2 methodology, spending 2 years learning preclinical basic sciences and 2 years in on-the-job training set in clinical environments, irrespective of students' chosen medical specialties. During the first 2 preclinical years, students generally experience traditional lectures, small group sessions, interactive laboratories, and regular multiple-choice examinations. While these methods help to build a foundation in basic clinical sciences for medical students, the rapid expansion of knowledge and widespread cross-disciplinary collaboration in science makes it difficult for educators to consistently keep content up to date and current within traditional curricula. As described earlier, however, this problem could be addressed by relying more heavily on LMS models, flipped classrooms that deliver lectures electronically and follow with interactive sessions, or other technological innovations that move away from the physical lecture hall. Many of the basic science lectures, such as physiology, can be adequately covered through online portals.

PRECLINICAL YEARS

Preclinical medical students utilize some technologies designed to improve pedagogical, informational, and heuristic aspects of their training; however, these technologies are largely limited to computer-based approaches and are not directed toward maximizing competency or the rapid production of highly capable physicians. As with general education in secondary and postsecondary universities, undergraduate and graduate medical programs typically employ basic computing and networking technologies to deliver curricular content. According to the Association of American Medical Colleges (AAMC) Institute for Improving Medical Education (2007), the most common uses of technology today in medical classrooms include computer-aided instruction (CAI), virtual patients, and human-patient simulation. As implied by the term, technology in the form of CAI among preclinical medical students is largely driven by the ubiquity of computers and mobile technology. From a pedagogical standpoint, medical school faculty can utilize CAI to improve delivery and augment their educational content. Assuming that all students own desktops, laptops, or mobile-computing systems, employment of e-learning and flipped classroom models are also becoming more common fixtures in medical education, although not across the full spectrum of accredited allopathic and osteopathic medical schools.

Medical schools now also heavily leverage mobile-computing platforms, such as tablets and smartphones, with some schools even providing new iPads or other mobile devices to students upon admission, with the devices often preloaded with software, textbooks, and other clinical tools to facilitate learning and collaboration. Such concepts build upon popular existing constructs of social media, such as Facebook, Twitter, and Skype, with students receiving push notifications or regularly interacting on a virtual basis with colleagues and staff via their mobile devices. From an informational standpoint, this basic technology also contributes to medical education as a means to organize and collect data, provide secure environments for student testing and evaluation, and create online student environments that enable surveys, personal data management, and data-sharing applications.

In terms of heuristic applications, technology is one of the biggest drivers for individual success in medical schools today. Also based on computing and online networks, students today have many opportunities to seek out information required during medical coursework beyond standard prescribed textbooks and primary resources. Wide online content now exists, aimed at distilling information down to the key topics that students must master for success in class and on national licensing examinations. Examples include online histology, anatomy, and pathology resources; free Youtube, Khan

Academy, Coursera, and other video content; paid packaged online lecture programs such as Osmosis, Pathoma, Online MedEd; online test question banks such as USMLE World, Kaplan, USMLE Rx; spaced-repetition electronic flashcard programs, such as Osmosis, Firecracker, or Anki; Wiki-style or GoogleDoc collaborative writing software; and picture- or story-based learning modules such as Sketchy Medical and Picmonic. These examples outline just a few of the resources available to today's preclinical medical student, with online subscription-based and free content expanding at a rapid pace. The widespread use of such services by students as they prepare for standardized examinations introduces new research questions, including the pitfalls and dangers associated with accuracy and reliability of material not officially sanctioned by accredited medical schools; the performance metrics of such students versus those who utilize only school-delivered content; and reassessment of financial burdens faced by students today.

CLINICAL YEARS, RESIDENCY, AND FELLOWSHIP

As medical students transition to their third and fourth years, the curriculum pivots and focuses on the acquisition of clinical skills to be learned on the job in hospital wards and outpatient clinics, under the supervision of resident and attending physicians. The UME curriculum in these clinical years does provide some geriatrics exposure, but this is not intensive in dedicated blocks of time, such as seen with pediatrics, obstetrics, or even neurology. Owing to traditional rotational requirements, faculty access, and resources, many medical schools simply sprinkle geriatrics content throughout the 4 years of medical school, instead of placing a core intensive block dedicated to geriatrics. While students may be tested on their abilities to clinically examine standardized patients during this time, the majority of clinical experience is built working with real patients and while rotating through the various hospital wards. Experiences during this phase of training are often highly variable from school to school, and even among trainees at the same school, depending on students' timing through various clinical blocks. Trainee evaluations are typically based on subjective evaluations by supervising physicians and objective scores on standardized shelf examinations in the various clinical sciences, offered by the National Board of Medical Examiners. Because much of the second half of medical school is spent directly engaged in patient care and participating in real clinical medical scenarios, the educational emphasis also typically shifts from book-based knowledge to a more practical study of clinical techniques, reasoning, and management skills. As such, the use of technology during this time of training still includes many of the heuristic examples for personal study outside of working hours; however, technological advancements applicable to these clinical years are mostly evident in the transition to simulation-based training.

Simulation-based training is one aspect of medical education that has been around for a while. However, from the early days of cardiopulmonary resuscitation (CPR) training on unrealistic plastic manikins of decades ago, modern simulation-based training has become much more sophisticated, with lifelike robots and models that mimic the behavior of real patients. As Motola, Devine, Hyun, Sullivan, and Issenberg described (2013), older simulation models were improved by emulating various other industries with rich histories of simulation training, including aviation, military, and space organizations, which continue to advance us toward new frontiers for medical education. As the AAMC defined it in 2007, the purpose of various simulation models in medical education is to "simulate patient care environments for instructional or assessment purposes" and to "simulate specific procedural tasks."

Given increased demands placed on today's medical trainees at all levels, and the greater emphasis placed on safety protocols and team-based medicine, simulation-based training serves as an efficient means to practice in realistic scenarios, yet without the risks of practicing techniques on live patients. As such, simulation-based training serves as the mainstay for clinical years and postgraduate training, demonstrating one critical area in which technology provides a means to demonstrate clinical competency and reinforce institutional protocols. Patient-simulation drills also serve to build teamwork and efficiency among staff members, prepare trainees for challenging clinical encounters, and improve patient safety. As Motola et al. describe (2013), significant efforts among medical educational researchers are currently directed toward evaluating ways in which simulation-based training can be more effectively integrated into modern training programs, and how more realistic and powerful simulation models can be developed: These efforts are likely to move from manikin-based and physical simulation toward AR and VR models, as computing and graphics-processing technologies advance.

CONCLUSION

Technological advances are dramatically changing medical education and real clinical medicine to involve mobile applications that can perform a wide range of diagnostic and clinical tests, information highly valuable to medical students and residents working in the hospital. For example, students, nurses, and other clinical staff can now perform funduscopic exams, collect temperature and pulse-oximetry data, and gauge neurological tremors and heart rates using the powerful computing technology and application-based flexibility of mobile smartphones. Smartphone applications and enhanced camera adapters allow even lay people to take funduscopic images as these products can be searched and purchased direct to consumer on the Internet. Physicians and pharmacists also have ready volumes of reference material and pharmaceutical dosing calculators at their fingertips. The wide array of mobile-platform applications that can aid in clinical examination, diagnosis, and treatment will continue to expand, as user feedback and innovations in engineering drive future advances in technology. Applications, phone-embedded sensor technology, and the ease of creating new applications and mobile sites creates a creative environment wherein new medical direct-to-consumer grade products and tools are created daily without validation or testing.

It is incumbent upon practitioners to stay current with new technologies, especially as they are utilized by their patient populations. These promising new tools offer new ways for both practitioners and patients, especially when used to augment traditional teaching methods, while enhancing learning, safety, and comprehension. However, more research is needed in order to identify which tools are most effective as educational instruments for various populations. Therefore, new research should focus on segmenting learning groups to ascertain which methods may produce the best outcomes.

Health technology is constantly advancing and health care practitioners must be ready to adapt as new tools are created. We must ensure our professions are well represented during the development of these tools and utilize them throughout our education. From emerging artificial intelligence technologies such as cognitive computing and "smart" manikins, to VR and AR, clinical representation is vital to ensure that these tools meet the needs of both practitioners and patients.

REFERENCES

AAMC Institute for Improving Medical Education. (2007). Effective use of educational technology in medical education: Colloquium on educational technology: Recommendations and guidelines for medical educators. Retrieved from https://members.aamc.org/eweb/upload/Effective%20Use%20of%20Educational.pdf

Abdullateef, B. N., Elias, N. F., Mohamed, H., Zaidan, A. A., & Zaidan, B. B. (2016). An evaluation and selection problems of OSS-LMS packages. *SpringerPlus, 5*(1), 1

Ahn, S. J. (2016). Virtual exemplars in health promotion campaigns: Heightened perceived risk and involvement to reduce soft drink consumption in young adults. *Journal of Media Psychology*, 1–13. doi:10.1027/1864-1105/a000184

Ahn, S. J., Johnsen, K. J., Moore, J. N., & Ball, C. (2016). Using virtual pets to increase fruit and vegetable consumption in children: A technology-assisted social cognitive theory approach. *Cyberpsychology, Behavior and Social Networking, 19*(2), 86–92.

Ahn, S. J., Johnsen, K. J., Robertson, T., & Basu, A. (2015). Using virtual pets to promote physical activity in children: An application of the youth physical activity promotion model. *Journal of Health Communication, 20*(7), 807–815.

Allain, P., Foloppe, D. A., Besnard, J., Yamaguchi, T., Etcharry-Bouyx, F., Le Gall, D., & Richard, P. (2014). Detecting everyday action deficits in Alzheimer's disease using a nonimmersive virtual reality kitchen. *Journal of the International Neuropsychology Society, 20*, 468–477.

American Association of Colleges of Nursing. (2015). Nursing faculty shortage. Retrieved from http://www.aacn.nche.edu/media-relations/FacultyShortageFS.pdf

Atreja, A., Mehta, N. B., Jain, A. K., Harris, C. M., Ishwaran, H., Avital, M., & Fishleder, A. J. (2008). Satisfaction with web-based training in an integrated healthcare delivery network: Do age, education, computer skills and attitudes matter? *BMC Medical Education, 8*(1), 1.

Behm-Morawitz, E., Lewallen, J., & Choi, G. (2016). A second chance at health: How a 3D virtual world can improve health self-efficacy for weight loss management among adults. *Cyberpsychology, Behavior, and Social Networking, 19*(2), 74–79.

Camacho, S. (2014). Augmented reality and simulation in dietetics education. *Journal of Nutrition Education and Behavior, 46*(4S), S127.

Cook, D. A., Levinson, A. J., Garside, S., Dupras, D. M., Erwin, P. J., & Montori, V. M. (2008). Internet-based learning in the health professions: A meta-analysis. *Journal of the American Medical Association, 300*(10), 1181–1196.

Cook, D. A., Levinson, A. J., Garside, S., Dupras, D. M., Erwin, P. J., & Montori, V. M. (2010). Instructional design variations in internet-based learning for health professions education: A systematic review and meta-analysis. *Academic Medicine, 85*(5), 909–922.

Cooke, M., Irby, D. M., & Obrien, B. C. (2010). *Educating physicians: A call for reform of medical school and residency*. The Carnegie Foundation for the Advancement of Teaching. Stanford, CA: Josey-Bass.

Coons, M. J., Roehrig, M., & Spring, B. (2011). The potential of virtual reality technologies to improve adherence to weight loss behaviors. *Journal of Diabetes Science and Technology, 5*(2), 340–344.

Dahlstrom, E., Brooks, D. C., & Bichsel, J. (2014). *The current ecosystem of learning management systems in higher education: Student, faculty, and IT perspectives*. Research report. Louisville, CO: ECAR.

Davis, A. (2015). Virtual reality simulation: An innovative teaching tool for dietetics experiential education. *The Open Nutrition Journal, 9*(Suppl. 1-M8), 65–75.

Davis, J., Chryssafidou, E., Zamora, J., Davies, D., Khan, K., & Coomarasamy, A. (2007). Computer-based teaching is as good as face to face lecture-based teaching of evidence based medicine: A randomised controlled trial. *BMC Medical Education, 7*(1), 1.

Drake, R. L. (2013). A retrospective and prospective look at medical education in the United States: Trends shaping anatomical sciences education. *Journal of Anatomy, 224*, 256–260. doi:10.1111/joa.12054

Ellis, R. (2009). Field guide to learning management systems. *ASTD Learning Circuits*. Retrieved from http://cgit.nutn.edu.tw:8080/cgit/PaperDL/hclin_091027163029.PDF

Ellis, R., & Calvo, R. A. (2007). Minimum indicators to quality assure blended learning supported by learning management systems. *Journal of Educational Technology and Society, 10*(2), 60–70.

Escárcega-Centeno, D., Hérnandez-Briones, A., Ochoa-Ortiz, E., & Gutiérrez-Gómez, Y. (2015). Augmented-sugar intake: A mobile application to teach population about sugar sweetened beverages. *Procedia Computer Science, 75*, 275–280.

Ferguson, C., Davidson, P. M., Scott, P. J., Jackson, D., & Hickman, L. D. (2015). Augmented reality, virtual reality and gaming: An integral part of nursing. *Contemporary Nurse, 51*(1), 1–4.

Flexner, A. (1910). *Medical education in the United States and Canada: A report to the Carnegie Foundation for the Advancement of Teaching*. Retrieved from http://archive.carnegiefoundation.org/pdfs/elibrary/Carnegie_Flexner_Report.pdf

García-Betances, R. I., Fico, G., Salvi, D., Ottaviano, M., & Arredondo, M. T. (2015). On the convergence of affective and persuasive technologies in computer-mediated health-care systems. *Human Technology, 11*(1), 71–93.

García-Betances, R. I., Jiménez-Mixco, V., Arredondo, M. T., & Cabrera-Umpiérrez, M. F. (2014). Using virtual reality for cognitive training of the elderly. *American Journal of Alzheimer's Disease and Other Dementias, 30*(1), 49–54.

García-Peñalvo, F. J., & Alier Forment, M. (2014). Learning management system: Evolving from silos to structures. *Interactive Learning Environments, 22*(2), 143–145.

Golden, A. G., Silverman, M. A., & Issenberg, S. B. (2015). Addressing the shortage of geriatricians: What medical educators can learn from the nurse practitioner training model. *Academic Medicine, 90*(9), 1236–1240. doi:10.1097/ACM.0000000000000822

Imam, B., & Jarus, T. (2014). Virtual reality rehabilitation from social cognitive and motor learning theoretical perspectives in stroke population. *Rehabilitation Research and Practice, 2014*, 1–11. doi:10.1155/2014/594540

Institute of Medicine of the National Academies. (2007). Retooling for an aging America: Building the health care workforce. Retrieved from http://www.nap.edu/catalog/12089.html

Johnston, J. D., Massey, M. P., & DeVaneaux, C. A. (2012). Innovation in weight loss programs: A 2-dimensional virtual-world approach. *Journal of Medical Internet Research, 14*(5), 186–195.

Keshavarz, B., Riecke, B. E., Hettinger, L. J., & Campos, J. L. (2015). Vection and visually induced motion sickness: How are they related? *Frontiers in Psychology, 20*(6), 472.

Ludmerer, K. M. (2010). Commentary: Understanding the Flexner report. *Academic Medicine, 85*, 193–196. doi:10.1097/ACM.0b013e3181c8f1e7

Luque-Moreno, C., Ferragut-Garcías, A., Rodríguez-Blanco, C., Heredia-Rizo, A. M., Oliva-Pascual-Vaca, J., Kiper, P., & Oliva-Pascual-Vaca, Á. (2015). A decade of progress using virtual reality for poststroke lower extremity rehabilitation: Systematic review of the intervention methods. *BioMed Research International*, 1–7. doi:10.1155/2015/342529

McMahon, D. D., Cihak, D. F., Gibbons, M. M., Fussell, L., & Mathison, S. (2013). Using a mobile app to teach individuals with intellectual disabilities to identify potential food allergens. *Journal of Special Education Technology, 28*(3), 21–32.

Microsoft Corporation. (2016). Microsoft HoloLens. Retrieved from https://www.microsoft.com/microsoft-hololens/en-us

Moskowitz, M. C. (2007). Academic health center CEOs say faculty shortages major problem. Retrieved from http://www.aahcdc.org/Portals/41/Series/Issue-Briefs/Faculty_Shortages_Major_Problem.pdf

Motola, I., Devine, L. A., Hyun, S. C., Sullivan, J. E., & Issenberg, B. (2013). Simulation in healthcare education: A best evidence practical guide. *Medical Teacher, 35*, e1511–e1530. Retrieved from http://www.tandfonline.com/doi/full/10.3109/0142159X.2013.818632

Oculus, V. R. (2016). Virtual reality. Retrieved from https://www3.oculus.com/en-us/rift

Oh, Y., Ouyang, A., Chockalingam, N., Chau, D., Broder, K., & Schulze, J. (2016). *A mixed reality medical device remote training tool for a WoundVAC* (Unpublished manuscript). La Jolla: University of California San Diego.

Padala, K. P., Padala, P. R., Malloy, T. R., Geske, J. A., Dubbert, P. M., Dennis, R. A., . . . Sullivan, D. H. (2012). Wii-Fit for improving gait and balance in an assisted living facility: A pilot study. *Journal of Aging Research, 2012*, 1–6. doi:10.1155/2012/597573

Patry, R., & Eiland, L. (2007). Addressing the shortage of pharmacy faculty and clinicians: The impact of demographic changes. *American Journal of Health-System Pharmacy, 64*(7), 773–775.

Reynolds, A. (2013). *Age-related differences in self-efficacy and the use of e-health supports for exercise behavior in adults* (doctoral dissertation). Retrieved from http://ufdcimages.uflib.ufl.edu/UF/E0/04/54/17/00001/REYNOLDS_A.pdf

Rothwell, E., Wong, B., Rose, N. C., Anderson, R., Fedor, B., Stark, L. A., & Botkin, J. R. (2014). A randomized controlled trial of an electronic informed consent process. *Journal of Empirical Research on Human Research Ethics, 9*(5), 1–7.

Ruiz, J. G., Mintzer, M. J., & Leipzig, R. M. (2006). The impact of e-learning in medical education. *Academic Medicine, 81*(3), 207–212.

Ruiz, J. G., Teasdale, T. A., Hajjar, I., Shaughnessy, M., & Mintzer, M. J. (2007). The consortium of e-learning in geriatrics instruction. *Journal of the American Geriatrics Society, 55*(3), 458–463.

Satterfield, H. (2015). Technology use in health education: A review and future implications. *Online Journal of Distance Education and e-Learning, 3*(2), 87–96.

Slobounov, S. M., Ray W., Johnson, B., Slobounov, E., & Newell, K. M. (2015). Modulation of cortical activity in 2D versus 3D virtual reality environments: An EEG study. *International Journal of Psychophysiology, 95*(3), 254–260.

Thibault, G. (2015). Technology in health professions education: 2015 annual report. Retrieved from http://macyfoundation.org/publications/publication/2015-annual-report-technology-in-health-professions-education

Trost, Z., & Parsons, T. D. (2014). Beyond distraction: Virtual reality graded exposure therapy as a treatment for pain-related fear and disability in chronic pain. *Journal of Applied Biobehavioral Research, 19*(2), 106–126.

Tsoupikova, D., Stoykov, N. S., Corrigan, M., Thielbar, K., Vick, R., Li, Y., . . . Kamper, D. (2015). Virtual immersion for post-stroke hand rehabilitation therapy. *Annals of Biomedical Engineering, 43*(2), 467–477.

Virtual Reality/Augmented Reality Association. (2016). Mission statement. Retrieved from http://www.thevrara.com

Virtual Reality Society. (2016). Virtual reality. Retrieved from http://www.vrs.org.uk/virtual-reality/what-is-virtual-reality.html

Zaharias, P., & Pappas, C. (2016). Quality management of learning management systems: A user experience perspective. *Current Issues in Emerging eLearning, 3*(1), 5.

Index